Case Studies in Eye Diseases and Disorders

Case Studies in Eye Diseases and Disorders

Editor: Emmie Hunter

AMERICAN
MEDICAL PUBLISHERS
www.americanmedicalpublishers.com

AMERICAN
MEDICAL PUBLISHERS
www.americanmedicalpublishers.com

Cataloging-in-Publication Data

Case studies in eye diseases and disorders / edited by Emmie Hunter.
p. cm.
Includes bibliographical references and index.
ISBN 979-8-88740-598-8
1. Eye--Diseases--Diagnosis. 2. Eye--Diseases--Treatment. 3. Eye--Abnormalities.
4. Eye--Care and hygiene. I. Hunter, Emmie
RE46 .D53 2023
617.7--dc23

American Medical Publishers,
41 Flatbush Avenue,
1st Floor, New York,
NY 11217, USA

ISBN 979-8-88740-598-8 (Hardback)

Contents

Preface

Over the recent decade, advancements and applications have progressed exponentially. This has led to the increased interest in this field and projects are being conducted to enhance knowledge. The main objective of this book is to present some of the critical challenges and provide insights into possible solutions. This book will answer the varied questions that arise in the field and also provide an increased scope for furthering studies.

Eye diseases and disorders encompass a wide range of conditions that can affect the vision and overall eye health of a person. A few of the common eye diseases are cataracts, glaucoma, macular degeneration, diabetic retinopathy, myopia, hyperopia and astigmatism. The diagnosis of these conditions might involve visual acuity tests, tonometry, dilated eye exams, and imaging techniques like optical coherence tomography (OCT) to provide detailed images of the eye structures. The management of eye diseases and disorders depends on the particular condition which has been diagnosed. Treatments may include corrective lenses or contact lenses to manage refractive errors, medications to control intraocular pressure in glaucoma, or surgical interventions like cataract extraction or retinal detachment repair. Early detection and intervention can often slow the progression of certain conditions and preserve vision. This book includes some of the vital pieces of works being conducted across the world, on various topics related to eye diseases and disorders. It will serve as a reference to a broad spectrum of readers.

I hope that this book, with its visionary approach, will be a valuable addition and will promote interest among readers. Each of the authors has provided their extraordinary competence in their specific fields by providing different perspectives as they come from diverse nations and regions. I thank them for their contributions.

Editor

1

Recurrence of Herpetic Keratitis after COVID-19 Vaccination: A Report of Two Cases

Ali Mahdavi Fard,[1] Jeffrey Desilets,[1] and Sangita Patel[1,2]

[1]*Ross Eye Institute, Department of Ophthalmology, Jacobs School of Medicine and Biomedical Sciences, State University at Buffalo, Buffalo, New York, USA*
[2]*Research and Ophthalmology Services, Veterans Administration of Western New York Healthcare System, Buffalo, NY, USA*

Correspondence should be addressed to Sangita Patel; sppatel@buffalo.edu

Academic Editor: Hiroshi Eguchi

Background. Recurrence of herpetic keratitis following vaccination has been documented following vaccination with the Zostavax, trivalent flu, hepatitis A, and rabies vaccines. The USFDA and WHO have acknowledged that the novel COVID-19 vaccines similarly have a risk of reactive immunologic-based inflammation, namely, myositis, pericarditis, and Guillain-Barré syndrome. *Case Presentation.* We present two patients with latent herpetic keratitis who experienced reactivation of keratitis within weeks of COVID-19 vaccination despite prolonged periods of prior latency. A 52-year-old healthy male with no herpes simplex virus (HSV) keratitis recurrences in two years developed visual decline and patchy stromal haze within 24-48 hours of receiving the second Pfizer-BioNTech (COVID-19 BNT162b2) vaccine. A 67-year-old female with chronic neurotrophic keratitis developed her most severe exacerbation of herpes zoster keratitis in over 10 years occurring 2-3 weeks after her first Moderna (mRNA-1273) vaccine, which was later complicated by bacterial superinfection. *Conclusions.* The COVID-19 vaccines work by generating both adaptive humoral and cellular immune responses in humans, including elevation of anti-spike neutralizing antibody titers, antigen-specific CD4+ and CD8+ T-cell responses, and increased levels of proinflammatory cytokines such as interferon gamma (IFNγ). The general activation of the T-cell-mediated immune response and proinflammatory cytokines such as IFNγ may underlie the role of the COVID vaccines in reactivation of herpetic stromal keratitis and the clinical findings in our reported cases.

1. Introduction

Following the historic rollout of the COVID-19 vaccines to the public in early 2021, the United States Food and Drug Administration and World Health Organization have acknowledged a low risk of certain forms of reactive immunologic-based inflammation, namely, myositis, pericarditis, and Guillain-Barré syndrome [1]. We present two patients with chronic herpetic keratitis and prolonged periods of prior latency who experienced reactivation of keratitis within weeks of vaccination.

2. Case 1

A 52-year-old healthy male had a longstanding history of herpetic keratitis of the right eye. The herpes simplex virus (HSV) stromal keratitis first occurred in 1992, and the patient experienced 3-4 episodes of reactivation per year in the right eye until 2010 after which the frequency decreased to one episode of reactivation every other year with the last episode in 2019. A typical episode would include pruritus, irritation, redness, and photophobia without vision changes and would last 2-3 weeks. These recurrences were treated with topical prednisolone acetate 1%, topical trifluridine, and oral antiviral (acyclovir or valacyclovir). Between episodes, he was maintained on oral antiviral prophylaxis and topical prednisolone acetate 1% 2-3×/week. The topical steroid was discontinued in 2017. The patient received the Zostavax varicella zoster vaccine in March 2020 without incident. He received the Pfizer-BioNTech COVID-19 vaccines (COVID-19 BNT162b2) in March 2021 and April 2021. Within 24-48 hours of receiving the second vaccination, the patient began to experience blurry vision in the right eye which he had not experienced during prior episodes of recurrence of herpetic keratitis. There was no associated pruritus, redness, irritation, or photophobia like his prior episodes. The patient had an eye exam two weeks after the initial symptoms and was found to have 20/40 visual acuity in the right eye with patchy stromal haze and confluent punctate epithelial erosions along the inferior cornea. The patient's prophylactic dose of acyclovir 800 mg daily was increased to 400 mg 5×/day, and topical trifluridine was prescribed at 5×/day in the right eye. One week later, the patient presented to our clinic and vision had declined to 20/60 with new nummular opacities at multiple stromal levels. Sector iris stromal atrophy was noted (Figure 1). Prednisolone acetate 1% drops 5×/day were started with improved vision within 2-3 days. The prednisolone acetate 1% drops were tapered gradually to fluorometholone 0.1%, and antiviral was switched to valacyclovir 500 mg once daily with maintained quiescence of the herpetic keratitis. This patient continues to be followed, and vision in the right eye has stabilized at 20/30.

3. Case 2

A 67-year-old female had a history of hypercholesterolemia, hypothyroidism, Hodgkin's lymphoma, and complicated herpes zoster ophthalmicus (HZO) of her left eye. She developed herpes zoster ophthalmicus in 1981 while completing chemotherapy for Hodgkin's lymphoma. At that time, she was hospitalized for 3 months with severe Guillain-Barré syndrome with full-body flaccid paralysis and respiratory compromise without intubation. She had severe ocular involvement which could not be fully evaluated due to her systemic status, and a left eye tarsorrhaphy was maintained through her hospitalization. Despite a severe initial course, with prophylactic bandage contact lens wear for neurotrophic corneal status and fluorometholone 0.1% drops once daily, the patient had maintained 20/40 visual acuity with a clear cornea for over 10 years prior to the current case presentation. The patient received the Zostavax shingles vaccine in 2017 and the Shingrix vaccine in 2019 and 2020 without ocular issues. She believed she experienced COVID-19 infection in March 2020 due to an illness with fever and cough and subsequent positive at-home COVID-19 antibody test but had no ocular issues at that time. The patient received the Moderna COVID-19 vaccines (mRNA-1273) in January 2021 and February 2021. She began to experience blurry vision, redness, and abnormal sensation in her left eye at the end of January 2021, just prior to her second COVID-19 vaccination. Her visual acuity in the left eye had

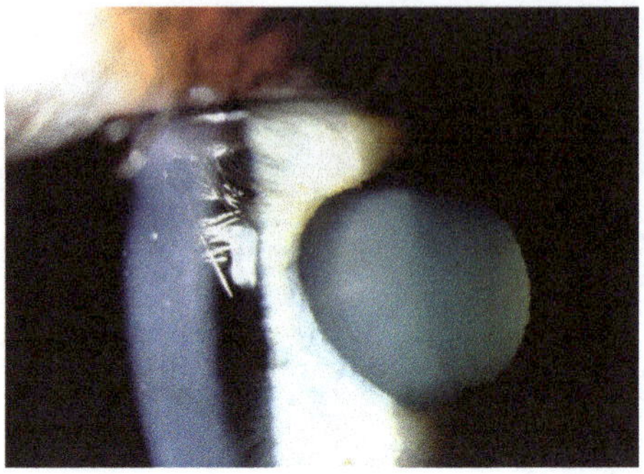

Figure 1: Slit lamp photograph of the right eye of the patient in case 1 depicting corneal stromal haziness and sectoral iris atrophy.

decreased to 20/150, and the corneal exam revealed a 1 × 0.5 mm corneal epithelial defect without infiltrate suggestive of herpetic epithelial keratitis. A bandage contact lens, oral valacyclovir 1 g twice daily, and ofloxacin 0.3% drops 4×/day were initiated with continuation of her baseline fluorometholone 0.1% once daily. A swab of the corneal lesion was submitted for evaluation for herpes simplex virus (1 and 2) and varicella zoster virus by qualitative polymerase chain reaction. The test results were inconclusive due to a low number of cells detected in the specimen by the endogenous control. A stromal infiltrate vs. herpetic stromal keratitis was present the subsequent week at which time bacterial corneal cultures were obtained. Cultures grew *Mycobacterium chelonae*, and amikacin drops 15 mg/mL with oral azithromycin 500 mg weekly for 5 weeks were started. While the ulcer resolved, the healing course was complicated by progressive stromal thinning, iritis, endotheliitis, and difficulty with corneal epithelial healing.

4. Discussion

There are multiple known triggers for reactivation of herpetic keratitis. Factors noted for reactivation of HSV keratitis include pyrexia, wind and sun exposure, trauma, and stress [2]. Recurrence of herpetic keratitis following vaccination has been reported following Zostavax vaccination [3]. In addition, reactivation of herpes zoster has been reported after the trivalent flu, hepatitis A, and rabies vaccines [4]. To the list of potential triggers for recurrent herpetic keratitis, we add the COVID-19 BNT162b2 and mRNA-1273 mRNA vaccines.

Recurrent herpetic stromal keratitis is typically the result of cell-mediated immunity against viral DNA antigens in the cornea, rather than active viral replication. Several studies have shown that during recurrent herpetic stromal keratitis, the T-cell profile is different from primary infection [5]. While cytotoxic T-cells are involved in primary disease [6], recurrent disease is most often associated with strong delayed-type hypersensitivity (DTH) responses [7]. The DTH response in recurrent herpetic stromal keratitis occurs as a result of developing an immune response against HSV-1 including antigen-specific CD4+ T-cells of both Th1 and Th2 subsets as well as HSV-1-specific CD8+ T-cells. Similar mechanisms of cell-mediated immunity against viral antigens in the cornea are responsible for the later manifestations of HZO [8]. In HSV stromal keratitis, the CD4+ T-cell production of inflammatory cytokines such as interferon gamma (IFNγ) also triggers pathogenic neutrophil infiltration [9].

Since the emergence of the COVID-19 pandemic, two mRNA-based vaccines, BNT162b2 and mRNA-1273, have been introduced that demonstrated a high efficacy rate with an acceptable safety profile for public administration against the SARS-CoV-2 virus. These vaccines work by generating both adaptive humoral and cellular immune responses in humans, including elevation of anti-spike neutralizing antibody titers, antigen-specific CD4+ and CD8+ T-cell responses, and increased levels of proinflammatory cytokines such as interferon gamma (IFNγ) [10]. While it is possible that the timing was a coincidence, the general activation of the T-cell-mediated immune response and proinflammatory cytokines such as IFNγ may underlie the role of the COVID vaccines in reactivation of herpetic keratitis and the clinical findings in our reported cases.

The COVID-19 vaccines have over 90% efficacy in preventing a disease that was responsible for about 2.6 million deaths worldwide during its first year alone; this medical advancement provides paramount protection to both the individual and society at large. For patients with HSV and VZV with history of ocular involvement, clinicians may wish to observe for ocular changes presenting around the time of vaccination. Patients may also be advised to self-monitor vision and ocular symptoms in the weeks following vaccination and to report any changes immediately.

Consent

Verbal patient consent was obtained for publication. No patient identifiable data is included in this case report.

Disclosure

The contents do not represent the views of the U.S. Department of Veterans Affairs or the United States Government.

References

[1] WHO, "Covid-19 vaccines," in *Safety Surveillance Manual second edition*, World Health Organization, Geneva, 2021.

[2] L. J. Al-Dujaili, P. P. Clerkin, C. Clement et al., "Ocular herpes simplex virus: how are latency, reactivation, recurrent disease and therapy interrelated?," *Future Microbiology*, vol. 6, no. 8, pp. 877–907, 2011.

[3] C. W. Hwang Jr., W. A. Steigleman, E. Saucedo-Sanchez, and S. S. Tuli, "Reactivation of herpes zoster keratitis in an adult after varicella zoster vaccination," *Cornea*, vol. 32, no. 4, pp. 508-509, 2013.

[4] R. Walter, K. Hartmann, F. Fleisch, W. H. Reinhart, and M. Kuhn, "Reactivation of herpesvirus infections after vaccinations?," *Lancet*, vol. 353, no. 9155, p. 810, 1999.

[5] T. L. Keadle, J. L. Morris, J. S. Pepose, and P. M. Stuart, "$CD4^+$ and $CD8^+$ cells are key participants in the development of recurrent herpetic stromal keratitis in mice," *Microbial Pathogenesis*, vol. 32, no. 6, pp. 255–262, 2002.

[6] E. Chang, L. Galle, D. Maggs, D. M. Estes, and W. J. Mitchell, "Pathogenesis of herpes simplex virus type 1-induced corneal inflammation in perforin-deficient mice," *Journal of Virology*, vol. 74, no. 24, pp. 11832–11840, 2000.

[7] T. L. Keadle, L. A. Morrison, J. L. Morris, J. S. Pepose, and P. M. Stuart, "Therapeutic immunization with a virion host shutoff-defective, replication-incompetent herpes simplex virus type 1 strain limits recurrent herpetic ocular infection," *Journal of Virology*, vol. 76, no. 8, pp. 3615–3625, 2002.

[8] K. H. Baratz, "The role of antiviral therapy after the resolution of acute herpes simplex keratitis or acute herpes zoster ophthalmicus," *Archives of Ophthalmology*, vol. 130, no. 1, pp. 108–110, 2012.

[9] A. M. Lobo, A. M. Agelidis, and D. Shukla, "Pathogenesis of herpes simplex keratitis: the host cell response and ocular surface sequelae to infection and inflammation," *The Ocular Surface*, vol. 17, no. 1, pp. 40–49, 2019.

[10] F. P. Polack, S. J. Thomas, N. Kitchin et al., "Safety and efficacy of the BNT162b2 mRNA Covid-19 vaccine," *New England Journal of Medicine*, vol. 383, no. 27, pp. 2603–2615, 2020.

2

Modification of the Intrastromal Ring Position according to Postimplant Visual and Refractive Failure: Report of Two Cases

Luis Izquierdo,[1] Josefina A. Mejías Smith,[2] Jose R. Lievano,[2] Ramón Sarquis,[2] and Maria A. Henriquez[3]

[1]*Head of Department of Cornea and Anterior Segment, Instituto de Ojos Oftalmosalud, Lima, Peru*
[2]*Research Department, Instituto de Ojos Oftalmosalud, Lima, Peru*
[3]*Head of Research Department, Instituto de Ojos Oftalmosalud, Av. Javier Prado Este 1142, San Isidro, Lima, Peru*

Correspondence should be addressed to Josefina A. Mejías Smith; josefina.mejias.smith@gmail.com

Academic Editor: Alexander A. Bialasiewicz

Objective. The following report presents the adaptation of an existing technique of intrastromal corneal ring (ICRS) implantation enabling repositioning of the ring position postoperatively to manage a refractive failure in two patients with keratoconus. *Methods.* In two cases, KeraRing and Ferrara nomograms had suggested different ring positions. To manage with the differences between the two nomograms, a longer corneal tunnel was created followed by the classic intervention to move the ring through the initial intrastromal corneal tunnel according to the topographic values. Once the first ring position has failed, the ring segment was repositioned along the longer corneal tunnel according to the postoperative outcome. *Results.* Significant improvement in both cases was observed in the best corrected visual acuity (BCVA), uncorrected visual acuity (UCVA), and root mean square (RMS) measured with Scheimpflug imaging (Pentacam; Oculus GmbH, Wetzlar, Germany). The participants were followed for one year. *Conclusion.* In patients with keratoconus which exhibit significant differences between KeraRing and Ferrara nomograms, a longer tunnel should be created to enable repositioning of the ring postoperatively if necessary, to avoid extracting the ring or changing it.

1. Introduction

Keratoconus is a noninflammatory, bilateral asymmetric eye disease in which the cornea progressively thins and forms a cone-like bulge. The disease typically involves the central two-thirds of the cornea; the apex of the cone usually centered just below the visual axis. The disease results in mild to severe impairment of visual function due to the development of progressive myopia and irregular astigmatism.

Keratoconus management depends on the progression and stage of the disease. In mild cases, it can be managed with crosslinking, eyeglasses, phakic lenses, photorefractive keratotomy (PRK), or contact lenses. In moderate cases, when the disease progression has stopped, the visual axis is clear and the patient's corrected-vision is not sufficient to perform his daily life activities and intracorneal ring segments (ICRS) can be used. Deep anterior lamellar keratoplasty (DALK) or penetrating keratoplasty (PK) can be used in severe cases when the visual axis is compromised by corneal scarring, best corrected visual acuity is 20/100 or worse, and the pachymetry is less than 300 um [1, 2].

The purpose of the implant is to reshape the corneal surface and improve tolerance to contact lenses and their related symptoms such as itching and eye dryness. Moreover, it can also delay or even prevent corneal transplantation.

ICRS are usually indicated for moderate keratoconus and high myopia cases, improving the best corrected visual acuity (BCVA), decreasing the keratometry values, remodeling the corneal topography, and delaying corneal keratoplasty [3–5]. Complications related to ICRS include extrusion, keratitis, corneal melting, perforations, and refractive failure [6]. Refractive failure is a term used to describe a poor postoperative outcome defined by a minimum loss of one line in uncorrected visual acuity (UCVA) or BCVA, an increase of two diopters of spherical equivalent, and an increase of 1 mm in the root mean square (RMS) [7].

To define both the meridian, the depth, and the implant area of the intrastromal ring segment, one must rely on the nomograms supplied by the manufactures of each ring [8, 9].

We performed implantations using both Ferrara and KeraRing nomograms. According to the KeraRing nomogram [8], the first step is to select the so-called reference meridian. If the best correction visual acuity (BCVA) is equal or greater than 0.5 logMAR, the refractive meridian (perpendicular to the refractive axis in negative) is selected; if the BCVA is less than 0.5 logMAR, the meridian of the coma is selected (perpendicular to the coma axis). The second step is to determine the type of corneal asymmetry considering the chosen meridian reference and the axial keratometric (curvature) map, followed by determining the slope area of one side of the selected reference meridian. According to this relation, four types of positions are described according to the percentage of unevenness area associated with the reference meridian.

For Ferrara nomogram the strategy is based on asphericity [9]. If the asphericity is less than -0.25 a 160° corneal segment is implanted on the topographically flatter axis; if the asphericity is between -0.25 and -1.25, two segments are implanted; if the asphericity is greater than -1.25, a 210° segment is implanted in the 90° axis; this classification continues dividing the cones into central or paracentral.

The following report presents the adaptation of an existing technique of intrastromal corneal ring (ICRS) implantation enabling repositioning of the ring position postoperatively to manage a refractive failure in two patients with keratoconus.

2. Case 1

A 27-year-old male with keratoconus presented at the Cornea and Anterior Segment Department with blurred vision that was difficult to correct with eyeglasses. In his right eye, his UCVA was 20/100 and his manifest refraction was -0.75-1.25 x 50° with BCVA of 20/30. In his left eye, his UCVA was 20/25 with -0.25-0.50 x 75° and BCVA of 20/20 (Figure 1(a)). ICRS was implanted in his right eye and crosslinking in his left eye.

The ICRS (KeraRing, Mediphacos, Belo Horizonte, Brazil) used in this study was a 160° segment ring made of polymethyl methacrylate (PMMA) implanted in the corneal tunnel (Figure 1(c)). Both ICRS nomograms, Ferrara and KeraRing, indicated different ring position (Figures 1(b)-1(d)), so a temporal 160°/200-micron ring was utilized. A femtosecond laser (Z6; Ziemer Ophthalmic Systems AG, Port, Switzerland) was used to make an incision at 114° (the steepest meridian), K1 42.3 D, and K2 47.4 D, and a 371um deep corneal tunnel was created (corresponding to 75% of the corneal thickness of 495 um at the thinnest point of the tunnel path), with a 355-degree length only 20 degrees more than the normal size of the ICRS. This longer channel allowed repositioning of the ring if necessary.

The thickness and degree of arc of the ICRS were selected and their location was planned according to the cone location on axial topography measured via Scheimpflug imaging (Pentacam; Oculus GmBH, Wetzlar, Germany), with a 5.5 mm diameter depending on the nomogram results.

Postoperative treatment included 0.3% topical tobramycin with 0.1% dexamethasone (Tobradex; Alcon, Fort Worth, TX, USA) four times a day for 2 weeks; the latter was then tapered over 4 weeks. Preservative-free artificial tear substitute (Lagricel Ofteno; Sophia, Guadalajara, Mexico) was used four times a day for 2 weeks.

Two months later the patient's UCVA was 20/100, his BCVA was 20/30, and manifest refraction was +1.50-1.75 x 10°, indicating a refractive failure. However, his RMS improved from 14.750 um to 10.346 um (Figure 1(e)).

According to the postoperative keratometric Scheimpflug map, the ring was moved 50 degrees counterclockwise according to the topographic results (Figure 1(d)). One-month after repositioning, the patient's UCVA was 20/25, his BCVA was 20/20, his manifest refraction was -0.50 x 90°, and his RMS had decreased to 5.392 um.

At a one-year follow-up, his right eye was UCVA 20/30-2, his manifest refraction was +1.00-2.00 x 90 degrees with BCVA of 20/20, and his RMS was 5.605 um (Figure 1(f)).

3. Case 2

A 26-year-old male presented at the Cornea and Anterior Segment Department with low vision in the right eye, which presented UCVA of 20/100 BCVA 20/30 and manifest refraction of -0.75-3.5 x 50°. His left eye had UCVA of 20/25, BCVA of 20/20, and manifest refraction of -0.25-0.50 x 75°. Keratoconus was diagnosed in both eyes; femto ICRS was indicated for the right eye and follow-up for the left eye (Figure 2(a)).

The two nomograms proposed, KeraRing and Ferrara, indicated different ring positions (Figures 2(b)-2(d)), so a temporal 160°/150-micron ring (Figure 2(c)) was utilized. A femtosecond laser (Z6; Ziemer Ophthalmic Systems AG, Port, Switzerland) was used to make an incision at 99.7° (the steepest meridian by topography), K1 42.5 D, and K2 46.1 D. Due to a pachymetry of 512 microns at the tunnel zone, a 371 um deep corneal tunnel (corresponding to 75% of the corneal thickness) was created with a 355-degree tunnel if repositioning was necessary.

Postoperative treatment included 0.3% topical tobramycin with 0.1% dexamethasone (Tobradex; Alcon, Fort Worth, TX, USA) four times a day for 2 weeks; the latter was then tapered over 4 weeks. Preservative-free artificial tear substitute (Lagricel Ofteno; Sophia, Guadalajara, Mexico) was used four times a day for 2 weeks.

Two months later, the patient's UCVA was 20/150, his BCVA was 20/40, and his manifest refraction was -1.00-2.00 x 50°, indicating a loss of one line of vision (Figure 2(e)). Additionally, his RMS decreased from 13.970 um to 11.327 um. The patient's outcome was not as planned, and his visual acuity was worse after the ICRS implantation. Therefore, the ring was moved 45 degrees counterclockwise in the tunnel according to the keratometric Scheimpflug map (Figure 2(d)).

One month after repositioning, the patient's UCVA improved to 20/40, his BCVA to 20/20, and his manifest refraction to +0.50-2.00 x 90°. His RMS decreased from 11.327 um to 8.275um.

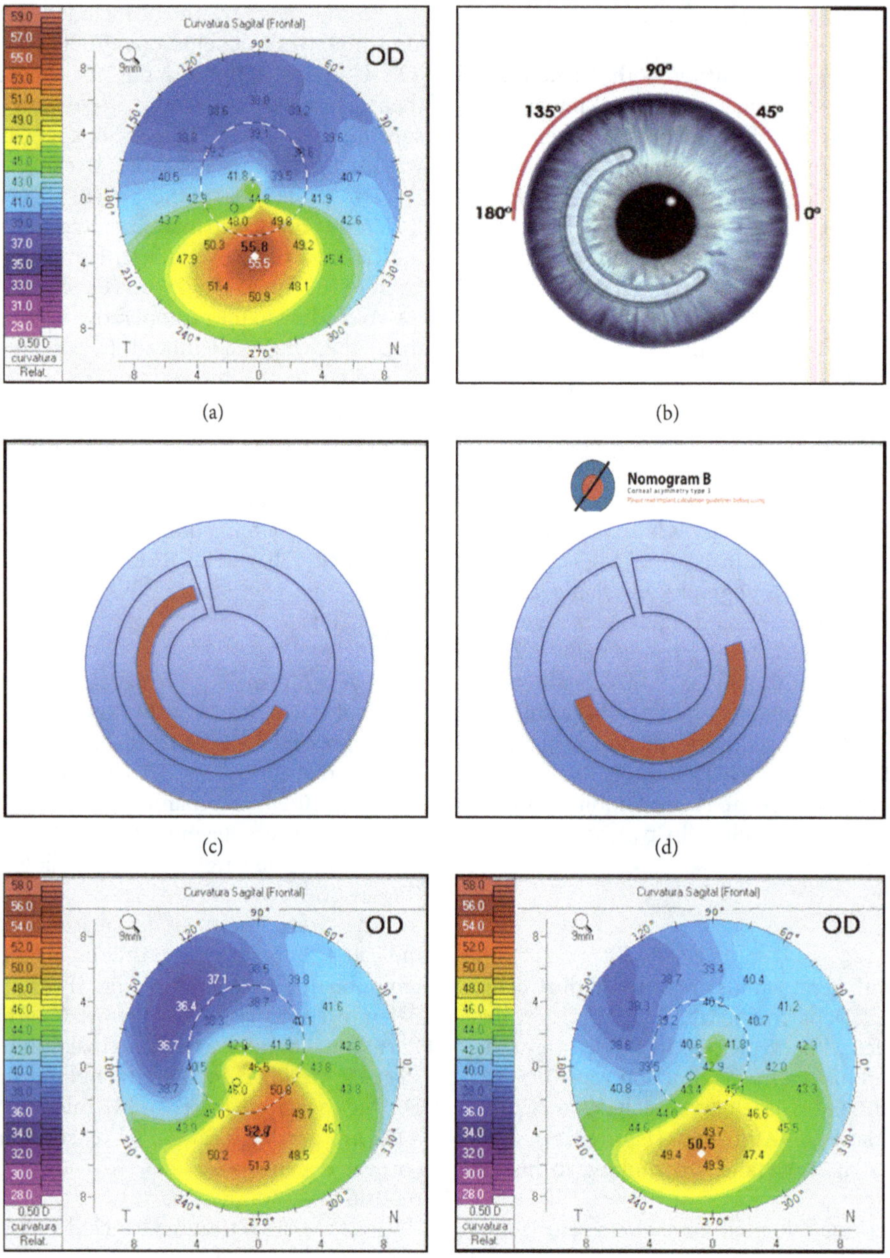

Figure 1: (a) Topography pretreatment. (b) Ferrara nomogram. (c) First intrastromal ring position. (d) KeraRing nomogram position. (e) One-month postimplantation ring position. (f) One-year postmodification ring position.

At a one-year follow-up, his right eye was UCVA 20/40-2, his manifest refraction was +0.50-2.00 x 90 with BCVA of 20/25+2, and his RMS was 7.569 um (Figure 2(f)).

4. Discussion

As indicated by the clinical data from both cases, the tunnel adaptation for the ICRS implantation has the potential to correct myopia, astigmatism, and corneal irregularity.

This adaptation provides opportunities to manage keratoconus to avoid refractive outcomes and ring explantation. The procedure is simple, has no additional cost, and can be used for manual or femtosecond tunnels.

Torquetti et al. evaluated 37 keratoconus eyes implanted with intrastromal corneal ring segments and described requirements for reintervention following overcorrection due to excessive flattening of the cornea with unsatisfactory results in all of the cases and limited improvement after the first procedure [10].

Coskunseven et al. [11] studied 50 eyes of patients with keratoconus using KeraRing ICRS and reported segment migration to the incision site in three eyes. To avoid melting,

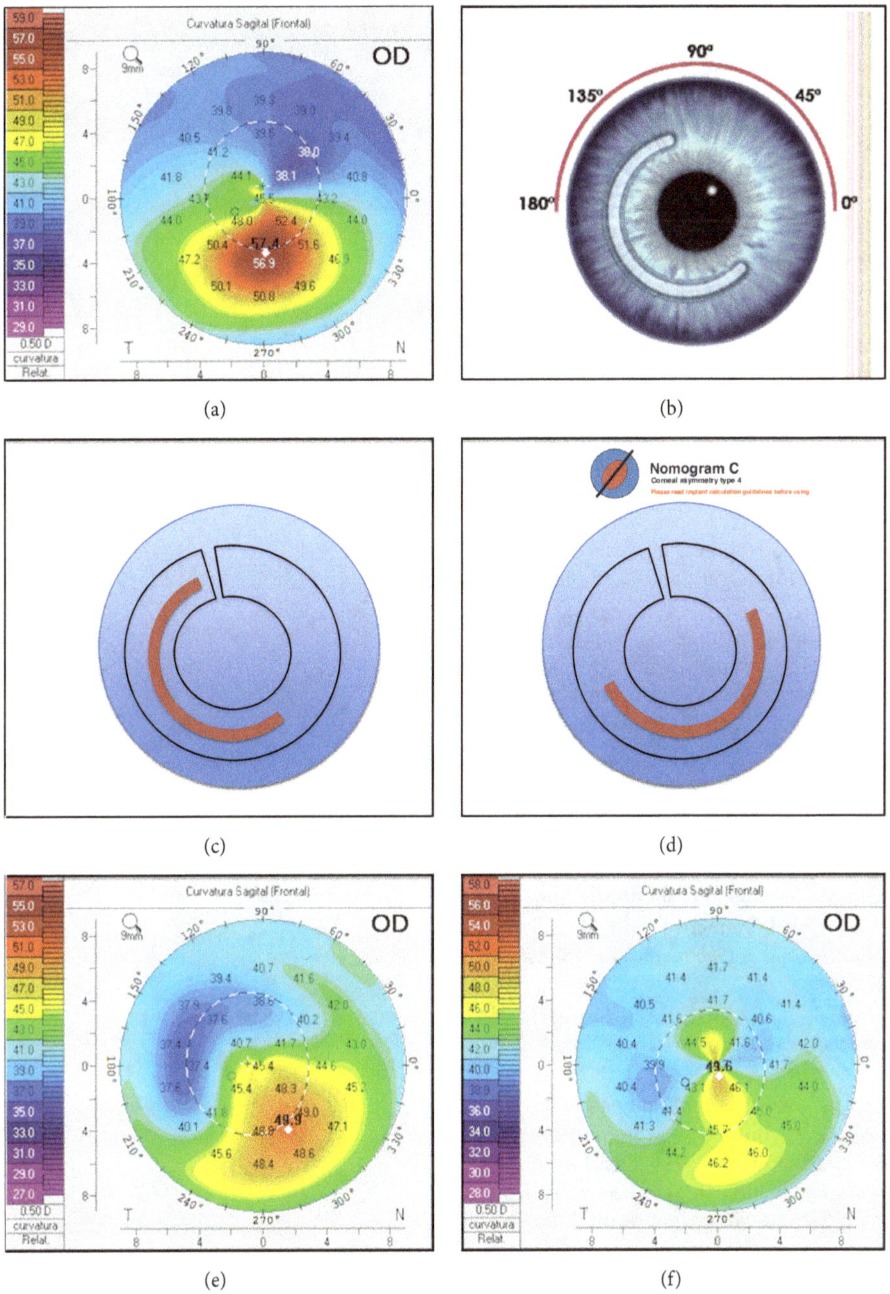

FIGURE 2: (a) Topography pretreatment. (b) Ferrara nomogram. (c) First intrastromal ring position. (d) KeraRing nomogram position. (e) One-month postimplantation ring position. (f) One-year postmodification ring position.

they repositioned the migrated segment away from the incision site with successful outcomes in all of the eyes. Heikal et al. reported no complications or need for ring repositioning in a 6-month follow-up of 20 patients [12].

Pokroy et al. [13] reported that 10% of keratoconic eyes with implanted ring segments needed adjustments (repositioning, exchange, or explantation) due to surgically induced astigmatism. The adjustment procedure was technically simple with no intraoperative complications.

Chan et al. [14] evaluated 3 case series of patients with previous insertion of 2 intrastromal corneal ring segments who underwent surgical removal and repositioning of the segments due to unsatisfactory visual and topographic outcomes. Although the results were good, the removal of the intrastromal ring and the creation of a new tunnel could have been avoided.

We believe when managing patients with significant differences between nomograms, a longer tunnel should be created to enable repositioning of the ring postoperatively if necessary. This technique may reduce the need in additional operations and improve the patient's refractive outcomes.

Disclosure

All of the authors attest that they meet the current ICMJE criteria for authorship.

References

[1] J. A. Gomes, D. Tan, C. J. Rapuano et al., "Global consensus on keratoconus and ectatic diseases," *Cornea*, vol. 34, no. 4, pp. 359–369, 2015.

[2] M. Belin and J. Duncan, "Keratoconus: the ABCD grading system," *Klinische Monatsblätter für Augenheilkunde*, vol. 233, no. 06, pp. 701–707, 2016.

[3] J. Colin, B. Cochener, G. Savary, and F. Malet, "Correcting keratoconus with intracorneal rings," *Journal of Cataract & Refractive Surgery*, vol. 26, no. 8, pp. 1117–1122, 2000.

[4] J. L. Alió, M. H. Shabayek, and A. Artola, "Intracorneal ring segments for keratoconus correction: long-term follow-up," *Journal of Cataract & Refractive Surgery*, vol. 32, no. 6, pp. 978–985, 2006.

[5] L. A. Beniz, G. H. Queiroz, C. F. Queiroz, W. L. Lopes, L. F. Moraes, and J. Beniz, "Intrastromal corneal ring segments delay corneal grafting in patients with keratoconus," *Arquivos Brasileiros de Oftalmologia*, vol. 79, no. 1, pp. 30–32, 2016.

[6] C. Ferrer, J. L. Alió, A. U. Montañés et al., "Causes of intrastromal corneal ring segment explantation: clinicopathologic correlation analysis," *Journal of Cataract & Refractive Surgery*, vol. 36, no. 6, pp. 970–977, 2010.

[7] A. Vega-Estrada, J. L. Alio, L. F. Brenner et al., "Outcome analysis of intracorneal ring segments for the treatment of keratoconus based on visual, refractive, and aberrometric impairment," *American Journal of Ophthalmology*, vol. 155, no. 3, pp. 575–584.el, 2013.

[8] "Keraring – Intraestromal Ring," MEDIPHACOS, http://mediphacos.com/en/products/corneal/keraring-anel-intraestromal/, 2019.

[9] "Nomogram," 2019, http://www.ajlsa.com/nomograma/.

[10] L. Torquetti, G. Ferrara, F. Almeida, L. Cunha, P. Ferrara, and J. Merayo-Lloves, "Clinical outcomes after intrastromal corneal ring segments reoperation in keratoconus patients," *International Journal of Ophthalmology*, vol. 6, no. 6, pp. 796–800, 2013.

[11] E. Coskunseven, G. D. Kymionis, N. S. Tsiklis et al., "One-year results of intrastromal corneal ring segment implantation (KerаRing) using femtosecond laser in patients with keratoconus," *American Journal of Ophthalmology*, vol. 145, no. 5, pp. 775–779, 2008.

[12] M. A. Heikal, M. Abdelshafy, T. T. Soliman, and A. M. Hamed, "Refractive and visual outcomes after Keraring intrastromal corneal ring segment implantation for keratoconus assisted by femtosecond laser at 6 months follow-up," *Clinical Ophthalmology (Auckland, N.Z.)*, vol. 11, pp. 81–86, 2017.

[13] R. Pokroy and S. Levinger, "Intacs adjustment surgery for keratoconus," *Journal of Cataract & Refractive Surgery*, vol. 32, no. 6, pp. 986–992, 2006.

[14] K. Chan and P. S. Hersh, "Removal and repositioning of intracorneal ring segments: improving corneal topography and clinical outcomes in keratoconus and ectasia," *Cornea*, vol. 36, no. 2, pp. 244–248, 2017.

Reactivation of Acute Retinal Necrosis following SARS-CoV-2 Infection

Monica P. Gonzalez,[1] Radames Rios,[1] Mariella Pappaterra,[1] Miguel Hernandez,[2] Allison Toledo,[3] Carmen Santos,[1] Andres Emanuelli,[1,3] Shree K. Kurup,[1,4] and Armando L. Oliver[1]

[1]*University of Puerto Rico, Medical Sciences Campus, Department of Ophthalmology, Paseo Dr. Jose Celso Barbosa, San Juan 00921, USA*
[2]*Ponce Health Sciences University School of Medicine, 388 Zona Industrial Reparada 2, Ponce, PR 00716, USA*
[3]*Emanuelli Research and Development Center, 452 Dr R Rivera Aulet Avenue, Suite 45 Arecibo, PR 00612-4368, USA*
[4]*Department of Ophthalmology & Visual Sciences, Case Western Reserve University, University Hospitals Cleveland Medical Center, 11100 Euclid Avenue, Cleveland, OH 44106, USA*

Correspondence should be addressed to Armando L. Oliver; armandoolivermd@gmail.com

Academic Editor: Benedetto Falsini

Purpose. To report on a case of reactivation of acute retinal necrosis following SARS-CoV-2 infection. *Methods.* Observational case report. *Observations.* A 32-year-old female with a distant history of left retinal detachment secondary to necrotizing herpetic retinitis complained of right-eye vision loss, pain, redness, and photophobia. An ophthalmological examination revealed findings consistent with acute retinal necrosis of the right eye. A polymerase chain reaction (PCR) analysis of the right vitreous was positive for herpes simplex virus type 2 (HSV-2). A coronavirus disease 2019 (COVID-19) screening test using reverse transcriptase- (RT-) PCR was positive for SARS-CoV-2 RNA. *Conclusions.* Our case suggests that COVID-19 may cause a latent HSV infection to reactivate, causing contralateral involvement in patients with a prior history of HSV-associated acute retinal necrosis.

1. Introduction

Acute retinal necrosis (ARN) is a rare posterior uveitis syndrome characterized by rapidly progressive vision loss that may affect both immunocompetent and immunodeficient patients of any age [1, 2]. ARN is characterized by discrete foci of retinal necrosis that progress rapidly in a circumferential fashion, with associated occlusive arterial vasculopathy and significant inflammation of the posterior and anterior segments of the eye [1]. It is most commonly associated with the varicella-zoster virus (VZV) and herpes simplex viruses 1 and 2 (HSV-1 and HSV-2) [3]. Common sequelae of the disease include retinal breaks, detachments, and macular edema; patients with ARN tend to have a guarded visual prognosis [3, 4]. Among the most feared ARN complications is contralateral involvement, which may lead to significant visual disability and blindness [3]. In a case series by Lei et al., 25 out of 30 patients with ARN developed the disease in the contralateral eye, most commonly within months of the initial presentation; however, a delayed involvement of the fellow eye, occurring after several years, was also described in a small subset of patients [5]. Prompt treatment with systemic acyclovir substantially reduces the risk of bilateral involvement [6]. Although long-term antiviral therapy with acyclovir may prevent ARN involvement in the fellow eye, its role remains undefined [6]. For ARN, the duration of secondary antiviral prophylaxis has not been thoroughly assessed; however, some important factors to consider are immune status and comorbidities [1, 7].

Herpesviruses are a large family of DNA viruses with high prevalence in the population [8]. It is estimated that approximately 90% of adults worldwide are infected with HSV-1, HSV-2, or both [8]. The lytic (active) and latent stages of these viruses ensure that, once infected, an individual will remain so throughout his or her lifetime [8]. When the virus enters the latent stage, a balance of various factors, including the continuous response of the adaptive immune system, is required for the virus to stay dormant [9]. The impairment of CD8+ T cell suppression of viral lytic gene expression could lead to an HSV recurrence [9]. The reactivation of herpesvirus-related infections, specifically of herpes zoster dermatitis, in patients with the coronavirus disease 2019 (COVID-19) superinfection, has recently been described, yet a precise mechanism for the said reactivation has only been hypothesized [10, 11].

SARS-CoV-2 causes COVID-19, whose symptoms include mild to severe respiratory illness and sundry systemic manifestations [12]. After entering the human body, SARS-CoV-2 binds to the angiotensin-converting enzyme 2 protein present on the host's pulmonary epithelial cells. Viral entry and fusion are then followed by a robust immune response involving the adaptive and the innate immune systems. This immunological cascade has been described to cause immune system dysregulation and to cause decreased lymphocyte counts, along with decreasing CD3, CD4, and CD8 T lymphocytes [13, 14].

The first description of the ocular manifestations of COVID-19 was reported by Wu et al. in a case series of 38 patients in which ocular findings were present in about 31.5% of the patients [15]. Wu et al. described the ocular manifestations of COVID-19 as conjunctival hyperemia, chemosis, and epiphora [15]. Marinho et al. reported the optical coherence tomography findings of 12 symptomatic patients with polymerase chain reaction- (PCR-) proven COVID-19 infection [16]. In their report, they described the presence of multiple hyperreflective retinal lesions at the ganglion cell and inner plexiform layers and cotton wool spots and microhemorrhages on a fundus exam [16].

To our knowledge, no prior cases of ARN reactivation after SARS-CoV-2 infection have been reported. We hereby report a case of a 32-year-old Hispanic female with a prior history of ARN in her left eye who presented with contralateral ARN after having been infected with SARS-CoV-2.

2. Case Report

A 32-year-old Hispanic woman reported sudden vision loss in her right eye (OD), associated with a 1-week history of pain, redness, and photophobia. She had a history of ARN in the left eye (OS), which had occurred 3.5 years prior. She had received treatment with IV acyclovir for 2 weeks, followed by oral valacyclovir, which she had discontinued 1 year before the current presentation. Her left ARN had caused rhegmatogenous retinal detachment, which resulted in the loss of light perception, despite the best surgical efforts. Her past medical history and review of systems were otherwise unremarkable. She was sexually active with her husband and had no history of alcohol or illicit drug abuse.

The best-corrected visual acuity was finger counting at 5 feet in OD; she had no light perception in OS. The intraocular pressure was 10 mmHg in OD and 5 mmHg in OS. Her right pupil was round and reactive to light; the left pupil was corectopic and unreactive, and a left afferent pupillary defect was present; finally, the left eye had atrophic phthisis bulbi. A slit-lamp exam of her right eye revealed diffuse conjunctival injection, punctate epithelial erosions, Descemet folds, and granulomatous keratic precipitates in Arlt's triangle. The anterior chamber had 1+ cells and flare, and the lens had 1+ nuclear sclerosis.

A dilated fundus exam of the right eye revealed 1+ vitritis, optic nerve edema, and retinal necrosis extending from 1 to 11 o'clock in zones 2 and 3 and in zone 1, sparing a small patch of the retina temporal to the optic disk (Figure 1(c)). The left eye revealed persistent retinal traction with fibrous tissue (Figure 1(d)). A fluorescein angiogram of the right eye revealed disk hyperfluorescence, macular and perivascular leakage, and severe peripheral capillary nonperfusion. The extraocular physical exam was unremarkable; in particular, she had normal vital signs, her lungs were clear to auscultation, her abdomen was soft to palpation, and her neurological status was unremarkable.

As her clinical findings were highly suggestive of ARN, she was admitted to the ward and treated with IV acyclovir (800 mg every 8 hours), topical prednisolone acetate 1% eye drops (4 times daily), and atropine sulfate 1% eye drops (3 times daily). A vitreous tap was performed, the resulting sample was sent for PCR analysis, and ganciclovir (2 mg/0.05 cc) was injected intravitreally. Forty-eight hours after commencing therapy, the infectious disease service switched her IV therapy to ganciclovir (380 mg IV every 12 hours).

Despite treatment, her clinical course continued to deteriorate, and after 4 days of therapy, she developed an inferior retinal detachment, which caused her visual acuity to drop to "hand motion." The patient was scheduled for a pars plana vitrectomy with a silicone oil tamponade to repair the retinal detachment, and as part of the preoperative workup, a SARS-CoV-2 PCR test was ordered. The following day, the patient's visual acuity was "light perception," and the partial retinal detachment had progressed to a total detachment.

Twenty-four hours later, the SARS-CoV-2 PCR test was reported as positive. No surgical management was pursued because of the patient's poor visual prognosis and positive SARS-CoV-2 test result. The patient continued to receive IV ganciclovir for 14 days. She was placed in an isolation room and received prophylactic anticoagulation with enoxaparin (40 mg subcutaneous every 12 hours) and iron supplementation to avoid COVID-19-associated complications. During her hospitalization, the patient had no COVID 19 associated symptoms and did not develop any other related complications.

The vitreous PCR test result was positive for HSV-2, confirming the diagnosis of HSV-2-associated ARN. Her serology results revealed positive HSV-1 IgG, HSV-2 IgG, CMV IgG, and VZV IgG. Toxoplasma antibodies (IgG and IgM), serum rapid plasma reagin, and human immunodeficiency

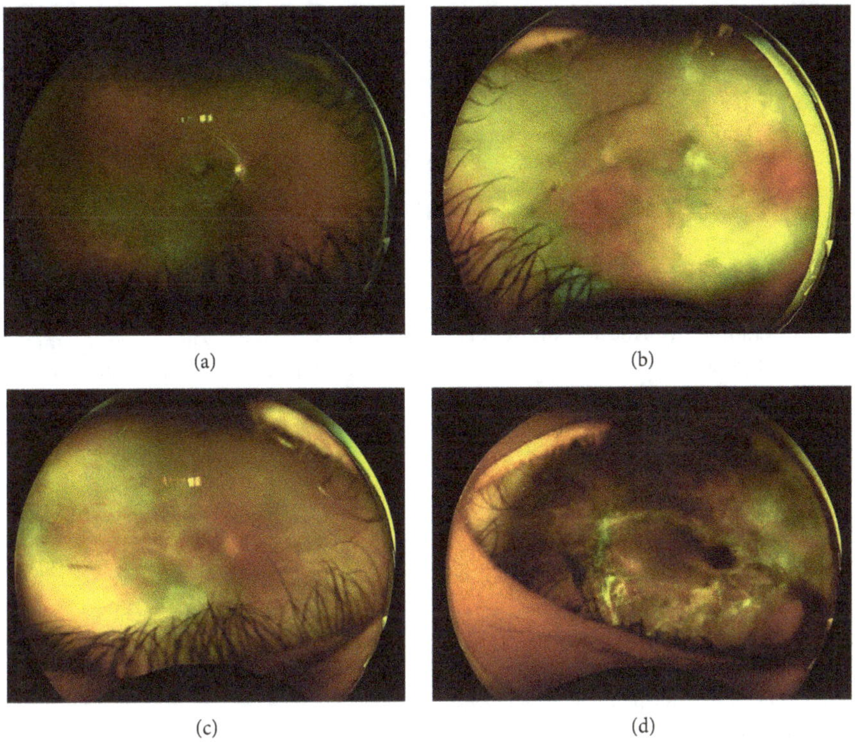

Figure 1: Ultra-widefield fundus photographs of the right (a, c) and left (b, d) eyes. Forty-three months prior to presentation, though the right eye remained uninvolved (a), the left eye developed extensive necrotizing retinitis involving over 80% of the retina. At presentation, the right eye (c) shows vitreous opacities, blurring of the disk margins, and retinal necrosis extending from 1 to 11 o'clock in zones 2 and 3 and diffusely in zone 1, sparing a small patch of the retina temporal to the optic disk. The left eye (d) has persistent retinal traction with fibrous tissue.

virus testing were all negative. The vitreous PCR was negative for HSV-1.

3. Discussion

The nature of the interaction between SARS-CoV-2 and other herpesviruses, such as HSV-2, remains uncertain. Following infection with SARS-CoV-2, a series of hyperinflammatory events occur, leading to immune system dysregulation at the cellular and molecular levels [13]. Tartari et al. reported on 4 patients who developed cutaneous zoster while being hospitalized for COVID-19, all of whom had decreased CD3+ CD8+ lymphocytes before the onset of zoster [10]. Cutaneous zoster reactivation has also been described in patients with asymptomatic COVID-19 [11]. COVID-19 and VZV coinfection, presenting as a trigeminal neuropathy, have also been reported in a 39-year-old immunocompetent man with very few COVID-19 symptoms [17]. The altered immune state that occurs following SARS-CoV-2 infection may potentially serve as the gateway for latent HSV-2 reactivation.

The bilateral involvement of ARN usually occurs within months of the initial presentation [5]. In our case, the reactivation in the fellow eye occurred 4 years after the initial presentation. Although contralateral involvement seldom occurs several years after the initial episode, in our patient, it may have been triggered by the secondary immune vulnerability caused by a SARS-CoV-2 superinfection [5]. Despite the fact that our patient was clinically asymptomatic, we hypothesize that SARS-CoV-2 may have caused decreased peripheral CD3+ CD8+ T lymphocyte counts, thus inhibiting both her regulatory mechanisms and her protection against latent HSV [18].

Patients who present with acute or reactivated diseases associated with immune system dysfunction, such as ARN, may warrant an evaluation for possible SARS-CoV-2 infection, at least during the remainder of the pandemic. In addition, patients with a personal history of conditions such as ARN, where patients may be vulnerable to immune system deregulation, should remain vigilant for potential reactivations in the setting of a SARS-CoV-2 RNA superinfection.

Due to the low recurrence rate of ARN, long-term antiviral therapy may not be a mainstay of clinical practice [19]. However, antiviral treatment has been shown to reduce the risk of developing bilateral ARN [6]. Therefore, in patients who have a history of ARN in 1 eye, the benefits of preventing a recurrence of ARN in the contralateral eye may outweigh the risks associated with long-term antiviral therapy. Given the altered immune state caused by COVID-19, patients with a prior history of ARN or any other ocular HSV manifestation may be at increased risk of disease reactivation and, therefore, should consider secondary antiviral prophylaxis during SARS CoV-2 infection.

4. Conclusion

Our case suggests that ARN reactivation may occur following COVID-19 infection. Ophthalmologists should be aware of the predisposition that COVID-19's impact on the immune system may induce the reactivation of HSV-related diseases. Secondary prophylaxis with systemic antiherpetic medications should be considered for patients with a prior history of vision loss due to ARN, particularly if they are suffering from COVID-19.

Consent

Consent to publish the case report was not obtained. This report does not contain any personal information that could lead to the identification of the patient.

Authors' Contributions

All authors attest that they meet the current ICMJE criteria for authorship.

References

[1] S. D. Schoenberger, S. J. Kim, J. E. Thorne et al., "Diagnosis and treatment of acute retinal necrosis: a report by the American Academy of Ophthalmology," *Ophthalmology*, vol. 124, no. 3, pp. 382–392, 2017.

[2] M. N. Muthiah, M. Michaelides, C. S. Child, and S. M. Mitchell, "Acute retinal necrosis: a national population-based study to assess the incidence, methods of diagnosis, treatment strategies and outcomes in the UK," *The British Journal of Ophthalmology*, vol. 91, no. 11, pp. 1452–1455, 2007.

[3] A. M. Williams, V. Q. Nguyen, B. W. Botsford, and A. W. Eller, "Bilateral acute retinal necrosis caused by two separate viral etiologies," *American Journal of Ophthalmology Case Reports*, vol. 18, 2020.

[4] J. G. Shantha, H. M. Weissman, M. R. Debiec, T. A. Albini, and S. Yeh, "Advances in the management of acute retinal necrosis," *International Ophthalmology Clinics*, vol. 55, no. 3, pp. 1–13, 2015.

[5] B. Lei, R. Jiang, Z. Wang, G. Xu, X. Wu, and M. Zhou, "Bilateral acute retinal necrosis: a case series," *Retina*, vol. 40, no. 1, pp. 145–153, 2020.

[6] D. A. Palay, P. Sternberg Jr., J. Davis et al., "Decrease in the risk of bilateral acute retinal necrosis by acyclovir therapy," *American Journal of Ophthalmology*, vol. 112, no. 3, pp. 250–255, 1991.

[7] A. L. Li, J. G. Shantha, S. Yeh, and H. F. Fine, "Update on the management of acute retinal necrosis," *Ophthalmic Surgery, Lasers & Imaging Retina*, vol. 50, no. 12, pp. 748–751, 2019.

[8] J. B. Suzich and A. R. Cliffe, "Strength in diversity: understanding the pathways to herpes simplex virus reactivation," *Virology*, vol. 522, pp. 81–91, 2018.

[9] K. P. Egan, S. Wu, B. Wigdahl, and S. R. Jennings, "Immunological control of herpes simplex virus infections," *Journal of Neurovirology*, vol. 19, no. 4, pp. 328–345, 2013.

[10] F. Tartari, A. Spadotto, C. Zengarini et al., "Herpes zoster in COVID-19-positive patients," *International Journal of Dermatology*, vol. 59, no. 8, pp. 1028-1029, 2020.

[11] M. L. Elsaie, E. A. Youssef, and H. A. Nada, "Herpes zoster might be an indicator for latent COVID 19 infection," *Dermatologic Therapy*, vol. 33, no. 4, article e13666, 2020.

[12] M. Latalska and J. Mackiewicz, "The implication of ocular manifestation of COVID-19 for medical staff and patients - systematic review," *Annals of Agricultural and Environmental Medicine*, vol. 27, no. 2, pp. 165–170, 2020.

[13] A. Tufan, A. Avanoğlu Güler, and M. Matucci-Cerinic, "COVID-19, immune system response, hyperinflammation and repurposing antirheumatic drugs," *Turkish Journal Of Medical Sciences*, vol. 50, no. SI-1, pp. 620–632, 2020.

[14] T. Li, Z. Qiu, L. Zhang et al., "Significant changes of peripheral T lymphocyte subsets in patients with severe acute respiratory syndrome," *The Journal of Infectious Diseases*, vol. 189, no. 4, pp. 648–651, 2004.

[15] P. Wu, F. Duan, C. Luo et al., "Characteristics of ocular findings of patients with coronavirus disease 2019 (COVID-19) in Hubei Province, China," *JAMA Ophthalmology*, vol. 138, no. 5, pp. 575–578, 2020.

[16] P. M. Marinho, A. A. A. Marcos, A. C. Romano, H. Nascimento, and R. Belfort Jr., "Retinal findings in patients with COVID-19," *Lancet*, vol. 395, no. 10237, p. 1610, 2020.

[17] A. C. A. de F. Ferreira, T. T. Romão, Y. S. Macedo, C. Pupe, O. J. M. Nascimento, and Fellow of the American Academy of Neurology (FAAN), "COVID-19 and herpes zoster co-infection presenting with trigeminal neuropathy," *European Journal of Neurology*, vol. 27, no. 9, pp. 1748–1750, 2020.

[18] F. Wang, J. Nie, H. Wang et al., "Characteristics of peripheral lymphocyte subset alteration in COVID-19 pneumonia," *The Journal of Infectious Diseases*, vol. 221, no. 11, pp. 1762–1769, 2020.

[19] C. P. Donovan, A. L. Levison, C. Y. Lowder, D. F. Martin, and S. K. Srivastava, "Delayed recurrence of acute retinal necrosis (ARN): a case series," *Journal of Clinical Virology*, vol. 80, pp. 68–71, 2016.

4

Stellate Nonhereditary Idiopathic Foveomacular Retinoschisis: Cataract Surgery

Sofie Van der Auwera[1] **and Oscar Kallay**[2]

[1]*Department of Ophthalmology, Antwerp University Hospital, Edegem, Belgium*
[2]*Centre Médical de l'Alliance, Braine l'Alleud, Belgium*

Correspondence should be addressed to Sofie Van der Auwera; sofie.vanderauwera@outlook.com and Oscar Kallay; oscar_kallay@yahoo.fr

Academic Editor: Stephen G. Schwartz

Purpose. We present the first case described in the literature of cataract surgery in a patient with stellate nonhereditary idiopathic foveomacular retinoschisis (SNIF). *Methods.* In this case report, we describe the extensive workup we did on our patient, including optical coherence tomography, fundus autofluorescence, fluo-angiography, full field electroretinogram, and genetic testing. We moreover describe the cataract surgery with clear lens extraction and implanting of a multifocal implant. *Results.* The refractive and lifestyle profile of our patient made implantation of multifocal intraocular implants the only solution for this case. During preoperative measurements, a SNIF diagnosis was suspected after optic coherence tomography imaging which led to an even more extensive workup of our patient and the diagnosis of stellate nonhereditary idiopathic foveomacular retinoschisis. We then proceeded to cataract surgery, which was performed safely and without any sequellae. *Conclusion.* Stellate nonhereditary idiopathic foveomacular retinoschisis (SNIF) is a relatively new disease entity. Only few cases in the literature describe this disease, and none of them describe cataract surgery in a patient with SNIF. We therefore describe the first known cataract surgery in such a case. Long term follow-up results show that the procedure can be performed safely. *Summary Statement.* We hereby present the first case described in the literature of cataract surgery of a patient diagnosed with stellate nonhereditary idiopathic foveomacular retinoschisis. A clear lens extraction with implantation of a multifocal intraocular implant was conducted with excellent postoperative results and a happy patient.

1. Introduction

Stellate nonhereditary idiopathic foveomacular retinoschisis is a rather new diagnosis in the retinal ophthalmology field. A few case reports about the disease entity have been published. Since little is known about SNIF, there is currently no data present about the postoperative status of anterior segment surgery with phacoemulsification in these patients. We hereby present a 51-year old woman with stellate nonhereditary idiopathic foveomacular retinoschisis who underwent a clear lens extraction for refractive needs and her 1-year follow-up.

2. Case Report

A 51-year old woman consulted for advice concerning refractive surgery. She had an intolerance to progressive glasses and suffered from daily work as a hairdresser. She was currently wearing monofocal glasses with a spherical correction of +3.50 on both sides, which resulted in a Snellen visual acuity (VA) of 20/30, without possible improvement and poor near vision. The autorefractor values were OD +4.00 (-1.25@97) and OS +3.75 (-0.50@90). Best corrected VA for near was Parinaud (P) 3 for both eyes. Clinical examination nor biomicroscopy did reveal any particulars. Fundoscopy was normal.

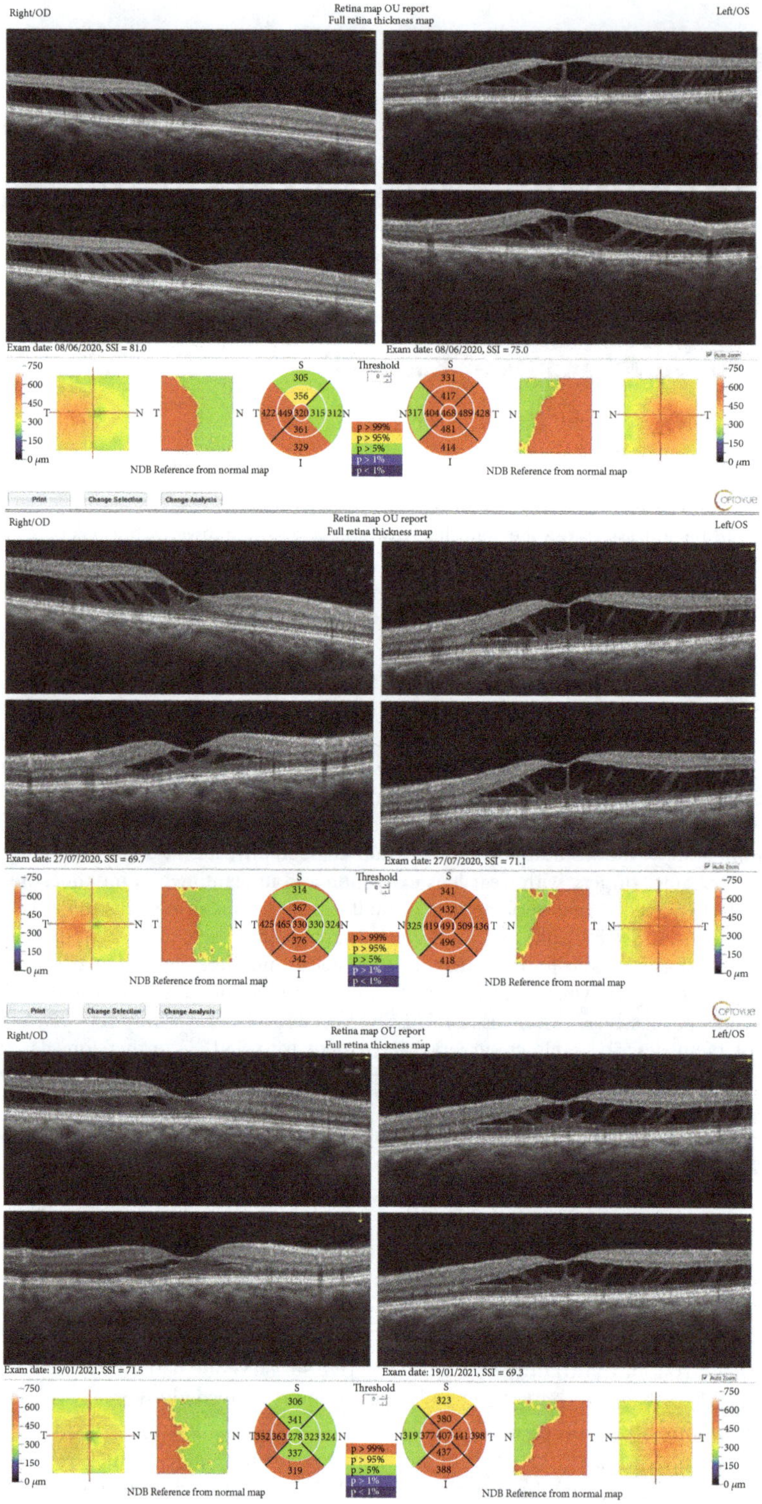

FIGURE 1: Bilateral OCT-imaging preoperative, 1 day postoperative and 6 months postoperative.

A macular optic coherence tomography (OCT) was performed which showed a bilateral stellate retinoschisis pattern between the outer plexiform layer and the outer nuclear layer. The schisis was located macular and was more widespread in the left eye. Figure 1.

Some additional tests were done to determine the origin of the retinoschisis. These tests included fundus imaging (Clarus®), fluo-angiography, and fundus autofluorescence. Each of these examinations showed normal macular anatomy and normal retinal vasculature without obstructions

Scot. ERG

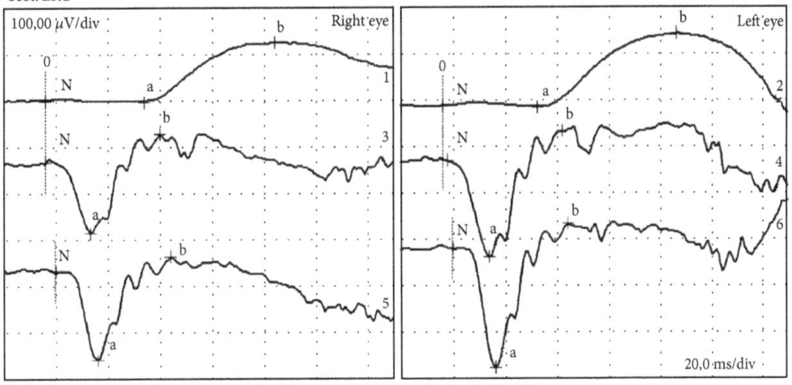

Step	a (ms)	b (ms)	a-wave (μV)	b-wave (μV)	Avgs.
1: OD DA 0.01	38,1	87,9	2,55	127,75	8,0
2: OS DA 0.01	36,3	90,5	2,17	159,32	8,0
3: OD DA 3.0	17,6	44,2	152,60	213,05	5,0
4: OS DA 3.0	18,2	46,0	206,78	269,42	5,0
5: OD DA 10.0	16,4	44,8	191,02	222,05	5,0
6: OS DA 10.0	16,4	44,2	257,16	310,15	5,0

Oscillatory-P.

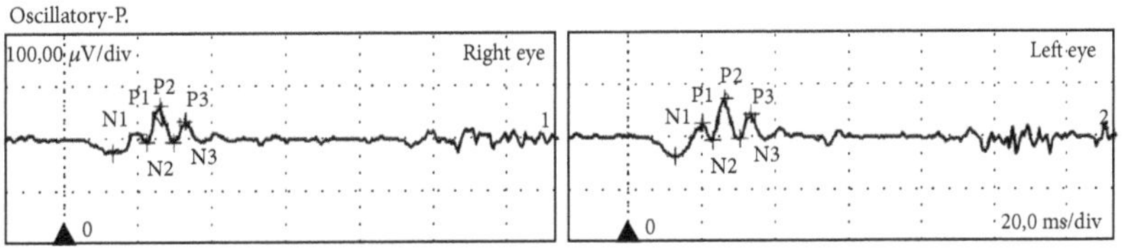

Step	N1 (ms)	P1 (ms)	N2 (ms)	P2 (ms)	N3 (ms)	P3 (ms)	OS1 (μV)	OS2 (μV)	OS3 (μV)	Avgs.
1: OD DA OP	13,5	19,9	22,6	26,1	29,9	33,1	36,35	67,82	37,60	2,0
2: OS DA OP	13,2	20,2	22,9	26,1	30,2	33,4	61,90	79,12	44,18	2,0

Phot.ERG

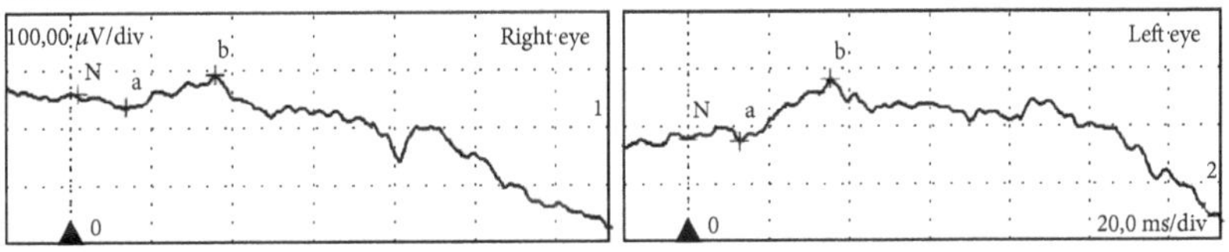

Step	a (ms)	b (ms)	a-wave (μV)	b-wave (μV)	Avgs.
1: OD LA 3.0	13,8	35,7	22,62	57,11	8,0
2: OS LA 3.0	13,2	35,4	4,56	109,78	7,0

30 Hz flicker

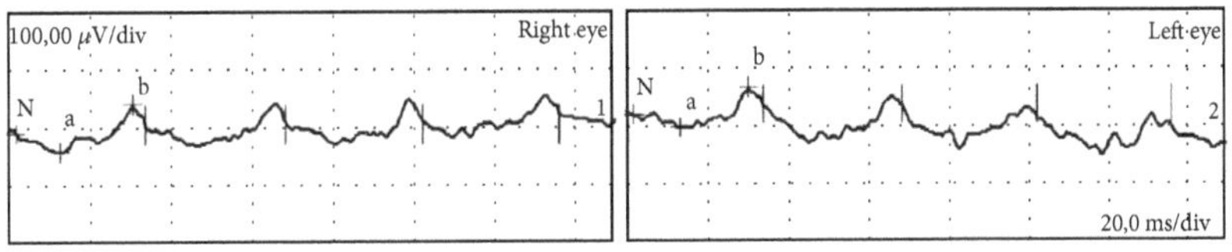

Step	a (ms)	b (ms)	a-wave (μV)	b-wave (μV)	Avgs.
1: OD LA 30 Hz	12,9	30,8	33,88	81,10	8,0
2: OS LA 30 Hz	13,5	30,5	25,63	69,15	8,0

Figure 2: Full field ERG results.

or hemorrhages. No exudates were visible. The optic disc had an estimated cup-disk ratio of 0,5 OD and 0,3 OS. A full-field electroretinogram (ff-ERG) was performed and showed some lowering in the amplitudes of the scotopic ERG, especially on the b-wave, but no electronegativity was seen. The photopic ERG showed higher amplitudes for the cones. These ERG-results correspond with the schisis seen on OCT, leaving the photoreceptors in contact with the outer nuclear layer (Figure 2). Blood samples for genetic testing were obtained, which showed our patient to be RS-1 negative. Thus excluding the possibility this retinoschisis was part of a known X-linked retinoschisis syndrome [1]. OCT-imaging in our patient parents showed a normal bilateral retina without schisis or other disease indications.

These additional results pointed towards the diagnosis of stellate nonhereditary idiopathic foveomacular retinoschisis (SNIF). SNIF is more often seen in female patients without hereditary mechanisms to explain the retinal disease. Typically, there is a rather low decrease in vision that does not cause any complaints. The schisis is, as suggested by its name, foveomacular without peripheral involvement. All of this pointed us in the direction of SNIF.

Being a hairdresser, a good vision for both near and far was necessary for the patient, but correction with multifocal glasses nor with contact lenses was tolerated. Because the refractive needs of our patient were not solvable with noninvasive refractive methods, we decided to take a leap and operate on our patient with SNIF.

When looking into literature, such an operation has not been described and thus was performed without knowing how the eye would react.

Phacoemulsification with a placement of multifocal implants was performed to meet the refractive demands of the patient. A superior scleral incision was used after which a manual capsulorhexis was performed. Phacoemulsification with the signature phaco machine was performed while using a linear flow. After removal of the clear lens and cleaning of the lens capsule, an implant was placed intracapsular. We used the AT LISA tri 839MP implant from Zeiss with bilateral +25.00D power. Peroperative lidocaine hydrochloride 1% and cefuroxime 10 mg/ml were used. A postoperative treatment regimen with dexamethasone eye drops, tobramycine eye drops, and indomethacin eye drops was prescribed.

The postoperative status led to a monocular vision of 1.2 (20/16) OD and 1.0 (20/20) OS, an improvement of, respectively, 2 and 3 lines on a standard Snellen vision chart, and a monocular near vision of P2 on both sides. Standard postoperative treatment with dexamethasone, tobramycine, and indometacine was augmented with nepafanac 3x/d to protect the retina from further damage. When consulting again after 6 months for a postoperative control, the vision had once again decreased to a best corrected Snellen VA of 0.7-2 (20/30) OD and 0.6 (20/30) OS and near vision P3 OD and P4 OS. At the 1-year postoperative control, the vision remained stable compared to the last control with no subjective complaints of decreased vision. Between both controls, autorefractor values remained stable as well with OD +0.75 (-0.75@94) and OS -0.25 (-0.25@150). The OCT images remained also stable (Figure 1). The patient was very happy in her daily work and private life with her eyesight.

3. Discussion

A stellate macular retinoschisis pattern in an RS1-negative patient in an eye without any other anatomical or functional defects is rather rare and can be classified as SNIF. Typically, this disease category represents stellate retinoschisis patterns in the foveomacular regions in an RS1-negative patient without a known family history of retinal diseases [2–5]. SNIF is a rather new diagnostic entity, with few case reports. Shimazaki and Matsuhashi [6] described a similar clinical entity as well. Most interestingly, the ERG-findings seem to be very similar between our case and theirs, with normal findings, but however a sensitive decrease of the b-wave. Their case describes a mother and daughter with the same type of retinoschisis in a SNIF pattern. In our case, however, additional OCT imaging of both parents was negative. Moreover, retinal abnormalities could be seen on fundoscopy in both women, which was not the case with our patient.

None of the described cases in literature underwent cataract surgery at the time. It is the first report of a phacoemulsification in a patient with SNIF. We had good postoperative results, without worsening of the schisis pattern. However, 1 patient is too few to draw any conclusions. We hope that when other cases in the literature age and their refractive need change, the results of the phacoemulsification procedures will be bundled and published.

Moraes et al. [7] did however perform a vitrectomy with phacoemulsification in a patient with SNIF and published about this some months after we treated our patient. They also concluded this procedure could be performed safely. They present postoperative results quite similar to ours, with no subjective decrease in vision and a good overall outcome. They did however not use a multifocal intraocular lens but a monofocal one.

We do agree with Ober et al. and Shimazaki and Matsuhashi that the disease entity described is a new clinical entity within the larger group of retinoschisis [2, 6]. We agree that further genetic testing of the uncoded parts of the RS-1 gene could help understand the etiology of such disease. Extensive screening of other family members could also be helpful, as well as the screening of (male) children of these patients. We think the ERG is an important test in the diagnostics of this type of retinoschisis, however, its exact interpretation is not fully understood [8]. We hope that with further evolving technologies in the field of electrophysiology.

4. Conclusion

We present a rather rare case of SNIF in a 51-year old female patient with bilateral disease in hyperopic eyes. Cataract surgery with clear lens extraction was performed, resulting in satisfactory postoperative results without worsening of the disease status. It is our opinion that operating on patients with SNIF can be performed safely, if all necessary precautionary measures are taken.

Additional Points

Summary Statement. We hereby present the first case described in the literature of cataract surgery of a patient diagnosed with stellate nonhereditary idiopathic foveomacular retinoschisis. A clear lens extraction with implantation of a multifocal intraocular implant was conducted with excellent postoperative results and a happy patient.

References

[1] T. Alitalo, T. A. Kruse, and A. de la Chapelle, "Refined localization of the gene causing X-linked juvenile retinoschisis," *Genomics*, vol. 9, no. 3, pp. 505–510, 1991.

[2] M. D. Ober, K. B. Freund, M. Shah et al., "Stellate nonhereditary idiopathic foveomacular retinoschisis," *Ophthalmology*, vol. 121, no. 7, pp. 1406–1413, 2014.

[3] D. Ahmed, M. Stattin, C. Glittenberg, I. Krebs, and S. Ansari-Shahrezaei, "Stellate nonhereditary idiopathic foveomacular retinoschisis accompanied by contralateral peripheral retinoschisis," *Retinal Cases and Brief Reports*, vol. 13, no. 2, pp. 135–140, 2019.

[4] M. Montano, M. D. Alfaro Dv Iii, M. A. Quiroz-Reyes et al., "Stellate unilateral nonhereditary idiopathic foveomacular retinoschisis: a multimodal imaging analysis and case report," *Retinal Cases and Brief Reports*, vol. 16, no. 4, pp. 439–443, 2022.

[5] J. B. Mandell, A. Y. Kim, A. Shahidzadeh, H. Ameri, C. A. Puliafito, and A. A. Moshfeghi, "Widefield OCT findings of a patient with stellate nonhereditary idiopathic foveomacular retinoschisis," *Ophthalmic Surgery, Lasers & Imaging Retina*, vol. 47, no. 8, pp. 774–777, 2016.

[6] J. Shimazaki and M. Matsuhashi, "Familial retinoschisis in female patients," *Documenta Ophthalmologica*, vol. 65, no. 3, pp. 393–400, 1987.

[7] B. R. Moraes, B. F. Ferreira, T. M. Nogueira, Y. Nakashima, H. P. Júnior, and E. C. Souza, "Vitrectomy for stellate nonhereditary idiopathic foveomacular retinoschisis associated with outer retinal layer defect," *Retinal Cases and Brief Reports*, vol. 16, no. 3, pp. 289–292, 2022.

[8] D. J. Creel, "Electroretinograms," *Handbook of Clinical Neurology*, vol. 160, pp. 481–493, 2019.

5

A Case Report of Purtscher-Like Retinopathy Secondary to *Pneumocystis jirovecii* Pneumonia in an Immunocompromised Patient

Alastair David Bezzina and Isaac Bertuello

Ophthalmology Department, Mater Dei General Teaching Hospital, Malta

Correspondence should be addressed to Isaac Bertuello; isaac.bertuello@gov.mt

Academic Editor: Kamal Kishore

To the best of our knowledge, we present the first case of a young adult male, on long-term immunosuppressive therapy following a live-donor kidney transplant, with Purtscher-like retinopathy (PLR) secondary to *Pneumocystis jirovecii* pneumonia (PCP). The patient had presented to a routine medical follow-up and complained of a few weeks' history of dyspnoea and tachycardia after minimal exertion followed by acute bilateral blurring of vision. Unfortunately, the patient did not respond to a trial of corticosteroid treatment and subsequently became severely visually impaired. This case report expands the aetiological spectrum behind PLR and helps portray the disease process which, in some cases, leads to severe ischaemic sequelae.

1. Introduction

PLR is an ischaemic retinopathy which occurs in the context of conditions other than trauma, which has been classically related to Purtscher's retinopathy (PR). PLR is thought to arise secondary to leucoaggregation in response to a variety of inflammatory aetiologies leading to arteriolar blockage and subsequent retinal ischaemia. As with other types of ocular vascular disorders, PLR presents with sudden loss of vision and on clinical examination one will observe cotton wool spots, intraretinal haemorrhages, and the pathognomonic "Purtscher flecken" which are areas of perivascular pallor representing inner retinal ischaemia [1]. Multiple aetiologies [2] have been associated with PLR in the literature but, to our knowledge, this case report describes the first case of PLR secondary to an opportunistic fungal infection in an immunocompromised patient.

2. Case Report

The patient in question is a 30-year-old Caucasian gentleman who was being followed up regularly by one of the local nephrology firms following a live-donor kidney transplant a few years back. The patient complained of a few weeks' history of dyspnoea and tachycardia on minimal exertion. He denied having other symptoms, but mild pitting lower limb oedema was noted on examination. The gentleman also complained of multiple patches of skin eruptions which had been slowly developing over the past 6 months.

His past medical and surgical history included chronic kidney disease secondary to meningococcal septicaemia at eight years of age. This progressed to end-stage chronic kidney disease at the age of twenty-one. He was first started on peritoneal dialysis and later converted to haemodialysis. At age twenty-eight, the patient received a live kidney transplant from his brother. Four months later, the transplanted kidney was biopsied after a rise in serum creatinine was noted. Histology showed mild tubulitis, suggesting early cell-mediated rejection, which led to the doses of his immunosuppressive medications to be increased.

At the time of presentation, the patient was on tacrolimus 3 mg twice daily, mycophenolate 720 mg twice daily, prednisolone 5 mg daily, omeprazole 20 mg daily, folic acid 5 mg daily, and bumetanide 0.5 mg daily. He had no known drug allergies. Family and social history were unremarkable.

Initial examination revealed a regular pulse rate of 95 beats per minute which increased to 120 beats per minute on walking, a blood pressure of 120/80 mmHg, and a SpO2 of 98% which remained stable on exertion. The patient was afebrile at the time of examination. Bilateral mild pitting oedema up to the ankles was present.

Initial investigations included laboratory tests which showed a normal neutrophil count of 8.30 ($4.30 - 11.40 \times 10^9$/L) with a lymphopenia of 0.74 ($2.10 - 3.60 \times 10^9$/L). Normocytic anaemia was present with a haemoglobin level of 11.0 g/dL (14.1–17.2 g/dL) and a haematocrit of 34.1% (40.4–50.4%). Platelet count was normal at 186 ($146 - 302 \times 10^9$/L). Creatinine was 120 μmol/L (59–104 μmol/L), which remained relatively stable since the renal transplant occurred, with a urea of 13.2 mmol/L (1.7–8.3 mmol/L) and an eGFR of 64 mL/min/1.73m^2. C-reactive protein and erythrocyte sedimentation rate were slightly elevated at 14.4 mg/L (0–5 mg/L) and 14 mm 1st hr (8–12 mm 1st hr), respectively. Natriuretic peptide (NT-proBNP) level was also slightly elevated at 147 pg/mL (5–125 pg/mL). Liver function tests were normal. The serum albumin had decreased slightly when compared to previous results at 34 g/L (32–52 g/L), previously 48 g/L, however, still in the normal range. The serum tacrolimus level was 8.8 ng/mL which was in range. Serological tests for toxoplasma and leishmania and the autoimmune screen were all negative. A virology screen was carried out which included polymerase chain reaction (PCR) tests for herpes simplex, varicella zoster, cytomegalovirus, Epstein-Barr virus, BK virus, COVID-19, and other viral respiratory pathogens, all of which turned out negative. The lactate dehydrogenase level was normal but beta-D glucan was detected at >523 pg/mL (positive > 80 pg/mL). Urinalysis and urine microscopy, culture, and sensitivity were all normal. An electrocardiogram showed a normal sinus rhythm at 90 bpm, and an echocardiogram excluded any cardiac pathology. Chest X-ray was unremarkable.

A few days after the nephrology team started their investigations, the patient presented to our eye emergency department complaining of sudden onset painless and rapidly progressive bilateral blurring of vision. Right eye visual acuity (VA) was 6/36, which improved to 6/36+1 with pinhole while the left eye VA was 6/60 and did not improve with pinhole. Pupils were both reactive with no RAPD. Ishihara colour testing was not possible as the patient could not read the test plate. Examination of the anterior segment was unremarkable. The intraocular pressures were 15 mmHg bilaterally. On dilated fundoscopy, the discs were unremarkable except for mild nasal blurring of the disc margins. Both maculae were surrounded by small patches of retinal pallor, cotton wool spots, and intraretinal haemorrhages were observed across the posterior pole and mid-periphery in both eyes (Figure 1). Optical coherence tomography (OCT) revealed bilateral hyperreflective patches at the level of the inner nuclear layer suggestive of paracentral acute middle maculopathy (Figure 2). Fluorescein angiography revealed an enlarged foveal avascular zone as well as early patchy hyperfluorescence (Figures 3 and 4). In view of a lack of history of trauma and the typical findings of perivascular patchy pallor, haemorrhages, and cotton wool spots, a diagnosis of PLR was made.

After discussion with the caring nephrology firm, it was agreed to wait for the CT-pulmonary angiogram (CTPA) before attempting a trial of steroids.

The CTPA excluded pulmonary embolism as the cause for dyspnoea and sinus tachycardia but showed faint diffuse ground glass changes which were more predominant in the perihilar areas. This was suggestive of pneumocystis pneumonia. PCR performed on bronchoalveolar lavage samples detected *Pneumocystis jirovecii* which confirmed the diagnosis of PCP. Tests for mycobacteria and galactomannan antigen were negative, and cytological analysis of the samples was unremarkable.

Given these findings, the tacrolimus dose was decreased in order to reduce the serum levels to 5-6 ng/mL, while mycophenolate was stopped temporarily. The PCP was treated with trimethoprim-sulfamethaxozole at 960 mg three times daily for a total of 21 days and then reduced to 480 mg daily indefinitely. A trial of pulsed methyl prednisolone was attempted to treat the PLR. This consisted of three doses of 250 mg IV methyl prednisolone over three days with omeprazole cover. This was followed by a course of oral prednisolone which was tapered down gradually. The patient was then left on a maintenance dose of 5 mg daily.

After commencing therapy, the dyspnoea and tachycardia resolved with PCP resolution also being confirmed on repeat CT Thorax. Patient was restarted on mycophenolate but on a lower dose of 360 mg twice daily, and the tacrolimus dose adjusted to maintain levels of around 5 ng/mL. His renal function and creatinine clearance remained stable all throughout. The patient was also seen by the dermatology team in view of the rash and was diagnosed with trichodysplasia spinulosa after histopathological analysis of a skin biopsy specimen revealed keratohyaline granules and a glass chromatic pattern. Even though viral immunostaining was negative, the patient responded well to empirical valganciclovir treatment, and the rash ultimately resolved.

Unfortunately, the ischaemia brought about by the PLR progressed as the patient continued losing his visual acuity. Four weeks postpresentation, the patient's VA was down to counting fingers eccentrically in both eyes. There was an increase in intraretinal haemorrhages and macular oedema on repeat fundoscopy (Figures 5–7). At that point, he was offered intravitreal bevacizumab injections but was not keen to commence such treatment. After a week, the patient accepted to undergo a trial of intravitreal bevacizumab in both eyes. The patient later developed bilateral neovascularisation at the disc (NVD) as well as a mild vitreous haemorrhage in the left eye. Bilateral pan-retinal photocoagulation was performed.

On examination, 4 weeks later, the condition was still worsening with florid NVDs present, and an epiretinal membrane had formed bilaterally. Further photocoagulation fill-in was performed.

Despite all our efforts, the VA had decreased to hand movements bilaterally at 4 months postpresentation. On fundoscopy of the right eye, one could observe a thickened posterior hyaloid and an extensive preretinal bleed which

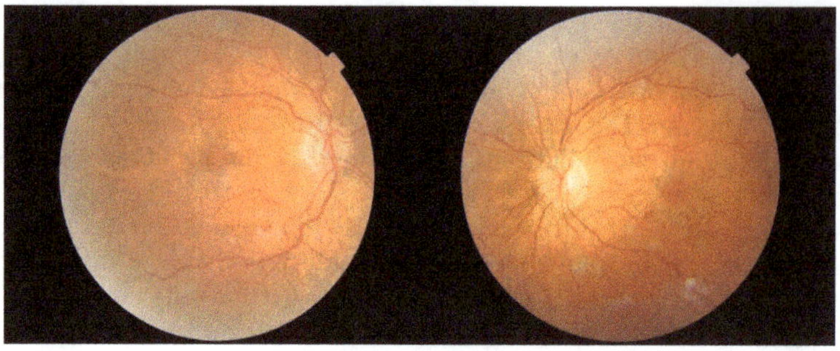

FIGURE 1: Fundal photos of the right and left eyes on presentation demonstrating intraretinal haemorrhages, cotton wool spots and Purtscher flecken with the characteristic clear zone between the lesions and the blood vessels.

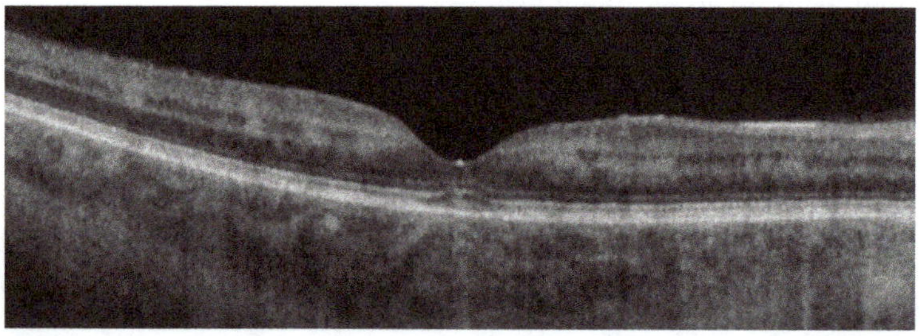

FIGURE 2: OCT B-scan at presentation demonstrating inner nuclear layer hyperreflectivity at the macula suggestive of paracentral acute middle maculopathy.

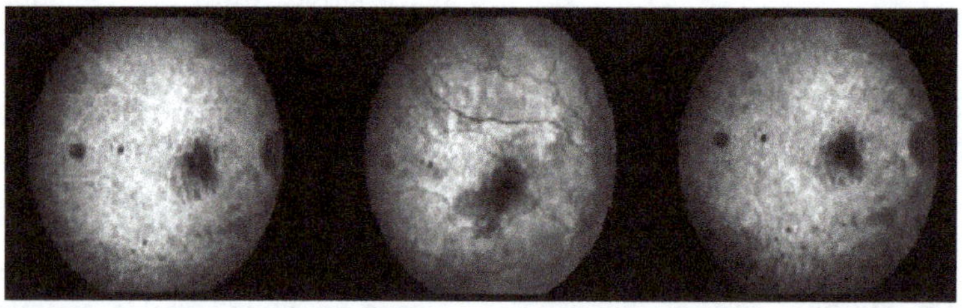

FIGURE 3: Fluorescein angiography of the right eye at presentation. One can observe the enlarged foveal avascular zone and patchy hypofluorescence in the early phases which suggest that the choroid is also involved in PLR.

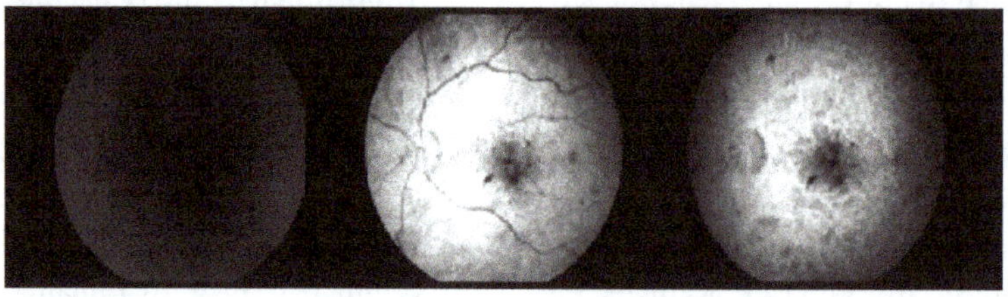

FIGURE 4: Fluorescein angiography of the left eye at presentation.

was obstructing the posterior pole view associated with a florid fibrovascular NVD (Figure 8) while in the left eye, there was a preretinal haemorrhage inferiorly as well as similar NVD plexus. A vitreoretinal opinion was obtained but due to the poor prognosis and high risk of surgery, it was agreed to proceed with further intravitreal bevacizumab injections and then consider surgery if there was no improvement.

The patient continued deteriorating with the visual field becoming more constricted and the VA decreasing to light perception in both eyes. At this point, it was agreed that surgery would not provide any benefit in view of the poor prognosis.

The patient is still being followed up in the outpatient clinic as he is at a high risk of neovascular glaucoma due to the extensive ischaemia affecting both retinas.

3. Discussion

To the best of our knowledge, this is the first reported case of PLR secondary to *Pneumocystis jirovecii* infection in an

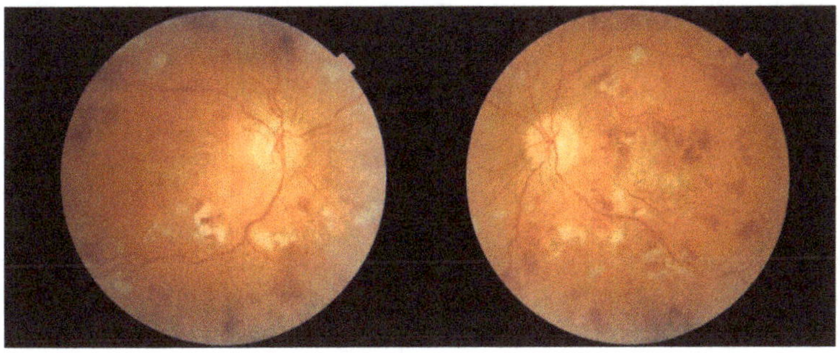

FIGURE 5: Fundal photos of the right and the left eyes 1-week postpresentation.

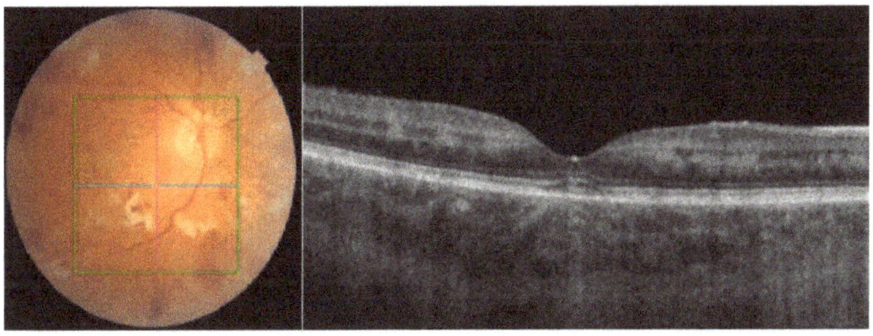

FIGURE 6: Fundal photo and OCT of the right eye 1-month postpresentation.

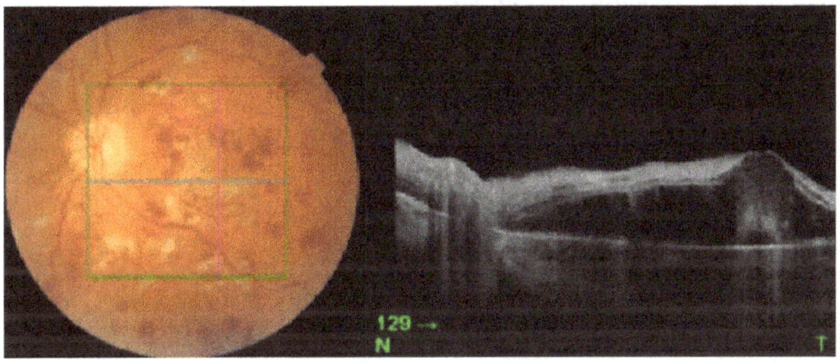

FIGURE 7: Fundal photo and OCT of the left eye 1-month postpresentation. An increase in cotton wool spots, intraretinal haemorrhages, and Purtscher's flecken was noted along with macular oedema which was confirmed on OCT.

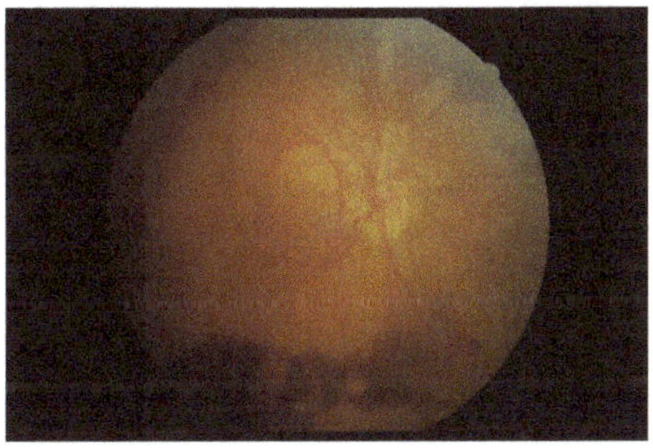

FIGURE 8: Fundal photo of the right eye 6-month postpresentation. Note: the florid NVD and inferior-lying preretinal haemorrhage.

immunocompromised patient. PR was originally described by Otmar Purtscher after examining the fundus of a patient who had previously sustained head trauma after a fall, describing the typical signs of retinal haemorrhages and areas of retinal pallor (later coined as Purtscher's flecken) [3]. According to data collected from the British Ophthalmic Surveillance Unit, the annual incidence of symptomatic PR and PLR totals to approximately 0.24 per million per year [4].

Similar to PR, PLR is a condition with similar clinical characteristics, albeit linked to other systemic issues other than the classical association to head and thoracic trauma. The diagnostic criteria selected by Miguel et al. in their systematic review on PR and PLR include the presence of Purtscher's flecken, cotton wool spots, retinal haemorrhages, coexisting systemic inflammation or recent trauma, and hypercomplementaemia [2]. Purtscher's flecken are areas of patchy perivascular retinal pallor with a typical sparing of the immediate perivascular representing small-calibre arteriolar blockage leading to inner retinal ischaemia [1]. Cotton wool spots are manifestations of blocked axoplasmic flow secondary to ischaemia and, although not pathognomonic in themselves, they are the most frequently reported fundal finding in PR and PLR alike [2].

PLR may mimic other conditions including retinal vein and arterial occlusions (which were ruled out based on the lack of fundoscopic findings and the appearance and behaviour of the initial fluorescein angiogram) as well as HIV retinopathy and viral retinitis which is also another important aetiology in immunocompromised patients. The mode of presentation, lack of retinitis on clinical examination, and negative viral PCR results helped exclude the latter differential diagnoses.

The pathogenesis of both PR and PLR is still being debated, but bilateral ischaemic ocular changes in the light of systemic disease suggest that a widespread thromboembolic phenomenon affecting small calibre vessels, namely, precapillary arterioles, is very likely [1]. The appearance of Purtscher's flecken, characterised by retinal pallor sparing the para-arterial area, suggests that intermediate-sized emboli are most likely responsible for this phenomenon as larger emboli would obstruct the larger tributaries creating the typical branch arterial occlusion phenotype [1]. Experimental models employing the injection of graded Ballotini beads injected via the common carotid artery were performed in 1965 by Ashton and Henkind who described a similar fundal appearance due to retinal arteriole embolization [5]. It has been postulated that PLR may be related to leucoaggregation and embolization secondary to hypercomplementaemia and increased complement activation, namely, complement 5a, secondary to systemic inflammation [1] whilst PR may be related to trauma-induced vascular endothelial damage which may lead to endothelin upregulation and ultimately fibrin and platelet aggregation leading to the formation of microthrombi [6]. Literature describing cases secondary to infection is scarce, but a report by Liang and Reichel in 2015 did report complement 5a hypercomplementaemia in a patient who developed PLR secondary to a gingival abcess [7] supporting the aforementioned hypothesis. Other sources of microemboli may include fat emboli released from long bones during surgery or after sustaining fractures [8] and air embolization following trauma [9].

Pneumocystis jirovecii is an opportunistic fungal infection which is again on the rise in view of an increase in patients requiring chemotherapy or immunomodulatory therapy to manage cancer or autoimmune conditions or who require immune suppression following solid organ transplantation as in this case [10]. The immunopathogenesis of *Pneumocystis jirovecii* infection is still debated, but studies using animal models revealed increased pulmonary macrophage-derived complement 3 release and subsequent cleavage and activation of complement 5 [11]. This, once again, supports the hypothesis suggesting that complement-driven leucoaggregation and embolization may be the cause behind PLR secondary to systemic inflammation.

The management of PR and PLR is a matter of ongoing debate. Multiple case reports have suggested faster resolution of PR and PLR following the administration of high-dose systemic corticosteroids, but results from the systematic review performed by Miguel et al., which assimilated multiple case reports and series over the years, concluded that there was no statistically significant difference in terms of visual outcome between patients who received corticosteroid treatment and those who were observed [2]. Corticosteroids are known to affect the complement system via an upregulation of C1 inhibitors, thus arresting the complement activation cascade leading to the activation of C5 [12] which might explain how timely administration of high-dose steroids may help in the management of PLR. Further studies are required to establish their efficacy, although the paucity of PLR cases will limit study design and strength. In this case, high-dose corticosteroids were contraindicated initially in view of the fungal aetiology.

Spontaneous visual recovery, to different degrees, has been described in both PR and PLR cases with the former usually having a better outcome [2]. According to Agrawal and McKibbin, findings such as outer retinal involvement on presentation and the presence of disc leakage and choroidal hypoperfusion as well as the extent of retinal ischaemia on initial fluorescein angiography have been associated with a poorer clinical outcome [1]. Similar to this case, neovascularisation secondary to the ischaemic drive posed by PR or PLR may occur as described in a few other cases [13, 14]. Although not commonly encountered, the ischaemic pathophysiology of PR and PLR would explain why such an event may occur and supports the microembolic theory behind both variants of the disease. Despite timely management using both pan-retinal photocoagulation and bevacizumab injections, the neovascularisation encountered in this case did not regress.

In conclusion, this case provides further evidence towards the association between systemic infection and the evolution of PLR as well as highlighting the risk of developing neovascularisation in such circumstances which can, at times, be resistant to mainstay laser and intravitreal therapies.

Authors' Contributions

Alastair David Bezzina contributed to the writing-reviewing and editing. Isaac Bertuello contributed to the writing-original draft preparation.

References

[1] A. Agrawal and M. A. McKibbin, "Purtscher's and Purtscher-like retinopathies: a review," *Survey of Ophthalmology*, vol. 51, no. 2, pp. 129–136, 2006.

[2] A. I. M. Miguel, F. Henriques, L. F. R. Azevedo, A. J. R. Loureiro, and D. A. L. Maberley, "Systematic review of Purtscher's and Purtscher-like retinopathies," *Eye*, vol. 27, no. 1, pp. 1–13, 2013.

[3] Ges OP-BDO, "1910 undefined. Noch unbekannte befunde nach schadeltrauma," 2022, https://ci.nii.ac.jp/naid/10011691104/.

[4] A. Agrawal and M. McKibbin, "Purtscher's retinopathy: epidemiology, clinical features and outcome," *The British Journal of Ophthalmology*, vol. 91, no. 11, pp. 1456–1459, 2007.

[5] N. Ashton and P. Henkind, "Experimental Occlusion of Retinal Arterioles (using graded glass Ballotini)," *British Journal of Ophthalmology*, vol. 49, pp. 225–234, 1965, https://www.ncbi.nlm.nih.gov/pmc/articles/PMC506101/.

[6] T. J. Harrison, C. O. Abbasi, and T. A. Khraishi, "Purtscher retinopathy: an alternative etiology supported by computer fluid dynamic simulations," *Investigative Opthalmology & Visual Science*, vol. 52, pp. 8102–8107, 2011.

[7] M. C. Liang, E. Reichel, and E. C. Wright, "Man referred for sudden onset decline in vision in left eye," 2015, https://www.healio.com/news/ophthalmology/20150516/j241_3310_32_news_print_1.

[8] D. Roden, G. Fitzpatrick, H. O'Donoghue, and D. Phelan, "Purtscher's retinopathy and fat embolism," *British Journal of Ophthalmology*, vol. 73, pp. 677–679, 1989.

[9] T. C. Burton, "Unilateral Purtscher's Retinopathy," *Ophthalmology*, vol. 87, no. 11, pp. 1096–1105, 1980.

[10] L. Patterson, P. Coyle, T. Curran, N. Q. Verlander, and J. Johnston, "Changing epidemiology of pneumocystis pneumonia, Northern Ireland, UK and implications for prevention, 1 July 2011-31 July 2012," *Journal of Medical Microbiology*, vol. 66, pp. 1650–1655, 2017.

[11] M. E. Lasbury, P. J. Durant, D. Tschang et al., "Expression and activation of complement protein and alveolar damage during pneumocystis pneumonia," *The Journal of Eukaryotic Microbiology*, vol. 53, no. s1, pp. S136–S137, 2006.

[12] E. Zimmermann-Nielsen, H. Grønbæk, J. F. Dahlerup, G. Baatrup, and O. Thorlacius-Ussing, "Complement activation capacity in plasma before and during high-dose prednisolone treatment and tapering in exacerbations of Crohn's disease and ulcerative colitis," *BMC Gastroenterology*, vol. 5, pp. 1–7, 2005.

[13] A. Chan, D. R. Fredrick, and T. Leng, "Neovascularization in Purtscher's retinopathy," *Clinical Ophthalmology*, vol. 5, p. 1585, 2011.

[14] M. Kuroda, A. Nishida, M. Kikuchi, and Y. Kurimoto, "Purtscher's retinopathy followed by neovascular glaucoma," *Clinical Ophthalmology*, vol. 7, pp. 2235–2237, 2013.

6

Bilateral Multiple Focal Choroidal Excavations in a Patient with Paroxysmal Nocturnal Hemoglobinuria (PNH)

Ping Huang, Tal Ben Ami, and Weiye Li

Department of Ophthalmology, Drexel University College of Medicine, 219 N. Broad Street, Philadelphia, PA 19107, USA

Correspondence should be addressed to Weiye Li; wl27@drexel.edu

Academic Editor: Nicola Rosa

Focal choroidal excavation (FCE) is an unusual configuration characterized by focal thinning and pitting of the choroid in the absence of staphyloma or scleral ectasia. The etiology and clinical implications of FCE are currently unknown. We report a case of bilateral multiple FCEs in a patient with a long history of paroxysmal nocturnal hemoglobinuria (PNH). Focal choriocapillaris thinning and hyperreflectivity of the adjacent outer nuclear layer were revealed by spectral domain optical coherence tomography, which suggests the occlusion of the choriocapillaries and secondary degeneration of the above photoreceptors. We hypothesize that thrombophilia in the condition of PNH played an important role in the formation of FCE. Although there is no histopathological evidence to support the association between the choroid changes and PNH, this case may offer new clues as for the etiology of FCE.

1. Introduction

Focal choroidal excavation is an unusual configuration of the choroid detected by spectral domain optical coherence tomography (OCT), which shows focal thinning and pitting of the choroid with an intact sclera. This clinical entity was first described in a case report by Jampol and colleagues in 2006 [1]. Later, Margolis et al. [2] reviewed 12 patients with similar choroidal contour and recommended to use the term focal choroidal excavation (FCE) for these OCT image findings. They also hypothesized that the FCE is a congenital posterior segment malformation. After this unique choroid contour was recognized, FCE has been reported to be associated with several different pathologies, such as polypoidal choroidal vasculopathy [3–5], central serous chorioretinopathy (CSCR) [6], choroidal neovascularization [7–9], blunt trauma [10], multiple evanescent white dot syndrome [11], and best vitelliform dystrophy [12].

The published reports were based on images by different modalities including OCT, fluorescein angiography (FA), fundus autofluorescence (FAF), and indocyanine green angiography (ICG). However, there are no histopathologic studies to support them. The etiology and clinical significance of FCE are still unclear.

We are reporting an observation of FCE in a patient with paroxysmal nocturnal hemoglobinuria (PNH). PNH is a rare acquired stem cell disorder characterized by chronic intravascular hemolysis and hemoglobinuria, an increased risk of thrombosis, and a variable degree of bone marrow failure [13]. It has been previously reported that PNH may cause retinal vascular occlusions [14]. There is one report describing bilateral central serous retinopathy in a patient with PNH [15].

Herein, we present a case with bilateral multiple focal choroidal excavations in a patient with PNH.

2. Case Report

A 54-year-old Chinese man presented in the clinic for a routine two-year ophthalmic examination. Past medical history is PNH. The patient was diagnosed with PNH at the age of 22. He is on Eculizumab (anti-complement factor 5 antibody) infusion which he started in 2007.

He was asymptomatic with best-corrected visual acuity of 20/40 on the right eye (spherical equivalent is +0.5), and 20/20 on the left eye (spherical equivalent is +0.25). Slit-lamp examination and intraocular pressures were normal. Posterior segment examination revealed subtle pigmentary changes temporal to the macula in both eyes (Figure 1). Enhanced depth imaging-OCT (EDI-OCT) of the macula was obtained and the entire posterior pole was also scanned. The OCT-detected multiple FCEs corresponded with the retinal

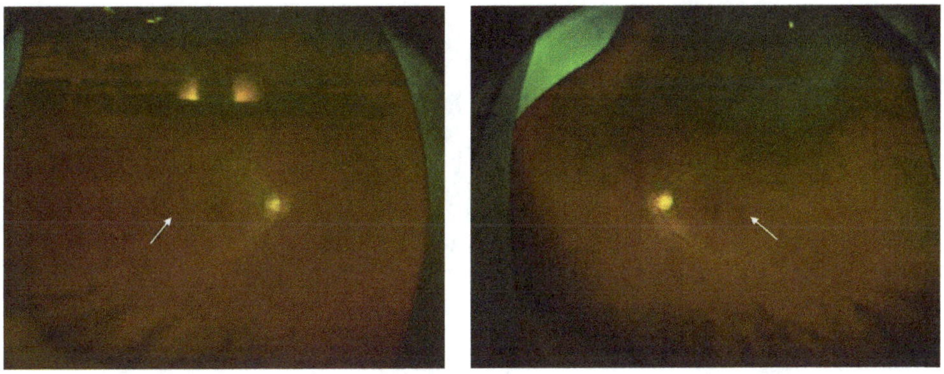

(a) (b)

FIGURE 1: Fundus color photo of (a) right eye; (b) left eye. Subtle pigmentary changes temporal to the macula (arrow).

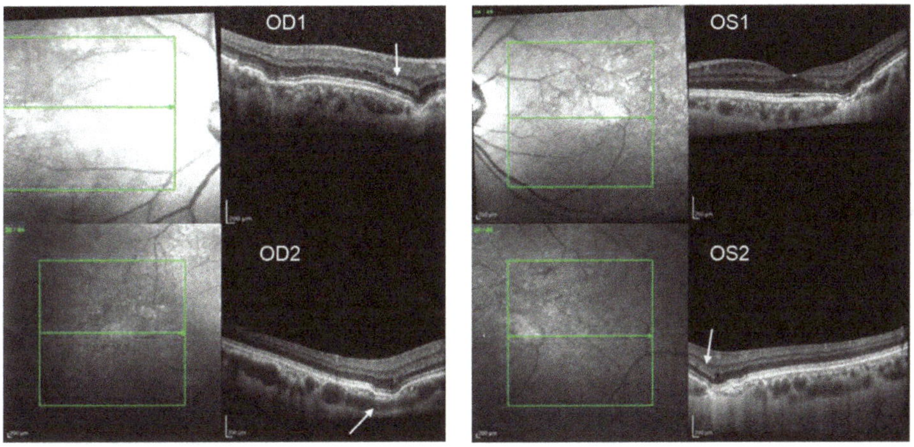

(a) (b)

FIGURE 2: EDI-OCT scan of posterior pole of right eye (OD) and left eye (OS). OD1: Multiple focal choroidal excavations were showed in one horizontal scan. The outer nuclear layers (ONLs) conformed to retinal pigment epithelium (RPE) alterations within the excavation. And the RPE layer followed the contour of the choroidal excavation. There is no RPE detachment and no separation between the photoreceptor and the RPE. One area (arrow) of outer nuclear layers (ONLs) beside the excavation became hyperreflective with a density similar to that of the outer plexiform layer (OPL). OD2: Choriocapillaris in the site of excavation (Arrow) is thinner with adjacent large blood vessels changes comparing to the surrounding choroid. OS1: Multiple FCE without involving the fovea. OS2: Similar hyperreflective ONLs revealed in the left eye beside of the FCE lesion (arrow).

pigmentary changes by infrared fundus photo in OCT (Figure 2). There was no FCE involving the foveal region. EDI-OCT showed the retinal pigment epithelium (RPE) layer complied with the contour of the choroidal excavation. And the outer nuclear layers (ONLs) conformed to the contour of the RPE within the excavation (Figure 2). There was no RPE detachment and no separation between the photoreceptor layers and the RPE. One area of ONL in proximity to the excavation demonstrated hyperreflectivity, similar to the reflectivity of the adjacent outer plexiform layer (OPL) (Figure 2 OD1 and OS2). The inner retinal layers from the OPL to the retinal nerve fiber layer were essentially undisturbed. Choriocapillaris thinning in the site of excavation was adjacent to large blood vessels as compared with the normal surrounding choroid layers without FCE (Figure 2 OD2). The sclerochoroidal junction was smooth and undisturbed without staphylomatous changes.

On FA, the FCE appeared to have normal fluorescence without leakage. No sign of neovascularization was found in the inner and subretinal space.

FAF photos of both eyes showed irregular hyper and hypo-autofluorescence in the macular area, which suggested some RPE loss or disturbance, which is corresponding to the locations of FCEs (Figure 3).

Humphrey Visual field testing in both eyes was performed twice. First was 24-2 Sita fast and the second was 10-2 Sita fast. But both of the visual field results were not reliable because of a high fixation loss.

The patient was observed without any intervention. The patient was followed up in 6 months with no changes of the symptoms, visual acuity, and the fundus exam.

3. Discussion

The case of bilateral FCEs we presented here is a 54-year-old Chinese male without any ocular disease. However, the patient has a significant systemic disease PNH. The formation of FCE in our patient might be associated with PNH.

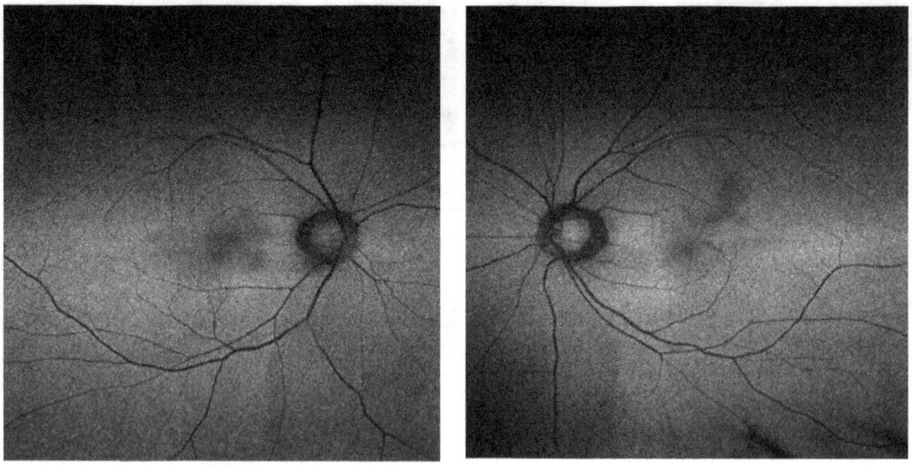

(a) (b)

Figure 3: Autofluorescence photo of (a) right eye and (b) left eye showed irregular hyper and hypofluorescence in the macular area, which suggested some retinal pigment epithelium loss or damage.

Thus far, our knowledge and hypothesis as for the etiology of FCE is based solely on multimodal imaging findings, especially OCT, however no histopathological analysis of this phenomenon has been performed.

Increasing cases of FCE have been discovered and reported since this characteristic feature was obtained by OCT. Some studies have hypothesized that FCE is a congenital choroidal abnormality, which may also be associated with other types of focal structural defects within the choroid [1, 16, 17]. Two studies reported the acquired FCE was identified following treatment of choroidal neovascular membrane with antiendothelial growth factor (antiVEGF) therapy [16, 18]. Some authors believed FCE lesions could represent scarring of the choroidal connective tissue from a previous inflammatory process [6, 19]. But our patient does not have any past ocular history of inflammation or neovascular membrane.

Based on the morphology on the OCT image, FCE was classified into two types: one is the conforming type which shows the outer retina conforms to the choroidal excavation with preservation of the junction between the photoreceptor tips and the retinal pigmented epithelium. Second is the nonconforming type which corresponds to FCEs with a separation between the photoreceptor tips and RPE, forming a subretinal space [20]. Some studies showed that the nonconforming type was significantly associated with visual symptoms and central serous chorioretinopathy [16, 21]. And CSCR progressed to nonconforming FCE after the subretinal fluid resolved in three cases [22]. Our patient has multiple lesions of FCE in each eye, and all the lesions are of the conforming type, which is consistent with his negative FA findings and minimal disturbed visual acuity.

Our patient presents unique features that have not been previously described. Most of the previously reported cases featured a single, unilateral FCE lesion [23]. Our patient's FCEs are multiple and bilateral, diffusely involving the posterior pole. Since our current OCT device cannot reliably obtain scans from peripheral retina, it is unknown if our patient has any peripheral FCE. To our knowledge, in most of the previously reported cases of FCE, patients are young and healthy without obvious systemic medical problems which might link to FCE formation. This is the first case reporting the bilateral FCE in a patient with PNH.

So far, there is no report describing choroidal changes including FCE with PNH. However, some authors suggested that the FCE lesion may be related to choroidal vascular ischemic process according to the characteristic focal thinning of the choroid [23]. Thrombophilia remains the leading cause of mortality in PNH. Thrombosis most often involves unusual sites of the venous system (cerebral, mesenteric, and hepatic veins) [24]. One case of retinal vascular occlusion was reported as the primary manifestation of PNH [14]. In that case, FA demonstrated multiple occlusions of retinal veins in the inferior macular region of both eyes. Since no OCT was done in that case, it is unknown if the patient had FCE or not. Our patient had one prior hospitalization for blurry vision and right-sided paresthesias in 2014. Neurologic examination, CT head, and MRI brain with contrast at that time were all negative. Carotid Doppler test revealed mild bilateral plaques. This episode suggests that this patient could experience a thrombosis attack. However, no evaluation was done by ophthalmology at that time. It is conceivable that the focal choroidal thinning of FCE in our patient is the sequela of choriocapillaris occlusions. In addition, the alterations of choriocapillaris in the site of excavation may lead to degeneration of adjacent photoreceptors, which appeared as a hyperreflective band in ONLs adjacent to the excavation area (Figure 2 OD1 and OS2).

In this case report, we presented an interesting rare case of bilateral multiple FCE in a patient with a long history of PNH. Although there is no histopathological evidence to confirm the association between the choroid changes and PNH, this case may offer new clues as for the etiology of FCE. We encourage obtaining multimodal imaging, especially OCT, in patients with PNH who develop visual disturbances, to look for further evidence and association between these peculiar lesions and PNH. This approach may provide us with better understanding of the clinical course, evolution, and the relationship between the FCE and PNH.

References

[1] L. M. Jampol, J. Shankle, R. Schroeder, P. Tornambe, R. F. Spaide, and M. R. Hee, "Diagnostic and therapeutic challenges," *Retina*, vol. 26, no. 9, pp. 1072–1076, 2006.

[2] R. Margolis, S. K. Mukkamala, L. M. Jampol et al., "The expanded spectrum of focal choroidal excavation," *Archives of Ophthalmology*, vol. 129, no. 10, pp. 1320–1325, 2011.

[3] W. Kabayashi, T. Abe, H. Tamai, and T. Nakazawa, "Choroidal excavation with polypoidal choroidal vasculopathy: a case report," *Clinical Ophthalmology*, vol. 6, pp. 1373–1376, 2012.

[4] E. A. T. Say, P. D. Jani, M. F. Appenzeller, and O. M. Houghton, "Focal choroidal excavation associated with polypoidal choroidal vasculopathy," *Ophthalmic Surgery, Lasers and Imaging Retina*, vol. 44, pp. 409–411, 2013.

[5] A. Okubo, K. Unoki, M. Sameshima, and T. Sakamoto, "Focal choroidal excavation with changes in shape and alterations of inner retina during long follow-up in an eye with polypoidal choroidal vasculopathy," *Clinical and Experimental Optometry*, vol. 98, no. 5, pp. 478–480, 2015.

[6] A. A. Ellabban, A. Tsujikawa, S. Ooto et al., "Focal choroidal excavation in eyes with central serous chorioretinopathy," *American Journal of Ophthalmology*, vol. 156, no. 4, pp. 673–683, 2013.

[7] H. Xu, F. Zeng, D. Shi, X. Sun, X. Chen, and Y. Bai, "Focal choroidal excavation complicated by choroidal neovascularisation," *Ophthalmology*, vol. 121, pp. 246–250, 2014.

[8] A. M. Haas, M. Stattin, D. Ahmed, I. Krebs, and S. Ansari-Shahrezaei, "Development of secondary choroidal neovascularization in focal choroidal excavation of punctate inner choroidopathy," *Ocular Immunology and Inflammation*, vol. 13, pp. 1–6, 2018.

[9] B. F. A. Ferreira, R. C. Preti, M. B. Schmidt, L. C. Zacharias, W. Y. Takahashi, and M. L. R. Monteiro, "Multimodal imaging of focal choroidal excavation complicated by choroidal neovascularization in a patient with angioid streaks and pseudoxanthoma elasticum," *Retinal Cases & Brief Reports*, p. 26, 2018.

[10] J. T. McCann, M. Y. Teke, B. C. S. Leong, and K. B. Freund, "Focal choroidal excavation following blunt trauma," *Ophthalmic Surgery, Lasers and Imaging Retina*, vol. 50, no. 3, pp. 187–191, 2019.

[11] H. Matsubara, E. Uchiyama, K. Suzuki, Y. Matsuda, and M. Kondo, "A case of focal choroidal excavation development associated with multiple evanescent white dot syndrome," *Case Reports in Ophthalmology*, vol. 9, no. 2, pp. 388–394, 2018.

[12] V. Kumar and K. Chatra, "Fibrotic pillar leads to focal choroidal excavation in Best vitelliform dystrophy," *Graefe's Archive for Clinical and Experimental Ophthalmology*, vol. 256, no. 11, pp. 2083–2087, 2018.

[13] S. T. Van Bijnen, W. L. Van Heerde, and P. Muus, "Mechanisms and clinical implications of thrombosis in paroxysmal nocturnal hemoglobinuria," *Journal of Thrombosis and Haemostasis*, vol. 10, no. 1, pp. 1–10, 2012.

[14] A. F. Scheuerle, N. Serbecic, and S. C. Beutelspacher, "Paroxysmal nocturnal hemoglobinuria may cause retinal vascular occlusions," *International Ophthalmology*, vol. 29, no. 3, pp. 187–190, 2009.

[15] K. Vahdani, G. Makrygiannis, H. Kaneshyogan, I. S. Sian, and O. Giasin, "Bilateral central serous retinopathy in a patient with paroxysmal nocturnal hemoglobinuria treated with deferoxamine," *European Journal of Ophthalmology*, vol. 26, no. 6, pp. e152–e154, 2016.

[16] C. S. Lee, S. J. Woo, Y. K. Kim et al., "Clinical and spectral-domain optical coherence tomography findings in patients with focal choroidal excavation," *Ophthalmology*, vol. 121, pp. 1029–1035, 2014.

[17] A. Shinojima, A. Kawamura, R. Mori, and M. Yuzawa, "Morphologic features of focal choroidal excavation on spectral domain optical coherence tomography with simultaneous angiography," *Retina*, vol. 34, pp. 1407–1414, 2014.

[18] R. C. Shah, M. Gopalakrishnan, A. Goyal, G. Anantharaman, and A. Sethia, "Focal choroidal excavation: cause or effect?," *Indian Journal of Ophthalmology*, vol. 67, no. 5, pp. 696–698, 2019.

[19] Y. Hashimoto, W. Saito, K. Noda, and S. Ishida, "Acquired focal choroidal excavation associated with multiple evanescent white dot syndrome: observations at onset and a pathogenic hypothesis," *BMC Ophthalmology*, vol. 14, no. 1, 135 pages, 2014.

[20] Y. Wakabayashi, A. Nishimura, T. Higashide, S. Ijiri, and K. Sugiyama, "Unilateral choroidal excavation in the macula detected by spectral-domain optical coherence tomography," *Acta Ophthalmology*, vol. 88, no. 3, pp. e87–e91, 2010.

[21] Z. Cebeci, Ş. Bayraktar, M. Oray, and N. Kır, "Focal choroidal excavation," *Turkish Journal of Ophthalmology*, vol. 46, no. 6, pp. 296–298, 2016.

[22] M. Suzuki, F. Gomi, C. Hara, M. Sawa, and K. Nishida, "Characteristics of central serous chorioretinopathy complicated by focal choroidal excavation," *Retina*, vol. 34, pp. 1216–1222, 2014.

[23] H. Chung, S. H. Byeon, and K. B. Freund, "Focal choroidal excavation and its association with pachychoroid spectrum disorders: a review of the literature and multimodal imaging findings," *Retina*, vol. 37, no. 2, pp. 199–221, 2017.

[24] C. Parker, M. Omine, S. Richards et al., "Diagnosis and management of paroxysmal nocturnal hemoglobinuria," *Blood*, vol. 106, no. 12, pp. 3699–3709, 2005.

7

Bilateral Anterior and Intermediate Uveitis with Occlusive Vasculitis as Sole Manifestation of Relapse in Multiple Sclerosis

Angelica Pedraza-Concha,[1] Karin Brandauer,[2] Alejandro Tello,[3] Carlos Mario Rangel,[4] and Christian Scheib[2]

[1]*Faculty of Medicine, Universidad Autónoma de Bucaramanga, Bucaramanga 680003, Colombia*
[2]*Augenklinik am Diakonissenkrankenhaus, Karlsruhe 76199, Germany*
[3]*Cornea and Anterior Segment Division, Centro Oftalmológico Virgilio Galvis, Bucaramanga 680003, Colombia*
[4]*Retina and Posterior Segment Division, Centro Oftalmológico Virgilio Galvis, Bucaramanga 680003, Colombia*

Correspondence should be addressed to Angelica Pedraza-Concha; angelicapedraza93@gmail.com

Academic Editor: Kevin J. Blinder

76-year-old female patient, with past medical history of relapsing-remitting multiple sclerosis manifested by retrobulbar optic neuritis in both eyes with an interval of one year between the first episode in the left eye and the one in the right eye and after three decades of remission, who consulted due to bilateral blurred and foggy vision. Subsequently, several differential diagnoses where ruled out. Diagnosis of bilateral anterior and intermediate uveitis with occlusive vasculitis attributed to a new relapse episode of multiple sclerosis was made, as the association between multiple sclerosis and intermediate uveitis is known, though the causal association is still questioned. This case shows how multiple sclerosis may only manifest with ocular involvement and exemplifies the broad spectrum of manifestations and complications, taking into account that ischemic areas from vasculitis and other comorbidities led to macular edema and unfortunately, prognosis became poorer. The complex course of the case enables emphasizing the responsibility role of the ophthalmologists in such systemic entities that may compromise the eye, in which suspicion of the disease and an adequate timing management approach is essential.

1. Introduction

The prevalence of multiple sclerosis (MS) in patients with any type of uveitis has been reported between 0,9 and 1,7%. On the other hand, prevalence of uveitis among patients with MS varies in a wide range though reaching very high frequency in some studies (between 0,65 and 36,7%) [1, 2]. Although causal association is still questioned, since the uvea has no myelin, an explanation of the relationship is their partially common embryonic neuroectodermic origin and association with HLA DR15 [2]. Other posterior segment condition, namely, retinal vasculitis, has been found between 10% and 35% of patients with MS, but retinal neovascularization, on the other hand, is an uncommon complication [3–5].

Furthermore, macular edema can complicate uveitis, in which most important risk factors are the severity and chronicity of the disease, aging, and smoking. The risk to develop cystoid macular edema (CME) related with intermediate uveitis is fourfold increased when the patient is a smoker [6].

Herein, we report the complex course of a patient with relapsing-remitting MS history, who was asymptomatic without receiving any treatment for more than 30 years and who presented a recurrence of the condition that manifested only with visual symptoms and ocular findings, only this time without affecting the optic nerve; consequently, turning out to be a diagnostic and management challenge.

2. Case Report

A 76-year-old, German, Caucasian female, with past medical history of relapsing-remitting MS (in remission for more than three decades), chronic obstructive pulmonary disease, hypertension, and heavy cigarette smoker, consulted to the

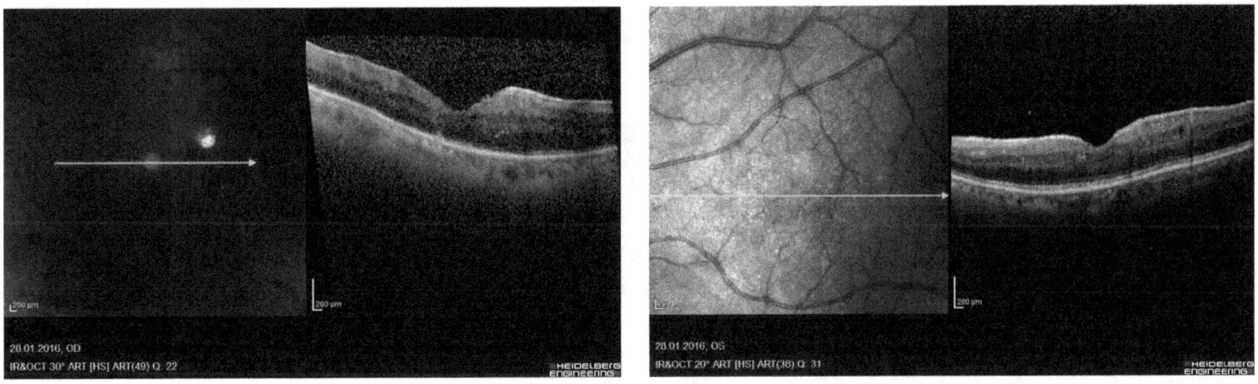

(a) (b)

FIGURE 1: (a) RE, inflammatory cells in vitreous humor, epiretinal membrane, preserved foveal architecture with parafoveal retinal thickening (mild macular edema), without cysts or serous detachment (b) LE, inflammatory cells in vitreous humor, epiretinal membrane without traction, preserved foveal architecture without cysts or serous detachment.

emergency department in 2016 referring increased glare and sudden fall of visual acuity (VA) on both eyes (OU) since a couple of days. Ophthalmological background was left eye (LE) amblyopia and retrobulbar optic neuritis in the LE in 1986 and in the right eye (RE) in 1987, which along with the findings in Magnetic Resonance Imaging (MRI) of the brain led to the diagnosis of MS. Both episodes were treated with Azathioprine but, since then, did not receive additional therapy. The patient denied additional neurological symptoms for the last 30 years. She had cataract surgery with intraocular lens (IOL) implantation in OU in 2012. She noted decreased vision in the RE around six months before consulting in 2016, and diagnoses of anterior uveitis and vitreous hemorrhage (VH) in the right eye (RE) were done elsewhere. However, the patient did not continue to attend the treating ophthalmologist and thus did not receive specific management. She consulted the emergency department two days after noticing a sudden and greater decrease in VA in OU.

Examination approach: VA in the RE was Counting Fingers and 0.32 in the LE (Snellen decimal scale), which did not improve with spectacles. Intraocular pressure (IOP) was 19 mmHg in the RE and 22 mmHg in the LE. Slit lamp examination revealed in OU marked inflammation in anterior chamber (cells 3+) and granulomatous endothelial precipitates. In addition, posterior synechia and precipitates on the IOL front surface were observed in the LE. Vitreous turbidity, vitreous cells and snowballs, and retinal vessels with mild sheathing and adjacent hemorrhages were found in OU.

B-scan Macular Optical Coherence Tomography (OCT) from the RE revealed inflammatory cells in vitreous humor, epiretinal membrane, and preserved foveal architecture, with parafoveal retinal thickening (mild macular edema), without cysts or serous detachment (Figure 1(a)). In the LE, inflammatory cells in vitreous humor, epiretinal membrane without traction, and preserved foveal architecture without cysts or serous detachment were revealed (Figure 1(b)). Fluorescein angiography showed on the RE blockage of choroidal fluorescence secondary to vitreous opacities, pronounced ischemic areas in inferotemporal arcade, collateral vessel formation, and leakage near the optic nerve head and along the retinal veins (periphlebitis) (Figure 2(a)). In the LE, blockage of choroidal fluorescence secondary to vitreous opacities, leakage in foveal area (macular edema (ME)) and along the retinal vessels, and staining of nasal retinal veins (periphlebitis) were shown (Figures 2(b) and 2(c)).

Neurological approach proved intact cranial nerves function, no paresis, no pyramidal tract signs, and adequate reflexes. MRI of the orbit exhibited no evidence of retrobulbar optic neuritis. Skull MRI revealed no evidence of acute inflammatory cerebral foci.

Paraclinical tests helped ruling out differential diagnosis. Sarcoidosis was excluded by normal serum angiotensin converting enzyme, and there were no relevant abnormalities on chest x-ray. Other diseases possibly associated with ocular signs were not likely on absence of systemic clinical findings, negative ANA, and ANCA, normal HbA1c (5,2%), and no heart rhythm abnormalities. Infectious etiologies such Syphilis, Bartonellosis, and Lyme disease were also ruled out. Regarding ischemic causes, Carotid Doppler showed no plaques, dissection, or stenosis. Furthermore, the absence of malignant suspicious lymphocytes (dysplasic, pleomorphic lymphocytes with elevated nucleus-cytoplasm ratio) in a vitreous sample from RE excluded ocular lymphoma (Masquerade syndrome). PCR tests in that sample were negative for Herpes simplex, Varicella Zoster, Cytomegalovirus, and Mycobacterium Tuberculosis. Eventually, given the exclusion of other possible etiologies, diagnosis was a bilateral anterior uveitis and intermediate uveitis with occlusive vasculitis and mild macular edema, attributable to a MS relapse.

Intravenous methylprednisolone, 250 mg q.i.d. for 5 days, was administered. Topical prednisolone was indicated, initially every hour, and then tapered gradually over around two months. Cyclopentolate b.i.d. was used for several weeks. This scheme led to improvement of the findings, but Dorzolamide/Timolol b.i.d. and Brimonidine t.i.d. had to be used to control IOP increase.

At discharge, 5 days after the admission, VA from the RE was 0.1 and 0.32 on the LE, which did not improve with

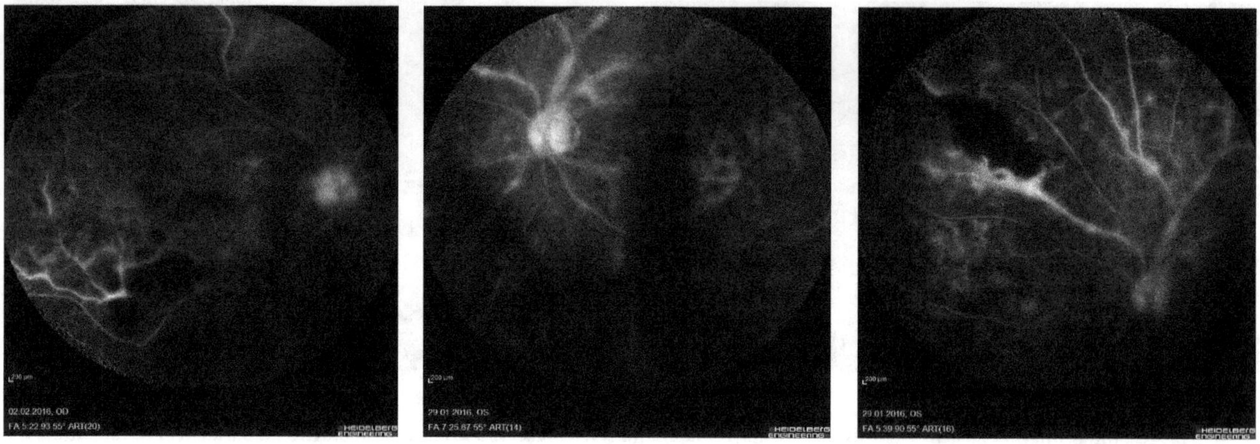

(a) (b) (c)

FIGURE 2: (a) RE, blockage of choroidal fluorescence secondary to vitreous opacities, pronounced ischemic areas in inferotemporal arcade, collateral vessel formation, and leakage near the optic nerve head and along the retinal veins. (b,c) LE, blockage of choroidal fluorescence secondary to vitreous opacities, leakage in foveal area along the retinal vessels, and staining of nasal retinal veins.

optical correction. IOP was normal in OU. Oral steroid taper schedule and hypotensive eye drops were prescribed. On the third month's control, even under daily oral steroids, bilateral vasculitis persisted. Consequently, interferon beta-1a (Rebif®) was initiated (44 mcg, 3 times per week, subcutaneously). On the sixth month's visit, CME was found in OU, despite the fact that she was receiving interferon beta-1a and 7.5 mg oral prednisolone. Bilateral subtenon injections of triamcinolone were performed. Two months later, CME persisted and a dexamethasone intravitreal implant (Ozurdex®) was injected in the RE and three months later in the LE as well.

Due to side effects with interferon beta-1a (Flu-like symptoms and depression), eight months after it was started, she was switched to peginterferon beta1-a (Plegridy®) 125 mcg injected subcutaneously every 2 weeks. A stable response to treatment was achieved, without inflammatory or neovascularization signs and improvement of CME for a couple of months. Nevertheless, due to persistence of ischemic findings in the retina (ischemic areas, collateral vessel formation, and mild macular edema reappearance) evidenced in fluorescein angiography image control, which possibly triggered recurrence of macular edema, despite having an adequate control of the inflammatory component, pan-retinal photocoagulation was performed in OU, in three sessions between 7 and 8 months after the initial consult, with satisfactory evolution. CDVA at the last check-up visit was 0.4 in the RE and 0.5 in the LE.

3. Discussion

In this patient with past medical history of relapsing-remitting MS, other causes of bilateral anterior and intermediate uveitis were ruled out, including viral infections (Herpes simplex, Varicella Zoster, and Cytomegalovirus), Sarcoidosis, and Systemic Lupus Erythematosus. Since vasculitis was present, further causes were also considered: Toxoplasmosis, Tuberculosis, Syphilis, and Borreliosis, but the results were also negative [1, 2, 5, 7].

Retinal vasculitis in MS occurs in a range of about 9-23% of the patients, and is almost exclusively limited to the veins [5]. Though rare, there are also cases in which MS presents only with retinal vessel affection and not even uveitis nor optical neuritis are present [5].

Intermediate uveitis itself has an overall favorable prognosis on absence of complications [2]; however when retinal vasculitis is present the possibility of developing CME and the risk of vision loss rises. Vasculitis may lead to areas of ischemia. Macular ischemia increases 4.4 times the risk of visual loss, and ischemia concerning ≥2 quadrants raises risks of neovascularization [4, 5]. Also, periphlebitis increases the risk of new relapsing events in the following 2 years [4, 7].

As for treatment approach, some authors have hypothesized that interferon beta might slow down the course of intermediate uveitis related to MS [8–10]. In the case we reported due to persistent bilateral vasculitis, interferon beta-1a was initiated 3 months after starting systemic and topical steroids. However bilateral CME developed and the patient initially required bilateral triamcinolone subtenon injection and then injection of dexamethasone intravitreal implant (Ozurdex®) in OU. Finally, due to persistent findings of retinal ischemia pan-retinal laser photocoagulation was performed in OU. The patient did not develop further complications of retinal ischemia, and in her nonamblyopic right eye the CDVA was preserved (0.4 in Snellen decimal scale) after the laser procedure.

Regarding diagnostic procedures, vitreous biopsy is not free of risks, and its use should be considered only when there is a significant doubt on the cause of the uveitis affecting the vitreous, especially when malignancy needs to be ruled out [11]. In this case, a vitreous biopsy performed in the RE using a 21G needle on a 1 ml syringe and was useful to rule out lymphoma (the immunophenotyping of the cells in the vitreous aspirate showed no evaluable lymphocyte population giving no indication of proliferation of lymphocytes). In addition, PCR results were negative for Herpes simplex, Varicella Zoster, Cytomegalovirus, and Mycobacterium Tuberculosis.

The VH initially found by an ophthalmologist elsewhere in the RE may be explained mainly due to retinal neovascularization secondary to the retinal ischemia, which in fact persisted in spite of dexamethasone intravitreal implant (Ozurdex®) and interferon, and pan-retinal photocoagulation was eventually required in OU.

This case exemplifies the broad spectrum of ocular manifestations and complications of MS. Given the background, ophthalmologists have great responsibility on suspicion of systemic diseases, such MS, when facing a patient with uveitis, since early diagnosis, therapy, and close follow-up play a significant role in prognosis [2, 12].

References

[1] T. G. Olsen and J. Frederiksen, "The association between multiple sclerosis and uveitis," *Survey of Ophthalmology*, vol. 62, no. 1, pp. 89–95, 2017.

[2] A. Hildebrandt and F. Mackensen, "Uveitis bei multipler SkleroseUveitis in multiple sclerosis," *Der Ophthalmologe*, vol. 111, no. 8, pp. 733–739, 2014.

[3] M. Patte, F. N. Rouher, D. Vernay, J-C. Delaire, and F. Bacin, "Vascularites rétiniennes proliférantes et sclérose en plaques. A propos d'un cas," *Journal Français D'Ophtalmologie*, vol. 26, no. 4, pp. 381–385, 2003.

[4] L. Sharief, S. Lightman, T. Blum-Hareuveni, A. Bar, and O. Tomkins-Netzer, "Clinical Outcome of Retinal Vasculitis and Predictors for Prognosis of Ischemic Retinal Vasculitis," *American Journal of Ophthalmology*, vol. 177, pp. 206–212, 2017.

[5] M. Fuest, G. Rößler, P. Walter, and N. Plange, "Retinale Vaskulitis als Erstmanifestation einer multiplen SkleroseRetinal vasculitis as manifestation of multiple sclerosis," *Der Ophthalmologe*, vol. 111, no. 9, pp. 871–875, 2014.

[6] J. E. Thorne, E. Daniel, D. A. Jabs, S. R. Kedhar, G. B. Peters, and J. P. Dunn, "Smoking as a risk factor for cystoid macular edema complicating intermediate uveitis," *American Journal of Ophthalmology*, vol. 145, no. 5, pp. 841–846.e2, 2008.

[7] J. Sepulcre, M. Murie-Fernandez, A. Salinas-Alaman, A. García-Layana, B. Bejarano, and P. Villoslada, "Diagnostic accuracy of retinal abnormalities in predicting disease activity in MS," *Neurology*, vol. 68, no. 18, pp. 1488–1494, 2007.

[8] F. Mackensen, E. Jakob, C. Springer et al., "Interferon versus Methotrexate in Intermediate Uveitis With Macular Edema: Results of a Randomized Controlled Clinical Trial," *American Journal of Ophthalmology*, vol. 156, no. 3, pp. 478–486.e1, 2013.

[9] M. D. Becker, "Interferon as a treatment for uveitis associated with multiple sclerosis," *British Journal of Ophthalmology*, vol. 89, no. 10, pp. 1254–1257, 2005.

[10] A. Heiligenhaus, B. Bertram, C. Heinz et al., "Stellungnahme der Deutschen Ophthalmologischen Gesellschaft, der Retinologischen Gesellschaft und des Berufsverbandes der Augenärzte Deutschlands zur intravitrealen Therapie des Makulaödems bei Uveitis (Stand: 02.07.2014)," *Klinische Monatsblätter für Augenheilkunde*, vol. 231, no. 09, pp. 929–936, 2014.

[11] H. Manku and P. McCluskey, "Diagnostic vitreous biopsy in patients with uveitis: a useful investigation?" *Clinical & Experimental Ophthalmology*, vol. 33, no. 6, pp. 604–610, 2005.

[12] C. Beisse, "Auge und multiple SkleroseEye and multiple sclerosis," *Der Ophthalmologe*, vol. 111, no. 8, pp. 708-708, 2014.

8

Delayed Vision Recovery after Carotid Vascular Surgery for Branch Retinal Artery Occlusion

Jessica Ruzicki,[1] Eric K. Chin,[2] and David Almeida[3]

[1]*Department of Ophthalmology, Kingston Health Sciences Centre, Queen's University, Kingston, ON, Canada*
[2]*Private Practice, Retina Consultants of Southern California, Redlands, California, USA*
[3]*Private Practice, Metrolina Eye Associates, Charlotte, North Carolina, USA*

Correspondence should be addressed to David Almeida; dalmeida@evolation-medical.com

Academic Editor: Kevin J. Blinder

Branch retinal artery occlusion (BRAO) is typically associated with irreversible vision and peripheral visual field loss. We report a case of a 62-year-old woman with a BRAO related to several cardiovascular risk factors. Our patient encountered gradual but significant vision recovery months following carotid artery endarterectomy for carotid stenosis.

1. Introduction

Branch retinal artery occlusion (BRAO) accounts for 38% of acute retinal artery obstruction cases [1]. In BRAO, obstruction of blood flow in the distribution of a branch of the central retinal artery leads to ischemia and reorganization of the retinal layers [2]. Concurrent or sequential cardiovascular events such as stroke or acute myocardial infarct can occur, and thus urgent systemic cardiovascular workup is often warranted [3].

Embolism is the most common cause of retinal artery occlusions with calcific plaques originating from the carotid artery as the primary source and less commonly the aortic arch or heart [3]. Patients with embolic BRAO have a higher frequency of acute cerebral infarctions along with a higher frequency of stenotic carotid arteries compared to arterial occlusions secondary to a nonembolic source [4]. Typical risk factors for embolic arterial occlusions include smoking, concurrent acute ischemic stroke, and carotid artery stenosis.

Various treatment modalities for BRAO have been proposed and reported including YAG laser embolysis and embolectomy, surgical embolus removal, and local fibrinolysis. Unfortunately, none of these have achieved an outcome better than natural history and each can be associated with serious complications [5].

Vision recovery after embolic BRAO is rare. Previously, we reported a case of surgical retinal embolectomy where retinal embolectomy successfully prevented vision loss [6]. Currently, there is little evidence of vision recovery after ocular or extraocular surgical intervention is done. Herein, we report a unique case of a patient with a BRAO who had dramatic but gradual visual improvement following carotid endarterectomy.

2. Case Presentation

A 62-year-old woman presented with a one-month history of sudden painless visual loss in the right eye. On examination, best corrected visual acuity (BCVA) was 20/20 in both eyes. Intraocular pressure was 21 mmHg in both eyes. Dilated funduscopic examination in the right eye revealed retinal emboli inferior to the optic disc obstructing a small arteriole associated with retinal ischemia (Figures 1(a) and 1(b)). The left eye was unremarkable. There was no prior past ocular history. The patient had hypertension and hypercholesterolemia and had an extensive smoking history.

Fluorescein angiography revealed delayed retinal perfusion along the inferior arcade in the right eye (Figures 1(c) and 1(d)). Optical coherence tomography showed normal foveal

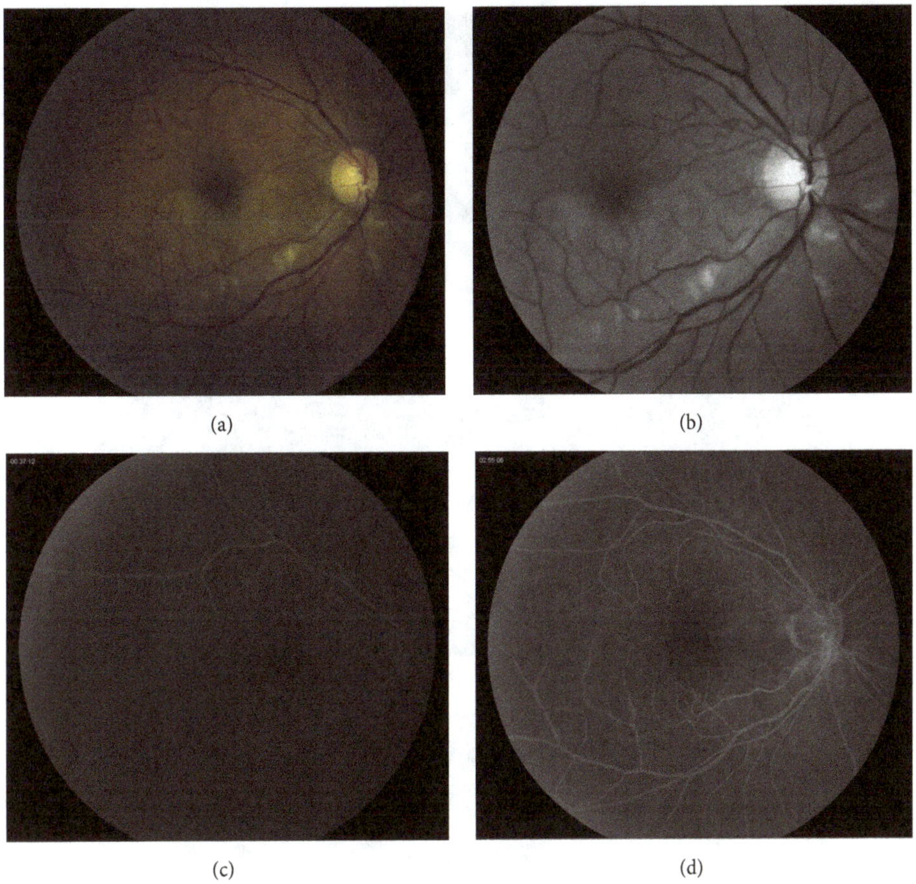

FIGURE 1: Color fundus photograph of the right eye at initial presentation where BCVA was 20/20 (a) demonstrating the site of occlusion with the emboli situated in a branch of the central retinal artery on the optic disc. Inferior retinal whitening was visible. Red free (b) photograph of the right eye at initial presentation. Fluorescein angiography at 37 seconds (c) showing delayed arterial filling along the inferior retinal vascular arcade. Fluorescein angiography at 2 minutes and 55 seconds (d) showing mild hyperfluroescence along the vessels emanating from the inferior optic nerve.

contour with inner retinal ischemia and thickening, consistent with an acute inferotemporal branch retinal artery occlusion (Figure 2(a)). The patient was started on Latanoprost at nighttime in the right eye to lower the intraocular pressure in hopes to increase reperfusion of the retina. An extensive cardiovascular workup was done, and significant carotid artery stenosis of less than 70% was found. She was started on plavix and aspirin by her cardiologist. The patient continued with BCVA 20/20 OU vision and persistent highly refractile peripapillary emboli; retinal ischemia resolved. Her OCT showed inner retinal atrophy (Figures 2(b) and 2(c)).

Unexpectedly, the patient presented with a three-day history of sudden painless visual loss OD a year and a half after her initial presentation. BCVA was counting fingers (CF) in the right eye. Fundus exam revealed new superotemporal retinal ischemia associated with two new emboli. OCT demonstrated thickening and hyperreflectivity of the inner retinal layers consistent with an acute BRAO OD (Figure 3(a)). The patient refused fluorescein angiography at that time. Urgent workup revealed worsening stenosis to 80% in her right common carotid artery. The vascular surgery referral prompted a right carotid endarterectomy with a carotid stent placement approximately two months following her presentation with acute vision loss.

After endarterectomy, vision in the right eye improved from counting fingers to 20/200 and 20/250 at 2 months and 6 months, respectively. Postoperatively, retinal whitening resolved and reduced intraretinal edema was noticed (Figure 3(b)). One year after endarterectomy, visual acuity was 20/30. The retinal swelling had resolved (Figure 3(c)).

3. Discussion

Our patient presented with a clinical picture consistent an embolic BRAO. However, there was significant and gradual improvement in her vision following carotid endarterectomy. Currently, there exists no evidence-based efficacious treatment for BRAO [3]. Our patient demonstrated a varying clinical course with loss of her central vision initially but her vision significantly improved following right carotid endarterectomy surgery.

Carotid endarterectomy has been studied for carotid stenosis; according to the most current Cochrane Review [7], participants defined as symptomatic had stenosis of the

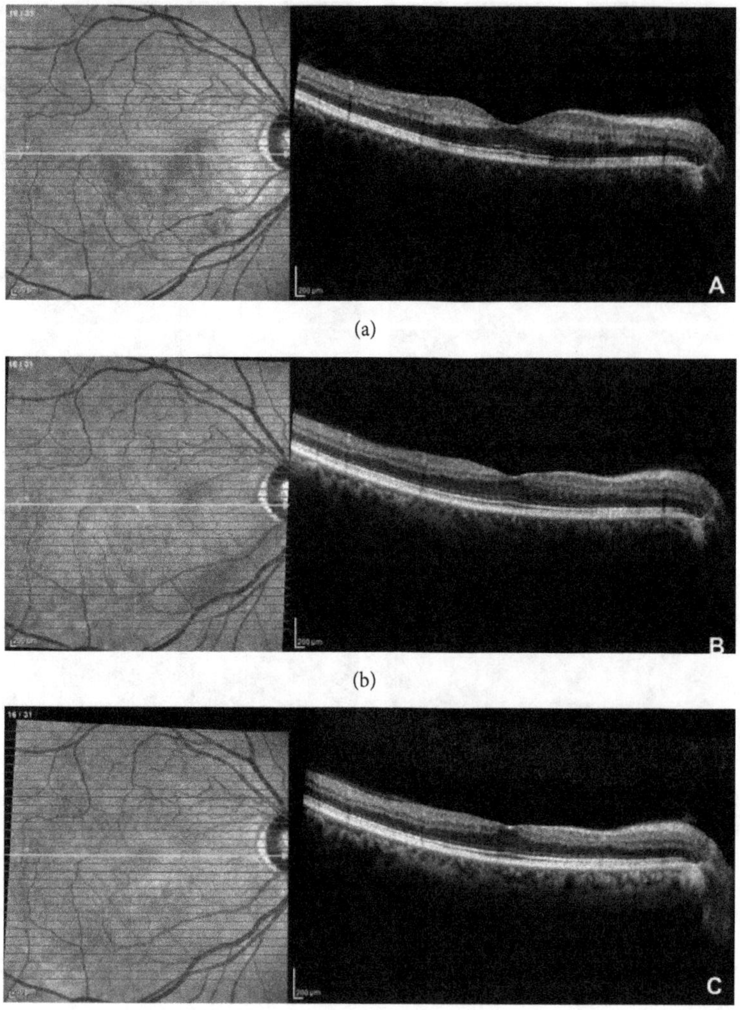

Figure 2: Optical coherence tomography showing acute inner retinal thickening and hyperreflectivity at the patient's initial presentation (a). Optical coherence tomography showing very mild thinning and atrophy of the inner retinal layers two and a half months (b) and six months after her initial presentation (c).

ipsilateral (symptomatic) internal carotid artery with recent TIA, nondisabling ischemic stroke, or retinal infarction. Current recommendations indicate that endarterectomy is beneficial for those symptomatic patients with 70% to 99% stenosis and of some benefit to those with 50 to 69% of stenosis (moderate-quality evidence). Further emboli can possibly be released during or after a carotid endarterectomy; therefore care must be taken to remove all of the debris from the intimal surface of the artery.

Dr. Hayreh and Dr. Zimmerman [8] have described an entity called "transient" central retinal arterial occlusion (CRAO) that is based on a sudden vision loss and classic fundus findings of CRAO but normal retinal circulation based on initial fluorescein angiography. An OCT angiography can be performed in unclear cases as well [3]; however this was not available at our institution. Dr. Hayreh and Dr. Zimmerman [8] concluded that CRAO spontaneous improvement in vision and visual field mainly occurs in the first 7 days if any visual recovery is to be seen. However, visual recovery is rare with arterial occlusions.

Experimental studies have shown that the retina suffers no damage with RAOs lasting less than 97 minutes; however, occlusions lasting longer than about 240 minutes cause irreversible retinal damage [9]. With CRAO, Hayreh SS et al. concluded that unless retinal circulation has returned to normal within 4 hours, treatment instituted more than four hours or even days after the onset of CRAO cannot typically achieve any improvement of vision [8].

Our case is unique in that our patient with cardiovascular risk factors had a BRAO with significant acute vision loss. Her endarterectomy was several months after her presentation with acute visual loss, and her vision improvement was gradually seen months after this extraocular intervention. Our case highlights the utility of urgent cardiovascular workup

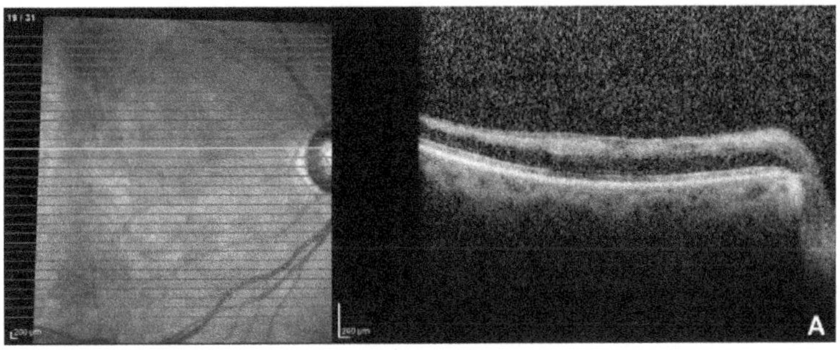

(a)

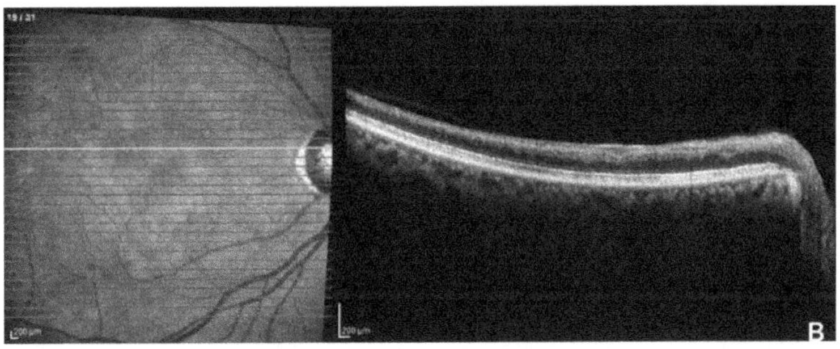

(b)

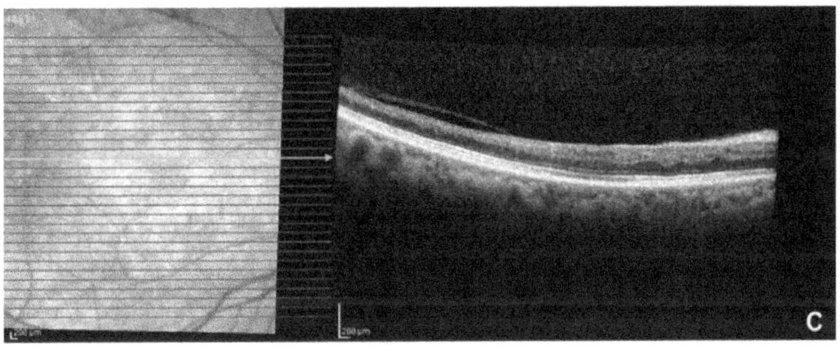

(c)

FIGURE 3: Optical coherence tomography showing inner retinal thickening and hyperreflectivity at the time of acute vision loss, a year and a half following her initial presentation where BCVA was CF (a). Optical coherence tomography imaging showing thinning and atrophy of the inner retina at six months (b) and one year after her acute vision loss secondary to BRAO (c).

and referral to a subspecialist pending further workup. Long-term vascular remodeling, especially prominent in former smokers, may lead to cardiovascular recovery as a protective recovery mechanism. The exact timing and threshold for endarterectomy in the setting of acute BRAO warrants further investigation.

Consent

Informed consent was provided by the patient.

References

[1] G. C. Brown and J. A. Shields, "Cilioretinal Arteries and Retinal Arterial Occlusion," *JAMA Ophtalmology*, vol. 97, no. 1, pp. 84–92, 1979.

[2] A. Stepanov, L. Hejsek, N. Jiraskova, A. Feuermannova, E. Rencova, and P. Rozsival, "Transient branch retinal artery occlusion in a 15-year-old girl and review of the literature," *Biomedical Papers*, vol. 159, no. 3, pp. 508–511, 2015.

[3] M. Dattilo, N. J. Newman, and V. Biousse, "Acute retinal arterial ischemia," *Annals of Eye Science*, vol. 3, 2018.

[4] K. H. Cho, C. K. Kim, S. J. Woo, K. H. Park, and S. J. Park, "Cerebral Small Vessel Disease in Branch Retinal Artery Occlusion," *Investigative Opthalmology & Visual Science*, vol. 57, no. 13, p. 5818, 2016.

[5] S. S. Hayreh, "Ocular vascular occlusive disorders: natural history of visual outcome," *Progress in Retinal and Eye Research*, vol. 41, no. 6, pp. 1–25, 2014.

[6] D. R. P. Almeida, Z. Mammo, E. K. Chin, and V. B. Mahajan, "Surgical embolectomy for fovea-threatening acute retinal artery occlusion," *Retinal Cases and Brief Reports*, vol. 10, no. 4, pp. 331–333, 2016.

[7] S. Orrapin and K. Rerkasem, "Carotid endarterectomy for

symptomatic carotid stenosis," *Cochrane Database of Systematic Reviews*, vol. 2017, no. 6, 2017.

[8] S. S. Hayreh and M. B. Zimmerman, "Central retinal artery occlusion: visual outcome," *American Journal of Ophthalmology*, vol. 140, no. 3, pp. 376.e1–376.e, 2005.

[9] S. S. Hayreh, P. A. Podhajsky, and M. B. Zimmerman, "Branch Retinal Artery Occlusion. Natural History of Visual Outcome," *Ophthalmology*, vol. 116, no. 6, pp. 1188–1194, 2009.

9

Bilateral Retinal Angiomatous Proliferation in a Variant of Retinitis Pigmentosa

G. Aloe,[1] C. M. De Sanctis,[1] C. Strafella,[2,3] R. Cascella,[3,4] F. Missiroli,[1] M. Cesareo,[1] E. Giardina,[2,3] and F. Ricci[1]

[1] Unit Retinal Pathology PTV Foundation, Tor Vergata University, Rome, Italy
[2] Department of Biomedicine and Prevention, Tor Vergata University, Rome, Italy
[3] Molecular Genetics Laboratory UILDM, Santa Lucia Foundation, Rome, Italy
[4] Department of Biomedical Sciences, Catholic University Our Lady of Good Counsel, Tirana, Albania

Correspondence should be addressed to G. Aloe; gianluca.aloe@alice.it

Academic Editor: Stephen G. Schwartz

Purpose. To describe the first case of bilateral retinal angiomatous proliferation (RAP) in a patient with a variant of retinitis pigmentosa (RP). *Case Report.* An 85-year-old man with RP presented with visual acuity decrease and metamorphopsia in the left eye (LE). Fundus examination revealed typical signs of RP in both eyes, associated with intraretinal macular hemorrhage in the LE. Multimodal imaging, using Colour fundus Photography, Fluorescein (FA), and Indocyanine Green Angiography (ICGA) as well as Spectral-Domain Optical Coherence Tomography (SD-OCT) and Optical Coherence Tomography Angiography (OCTA), revealed a type 3 neovascular lesion in the involved eye. Genetic testing (NGS analysis) was performed to search for genetic variants correlated with the disease phenotype displayed by the patient. The patient was treated with intravitreal injections of bevacizumab, according to a fixed protocol of bimonthly injections plus a booster dose at second month. After 9 months, he was referred for visual acuity decrease and metamorphopsia in the fellow eye, where SD-OCT/OCTA showed a type 3 neovascular lesion in the right eye (RE). He was scheduled for intravitreal injections of bevacizumab. In both eyes, treatment with intravitreal bevacizumab was successful.

1. Introduction

Retinitis pigmentosa (RP) is a complex of inherited retinal dystrophies characterized by the loss of photoreceptors and characterized by retinal pigment deposits in the peripheral retina with a relative sparing of the central retina. The most common form of RP is a rod-cone dystrophy, in which there is a primary degeneration of the photoreceptor rods, with secondary degeneration of cones, thus leading to night blindness, followed by the progressive loss in the peripheral visual field in daylight, and eventually blindness after several decades [1]. Retinal angiomatous proliferation (RAP), also referred to type 3 neovascularization, is a common neovascular lesion type occurring in age-related macular degeneration (AMD). It was first described by Yannuzzi et al in 2001 and it is characterized by intraretinal neovascularization with proliferation of intraretinal capillaries within the deep retinal layers, producing intraretinal and superficial retinal hemorrhages that can evolve toward a subretinal neovascularization and choroidal neovascularization (CNV) [2].

CNV is very rarely associated with RP [3]. To date, two cases of RP with RAP have been reported in literature, but those cases were not genetically characterized. Our study represents the first description of a bilateral type 3 neovascularization in a patient with RP genetically determined.

2. Case Report

An 85-year-old with RP was referred to our center in April 2016 for decrease in visual acuity and metamorphopsia in the left eye (LE) for a few weeks. The patient had the clinical diagnosis of retinitis pigmentosa from the age of 15 years old and for this reason did not do military service. He reported a history of night blindness and narrowing of the subjective visual field in both eyes with a recent visual impairment in the LE. Best corrected visual acuity was 0.1 LogMAR (80 LN) in the right eye (RE) and 0.7 LogMAR (50 LN) in the LE. The visual field test was not reliable due to the poor collaboration of the patient.

Fundus examination revealed arteriolar attenuation, peripapillary atrophy, optic disc pallor, macular edema and typical retinal pigment deposits involving the midperipheral retina (bone spicules) of both eyes, associated with intraretinal hemorrhage in the macular region of the LE.

Fluorescein angiography (FA) (Heidelberg Retina Angiograph II, Heidelberg Engineering, Heidelberg, Germany) revealed a continuous retinal-retinal anastomosis and the presence of well distinct area of intense leakage temporally to the fovea corresponding to the neovascularization with a late pooling of dye due to intraretinal cystoid edema [2]. In the fellow eye, FA showed late pooling due to cystoid macular edema.

Indocyanine green angiography (ICGA) (Heidelberg Retina Angiograph II, Heidelberg Engineering, Heidelberg, Germany) revealed a well-distinct "triangular shape" area of intense hypercyanescence ("hot spot") corresponding to the neovascularization and a feeder and draining vessel, pathognomonic for RAP. In the fellow eye, ICGA did not show any signs of neovascularization.

Spectral-Domain Optical Coherence Tomography (SD-OCT) (Spectralis HRA OCT; Heidelberg Engineering, Heidelberg, Germany) in correspondence of the hyperfluorescent area of the LE revealed a hyperreflective intraretinal lesion located at the outer retinal layers apparently connected with the sub-RPE space, characterized by intraretinal and subretinal exudation and intraretinal fluid [4]. In the fellow eye, SD-OCT showed epiretinal membrane with cystoid intraretinal fluid.

Optical Coherence Tomography Angiography (OCTA) (Optovue, Inc., Freemont, CA, USA) is a rapid, noninvasive technique that showed clearly the intraretinal neovascularization with capillary proliferation and retinal-retinal anastomoses [5].

In the segmentation of deep capillary plexus, OCTA revealed a high- flow third- order vessel descending into a tuft-shaped high-flow lesion toward the outer retinal layers, characterized by a retinal-retinal anastomosis and bordering the sub-RPE space [6] (Figure 1).

Taking into consideration the clinical picture of patient we decided to perform a genetic testing to search for genetic variants, which may be correlated with the RP-like phenotype observed in the patient. To this purpose, the patient was asked to sign an informed consent and to give a saliva sample for genetic testing [7]. The DNA was extracted using MagPurix Tissue DNA Extraction Kit and MagPurix Automatic Extraction System (Resnova) according to the manufacturer's instructions. Samples were sequenced by Next-Generation Sequencing (NGS) with Ampliseq DNA protocol and Ion Torrent S5 system. In this case, the panel contains 24 genes, which are associated with different anterior and posterior segment eye disorders, including Glaucoma, Retinitis Pigmentosa [8, 9].

NGS analysis revealed the presence of two missense variants (namely, NM_001193300: c.1265C>T and NM_001142564: c.1162T>C) located in SEMA4A (1q22) and in CNGA1 (4p12), respectively. In particular, SEMA4A encodes a member of semaphorin family of transmembrane proteins and modulate the transport of retinoid-binding proteins in RPE cells (REF4). CNGA1 codes for the homonymous protein that is crucial for phototransduction pathway [9]. The c.1265C>T variant (rs145228550) was found at the heterozygous state and resulted in an amino acid change (p.Thr422Ile). Multiple computational evidence predicted no impact on the gene or gene product, although it has a very low frequency (ExAc:0.00005) in the general population. The c.1162T>C variant (rs914018863) was detected at the homozygous state and caused an amino acid change (p.Tyr388His). Interestingly, c.1162T>C has a very low frequency (GnomAD <0.00001) and the prediction analysis reported a potential deleterious effect on the gene or gene product. Although c.1265C>T and c.1162T>C are located within two genes associated with retinal disorders including autosomal recessive RP, these variants are not described in literature and there are no functional assays demonstrating their real pathogenic effect. These variants are therefore classified as Variants of Uncertain Significance (VUS, class 3) according to the ACMG guidelines [10], meaning that such variants cannot be certainly classified as benign or pathogenic at the moment. Therefore, these results cannot be utilized to provide a genetic explanation to RP-associated phenotype observed in the patient, although the identified VUS may be revisited along with further investigations which may increase the knowledge concerning their clinical implications.

Successively, the patient was screened for AMD-related variants, in order to estimate the genetic susceptibility to disease, considering the observation of a neovascular lesion and the advanced age of the patient. In particular, three polymorphisms were tested, namely rs1061170 (T/C), rs10490924 (G/T) and rs2227306 (C/T) [11, 12]. They are located in CFH (1q31), ARMS2 (10q26) and IL8 (4q13) genes, respectively, which are known to be three major contributors to genetic susceptibility to AMD among Italian and worldwide populations [13, 14]. The test was performed by TaqMan assay using a 7500 Fast Real Time PCR device (Applied Biosystems) according to the manufacturer's instructions. Results were interpreted using Sequence Detection System 2.1 software (Applied Biosystems). The screening test revealed that the patient is heterozygous for the ARMS2 (G/T), IL-8 (C/T) and wild-type for CFH (T/T) polymorphisms, meaning that the patient is approximately 5 times more likely to develop AMD during his lifetime. These results highlighted therefore a genetic predisposition to develop AMD in the patient, which is consistent with the presence of a type 3 neovascularization.

We decided to treat the patient with 3 consecutive monthly intravitreal injections of bevacizumab adopting the Treat and Extend (TE) strategy after the loading phase.

In January 2017, 9 months later the first visit, patient referred for sudden visual acuity impairment in the fellow eye. Best corrected visual acuity decreased from 0.1 LogMAR 80 LN to 1.0 LogMAR 35 LN.

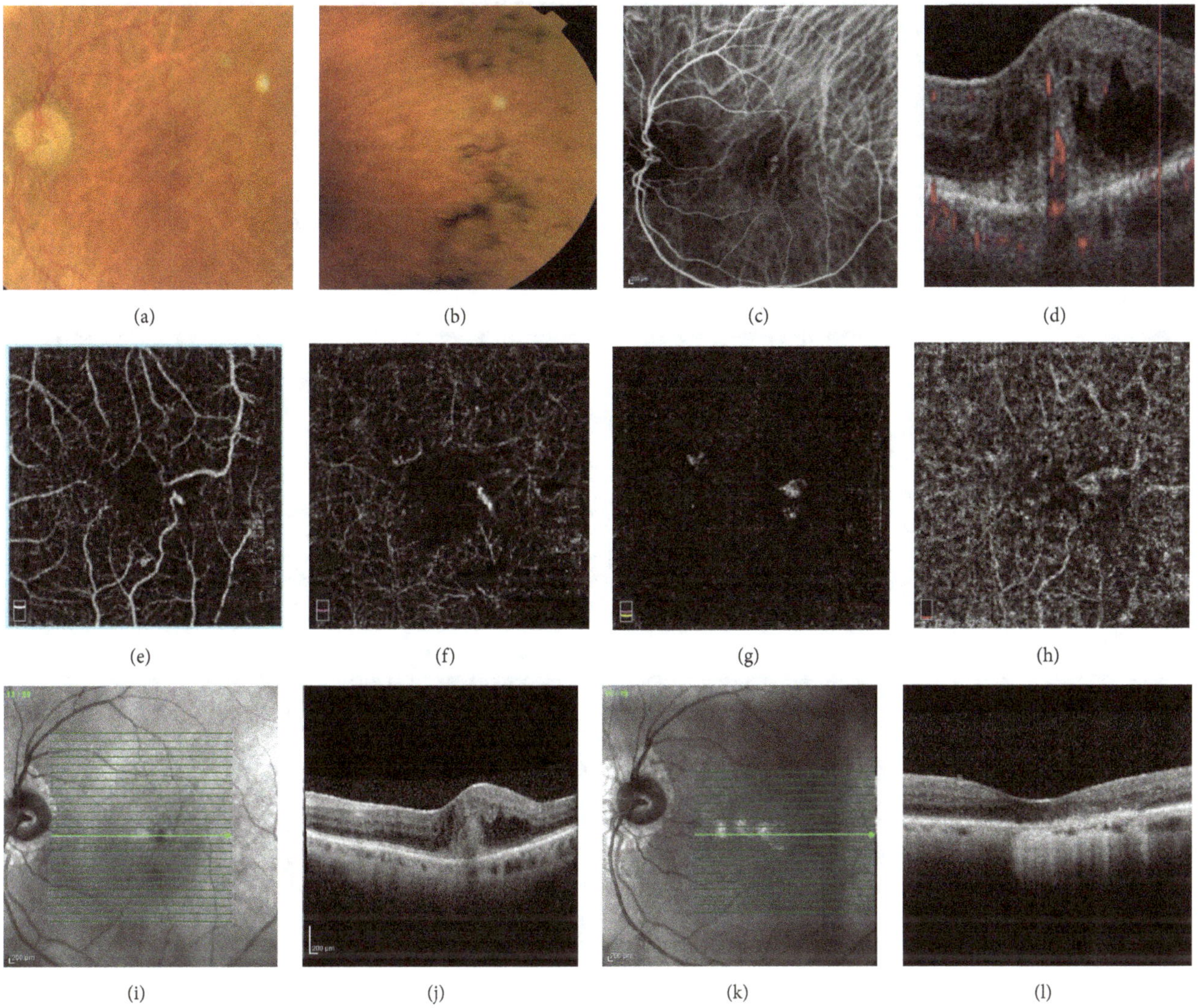

FIGURE 1: (a)-(b) Colour fundus photography showed arteriolar attenuation, peripapillary atrophy, optic disc pallor, macular hemorrhage and typical retinal pigment deposits (bone spicules) involving the mid-peripheral retina (c) Indocyanine green angiography (ICGA) revealed a well-distinct "triangular shape" area of intense hypercyanescence ("hot spot") corresponding to the neovascularization (d) B-Scan optical coherence tomography angiography revealed high-flow intraretinal neovascularization originated in the superficial layer descending into a tuft-shaped lesion toward the sub-RPE space. (e)–(h) Optical Coherence Tomography Angiography images (6 × 6 mm) revealing the progression of the tuft-shaped lesion from the superficial layer to choroid capillary. (e) Superficial capillary plexus segmentation. (f) Deep capillary plexus segmentation. (g) Outer retinal layer segmentation. (h) Choriocapillaris segmentation. (i)–(j) Spectral Domain-Optical Coherence Tomography at baseline. (k)–(l) Spectral Domain-Optical Coherence Tomography after treatment.

Fundus examination revealed macular hemorrhage, exudates and intraretinal edema in the right eye (RE); these clinical findings supported the diagnosis of type 3 CNV in the RE that was then confirmed by SD-OCT and OCTA imaging. OCTA showed clearly two distinct intraretinal neovascularizations located in the segmentation of choroid capillary, both bordering the sub-RPE space (Figure 2). We administered intravitreal injections of bevacizumab in the fellow eye. The patient received 10 intravitreal injections in the LE and 5 in the RE, with an improvement of 10 LN in visual acuity in both eyes.

To date, we decided to stop the anti-VEGF therapy because SD-OCT did not show any CNV activity in both eyes.

3. Discussion

CNV rarely occurs in patients affected by RP [15]. Only few cases of CNV have been described in the literature [15–19]. To date, two case of RP with RAP have been reported [19, 20]. Nagao et al firstly described a case of RP associated with RAP. Recently Sayadi et al reported another similar case of type 3 neovascularization associated with RP.

The underlying pathogenesis of RP-associated CNV remains uncertain. Malik et al hypothesized that retinal pigment epithelium changes, constantly present in retinitis pigmentosa, associated with concomitant photoreceptor cell involvement and chorio-capillaris damage could lead to

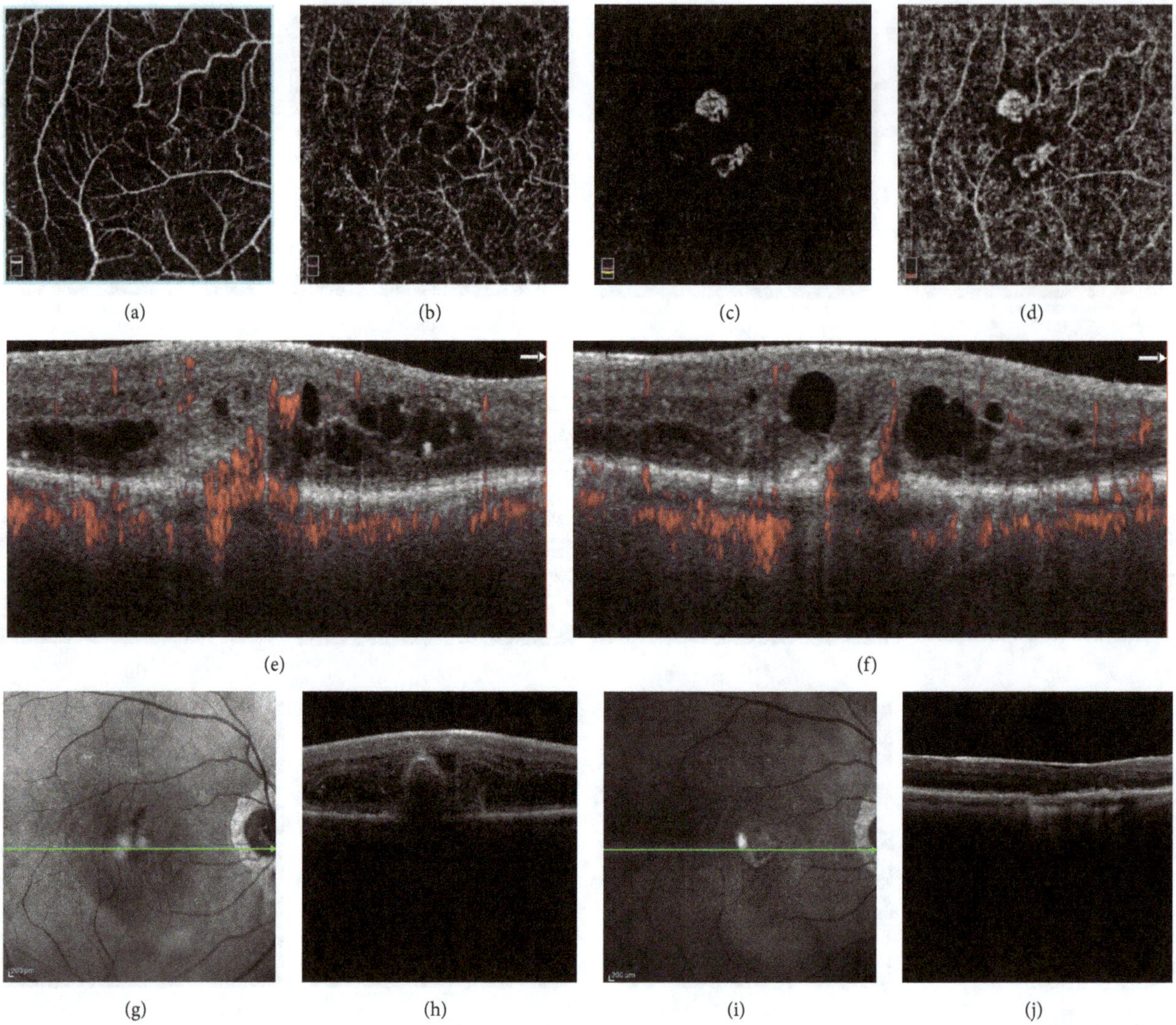

FIGURE 2: (a)-(d) Optical coherence tomography angiography images (6 × 6 mm) revealed the progression of the tuft-shaped lesion from the superficial layer to choroid capillary. (a) Superficial capillary plexus segmentation. (b) Deep capillary plexus segmentation. (c) Outer retinal layer segmentation. (d) Choriocapillaris segmentation. (e)-(f) B-Scans optical coherence tomography angiography showed clearly two distinct intraretinal neovascularizations originated in the superficial layer descending into a tuft-shaped lesion toward the sub-RPE space, respectively above (e) and under (f) the fovea. (g)–(h) Spectral Domain-Optical Coherence Tomography at baseline. (i)–(j) Spectral Domain-Optical Coherence Tomography after treatment.

development of CNV [3]. We decided to perform genetic analysis to search for genetic variants correlated with the disease phenotype displayed by the patient.

Genetic testing revealed the presence of two variants (c.1265C>T and c.1162T>C) in *SEMA4A* and *CNGA1*, respectively. Both genes are known to be associated with autosomal recessive RP. However, the clinical significance of these variants is ambiguous, and cannot be utilized to provide a certain genetic diagnosis of RP in this case. Further studies will be probably decisive to clarify the genetic background of peculiar phenotypes and of RP in general.

Concerning the AMD screening, the patient revealed a moderate risk to develop the disease (heterozygous genotypes for *ARMS2* and *IL-8* susceptibility variants). *ARMS2* and *IL-8* have also been associated with angiogenesis, Extra-Cellular Matrix (ECM) organization, alteration of Bruch's membrane, inflammatory and immune response overactivation observed in AMD [13, 14]. In addition, recent studies suggested that *SEMA4A* may play a critical role in immune response activation and angiogenesis [10]. Interestingly, previous studies correlated a decreased expression of *CNGA1* and other phototransduction related-genes to more severe AMD, especially the neovascular form of disease [14, 21]. Whether the identified VUS will be classified as pathogenic or not, *SEMA4A* and *CNGA1* share some biological pathways with *ARMS2* and *IL*-8, suggesting that these genes may interact together and contribute to increase the susceptibility to develop neovascular lesions, which may be more facilitated to grow in RP cases because of photoreceptor cells degeneration, RPE changes and choriocapillaris damage.

Our study represents the first description of a bilateral type 3 neovascularization in a patient with RP genetically determined.

Because of the rarity of the condition, limited experience about the effective treatment for RP-related CNV has been accrued. Laser photocoagulation [15], photodynamic therapy [16], and intravitreal injections [3, 18] have been proposed as available therapies for CNVs complicating RP. Intravitreal bevacizumab has been reported to be effective for CNV stabilization in patients with RP. Malik et al reported a successful treatment of CNV in RP with a single intravitreal bevacizumab injection [3]. Nevertheless, Battaglia Parodi et al reported a longer period of treatment to achieve CNV stabilization in patients with RP [18]. Recently Sayadi et al reported a case of type 3 neovascularization associated with RP treated with 8 intravitreal injections of ranibizumab during the first year of follow-up, suggesting that anatomical stabilization of RP-related CNV may be difficult to reach.

Despite the rarity of condition, we reported to date the first case of development of a bilateral type 3 neovascularization associated with RP. Given the age of the patient, we cannot certainly exclude that the simultaneous presence of the two pathologies shown by the patient (RP and CNV) may be purely coincidental. Further research is required to examine the mechanism associating these two conditions and to establish the effective treatment for RP-related CNVs.

References

[1] C. Hamel, "Retinitis pigmentosa," *Orphanet Journal of Rare Diseases*, vol. 1, article no. 40, 2006.

[2] L. A. Yannuzzi, S. Negrão, T. Iida et al., "Retinal angiomatous proliferation in age-related macular degeneration," *Retina*, vol. 21, no. 5, pp. 416–434, 2001.

[3] A. Malik, S. Sood, and S. Narang, "Successful treatment of choroidal neovascular membrane in retinitis pigmentosa with intravitreal bevacizumab," *International Ophthalmology*, vol. 30, no. 4, pp. 425–428, 2010.

[4] R. Brancato, U. Introini, L. Pierro et al., "Optical coherence tomography (OCT) in retinal angiomatous proliferation (RAP)," *European Journal of Ophthalmology*, vol. 12, no. 6, pp. 467–472, 2002.

[5] K. K. Dansingani, J. Naysan, and K. B. Freund, "En face OCT angiography demonstrates flow in early type 3 neovascularization (retinal angiomatous proliferation)," *Eye*, vol. 29, no. 5, pp. 703–706, 2015.

[6] A. Miere, G. Querques, O. Semoun, A. El Ameen, V. Capuano, and E. H. Souied, "Optical coherence tomography angiography in early type 3 neovascularization," *Retina*, vol. 35, no. 11, pp. 2236–2241, 2015.

[7] R. Cascella, L. Stocchi, C. Strafella et al., " Comparative analysis between saliva and buccal swabs as source of DNA: lesson from *HLA-B*57:01* testing ," *Pharmacogenomics*, vol. 16, no. 10, pp. 1039–1046, 2015.

[8] R. Cascella, C. Strafella, C. Germani et al., "The genetics and the genomics of primary congenital glaucoma," *BioMed Research International*, vol. 2015, Article ID 321291, 7 pages, 2015.

[9] S. K. Verbakel, R. A. van Huet, C. J. Boon et al., "Non-syndromic retinitis pigmentosa," *Progress in Retinal and Eye Research*, vol. 66, pp. 157–186, 2018.

[10] D. Ito and A. Kumanogoh, "The role of Sema4A in angiogenesis, immune responses, carcinogenesis, and retinal systems," *Cell Adhesion & Migration*, vol. 10, no. 6, pp. 692–699, 2016.

[11] R. Cascella, C. Strafella, G. Longo et al., "Assessing individual risk for AMD with genetic counseling, family history, and genetic testing," *Eye*, vol. 32, no. 2, pp. 446–450, 2018.

[12] F. Ricci, G. Staurenghi, T. Lepre et al., "Haplotypes in IL-8 gene are associated to age-related macular degeneration: a case-control study," *Plos One*, vol. 8, no. 6, Article ID e66978, 2013.

[13] R. Cascella, C. Strafella, G. Longo et al., "Uncovering genetic and non-genetic biomarkers specific for exudative age-related macular degeneration: significant association of twelve variants," *Oncotarget*, vol. 9, no. 8, pp. 7812–7821, 2018.

[14] R. Cascella, C. Strafella, V. Caputo et al., "Towards the application of precision medicine in age-related macular degeneration," *Progress in Retinal and Eye Research*, vol. 63, pp. 132–146, 2018.

[15] F. Marano, A. F. Deutman, A. Leys, and A. L. Aandekerk, "Hereditary retinal dystrophies and choroidal neovascularization," *Graefe's Archive for Clinical and Experimental Ophthalmology*, vol. 238, no. 9, pp. 760–764, 2000.

[16] R. Iwakiri, S. Okinami, and A. Hirata, "Two cases of retinitis pigmentosa associated with choroidal neovascularization," *Nippon Ganka Gakkai zasshi*, vol. 111, no. 8, pp. 606–611, 2007.

[17] J. Y. Cheng and K. H. Adrian, "Photodynamic therapy for choroidal neovascularization in stargardt disease and retinitis pigmentosa," *Retinal Cases & Brief Reports*, vol. 3, no. 4, pp. 388–390, 2009.

[18] M. B. Parodi, U. D. Benedetto, K. A. Knutsson et al., "Juxtafoveal choroidal neovascularization associated with retinitis pigmentosa treated with intravitreal bevacizumab," *Journal of Ocular Pharmacology and Therapeutics*, vol. 28, no. 2, pp. 202–204, 2012.

[19] Y. Nagao, Y. Hiramoto, and K. Takahashi, "A case of retinitis pigmentosa with retinal angiomatous proliferation," *Nippon Ganka Gakkai zasshi*, vol. 115, no. 2, pp. 147–150, 2011.

[20] J. Sayadi, A. Miere, E. Souied, and S. Cohen, "Type 3 neovascularization associated with retinitis pigmentosa," *Case Reports in Ophthalmology*, vol. 8, no. 1, pp. 245–249, 2017.

[21] A. M. Newman, N. B. Gallo, L. S. Hancox et al., "Systems-level analysis of age-related macular degeneration reveals global biomarkers and phenotype-specific functional networks," *Genome Medicine*, vol. 4, no. 2, article no. 16, 2012.

10

Keratoconus with Central Serous Chorioretinopathy: A Rare Combination

Anastasia Tsiogka[1] **Apostolos Gkartzonikas,**[1] **Konstantinos Markopoulos,**[1] **Iordanis Georgiou,**[1] **and George L. Spaeth**[2]

[1]*Department of Ophthalmology, 401 General Military Hospital, 3 P. Kanellopoulou Street, Athens 11525, Greece*
[2]*Department of Ophthalmology, Wills Eye Hospital, 840 Walnut St, Philadelphia, PA 19107, USA*

Correspondence should be addressed to Anastasia Tsiogka; anastasiatsi@med.uoa.gr

Academic Editor: Vishal Jhanji

Keratoconus and central serous chorioretinopathy are two rare diseases. They can occur together in some individuals. We report a case of a 48-year-old man, who presented to our clinic with decreased visual acuity on his left eye. Physical examination, biomicroscopy, corneal topography, and optical coherence tomography revealed keratoconus and central serous chorioretinopathy. We discuss the possible connection between these two conditions.

1. Introduction

Keratoconus causes visual loss due to increasing irregular corneal astigmatism and affects 86 in 100,000 people [1]. It is an idiopathic, noninflammatory, progressive corneal ectasia characterized by bilateral, usually asymmetric thinning of the cornea [2]. The onset typically is in teenage years, and it is much less common in middle-aged and elderly individuals [3, 4]. While it often presents as an isolated condition, keratoconus may also be associated with many systemic disorders and/or ocular diseases [5].

Central serous chorioretinopathy (CSC) is a major cause of vision threat among middle-aged male individuals [6]. It is a secondary idiopathic serous neurosensory detachment, believed to be due to a leakage of fluid from the choroid through tight junctions between adjacent retinal pigment epithelial cells (RPE) [7]. Its precise pathogenesis is unknown, but there are some possible risk factors relating to the occurrence of CSC, such as H. pylori infection, steroid use, sleep disorders, autoimmune disease, psychotropic medication use, and type-A behavior [8]. To the best of our knowledge, no association between CSC and corneal diseases has been described. Here, we present the case of a patient with keratoconus and central serious chorioretinopathy (CSC).

2. Case Report

2.1. History. A 48-year-old male was referred to our ophthalmology clinic with decreased visual acuity on the left eye. His medical history included Crohn's disease since 2005, seasonal allergic rhinoconjunctivitis, and prostate cancer status post prostatectomy in 2016. He had been treated with methylprednisolone intermittently therapy for the last 4 years. Five years ago, he had an episode of episcleritis treated with dexamethasone (1%) drops. He was very anxious. His family history was unremarkable.

2.2. Measurements

2.2.1. Entrance Tests, Refraction, and Binocularity. Best corrected distance visual acuity was 10/10 in the right eye and 2/10 in the left eye (Snellen chart). Ocular motility was normal. Visual fields were intact to confrontation visual field exam (Donders' test). His pupils were equal, round, and reactive to light, with no afferent pupillary defect. Color vision discrimination, using the Ishihara color vision test, showed normal color vision in each eye. The red-cap color comparison was equal between the two eyes. Automated keratometry revealed of -1.00 sph and -1.50 cyl at 90° in the right eye and -5.00 cyl at 120° in the left eye.

2.2.2. Biomicroscopy. The eyelids, eyelashes, conjunctiva, iris, and anterior chamber appeared normal. Anterior segment biomicroscopy showed mild corneal thinning inferior to the pupil in the left eye. There were no other signs of keratoconus (Fleischer's ring, Vogt's striae, Rizzuti's sign, oil drop). There was no stromal edema or corneal opacities in either eye. He had incipient posterior subcapsular cataract in both eyes. Fundus examination of both eyes was normal. Vitreous, optic nerves, vasculature, and peripheral retina in both eyes were unremarkable and normal for his age. The intraocular pressure (as measured by Goldmann applanation tonometry) was 30 mmHg in the right eye and 28 mmHg in the left eye.

2.2.3. Corneal Topography and Optical Coherence Tomography (OCT). The anterior surface corneal topography of the left eye showed normal K1 and K2 values, but the difference between Kmax-K2 was >1D. For the right eye, the simulated minimum keratometry reading had normal K1 and K2 values and the difference between Kmax-K2 was abnormal as the left eye. Secondary, Kmax (do)-Kmax (so) was >2D. Corneal pachymetry measurements at the thinnest locations were 477 microns and 504 microns for the left and right eye, respectively (Figure 1).

The OCT examination demonstrated fluid accumulation between the interdigitation zone (IZ) and the retinal pigment epithelium (RPE) as well as increased choroidal thickness. The junction between photoreceptor inner and outer segments (IS/OS) was not detected in the detached neurosensory retina. The outer photoreceptor layer of the detached neurosensory retina above the clear subretinal space was irregularly thickened and granulated (Figure 2(a)). The retinal thickness ILM was increased in the horizontal meridian (Figure 2(b)).

Clinical findings were characteristic of keratoconus, central serious chorioretinopathy, and elevated intraocular pressure, as a result of steroid therapy.

2.3. Treatment. Aldosterone antagonists are effective in decreasing subretinal fluid and improving visual acuity in patients with CSC [9]. We prescribed the selective aldosterone antagonist eplerenone which is associated with a favorable side effect profile. Beta blockers are not the most potent medication of IOP lowering, but they are efficacious, well tolerated by most patients and a low cost-effective choice, making them a good choice as a first-line agent in case of the absence of any contraindications. They induce b receptor blockage which lowers aqueous humor formation and secretion especially during daytime [9, 10]. Timolol is one of the most popular and prescribed antiglaucoma beta blocker agents, as a first-line drug in most forms of open angle glaucoma and ocular hypertension [11]. Our patient had elevated IOP due to chronic use of systemic steroids as part of treatment for his Crohn's disease. Given the necessity for ongoing steroid therapy, we elected to prescribe timolol to lower IOP (probably steroid responder). Spectacles were, also, prescribed for keratoconus to improve his vision [3].

3. Discussion

This case report demonstrates the coexistence of keratoconus and central serous chorioretinopathy to the left eye of a 48-year-old Caucasian male with Crohn's disease. Keratoconus and CSC are diseases that affect different parts of the eye.

Keratoconus may be associated with many systemic disorders such as diabetes, asthma, Down syndrome, collagen vascular disease, and sleep apnea [12]. There are some strong associations between keratoconus and several autoimmune diseases and allergic disorders [13]. Furthermore, patients with inflammatory bowel diseases may have an increased risk of keratoconus [14].

The main treatment of inflammatory bowel disease is corticosteroids. They are administered topically, orally, or intravenously and rapidly and consistently improve moderate to severe active ulcerative colitis and Crohn's disease [15]. There is no known association between corticosteroids and keratoconus. In vitro trials of dexamethasone on human cornea showed that dexamethasone significantly increases keratocyte proliferation, but it also induces apoptosis of cultured keratocytes at any concentration [16]. Keratocyte apoptosis is associated with keratoconus, in which keratocyte density is lower compared to healthy controls [17, 18]. On the other hand, central serous chorioretinopathy has been associated with most routes of steroid administration. The majority of the literature on CSC and steroid medication suggests a significant association [19]. At the current time, the pathophysiology of CSC is poorly understood [11].

To our knowledge, there is no direct association between these two conditions. The subfoveal choroid is diffusely thickened in patients with CSC likely because of the choroidal vascular dilatation [20, 21]. In addition, the subfoveal choroid in keratoconus eyes is thicker than that in healthy population [22, 23].

A genetic disorder could better explain the coexistence of keratoconus and central serous chorioretinopathy, especially in predisposed individuals. Keratoconus is associated with extensive alteration in the expression of genes coding collagen type IV, fibronectin, laminin, lysyl oxidase, and tissue inhibitor of metalloproteinase 3 (TIMP-3) involved in cell matrix, cell-cell interactions, massive changes of the cytoskeleton, extracellular matrix remodeling, and transmembrane signaling [24, 25].

The TIMPs are multifunctional proteins, with different cellular effects which are not well understood. TIMP-3 is the only TIMP protein that binds tightly to the extracellular matrix [26]. Immunohistochemistry showed TIMP3 immunostaining was dense, specifically localized in Bruch's membrane and some choroidal vascular basement membranes [27]. Increased expression of TIMP3 could contribute to the activation of apoptotic cell death processes through restructuring of the architecture, and disruption of photoreceptor—matrix interactions. Altered expression of TIMP-3

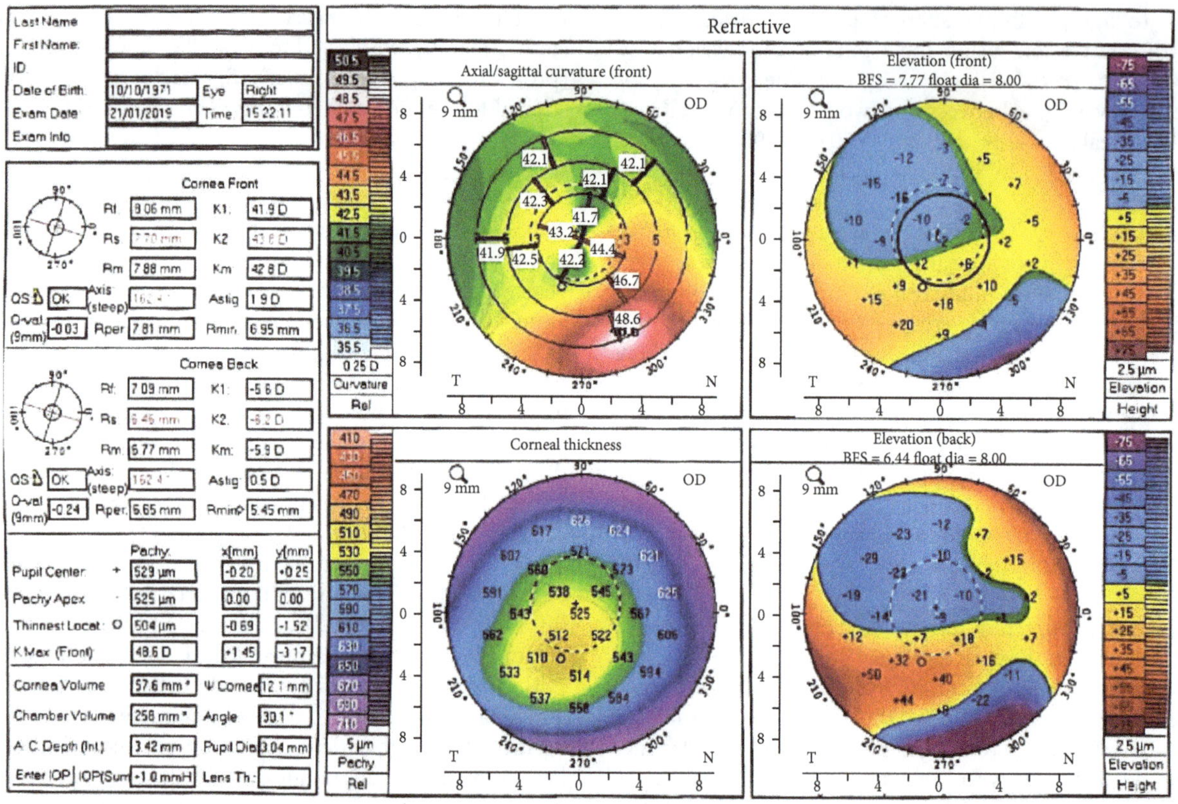

(a)

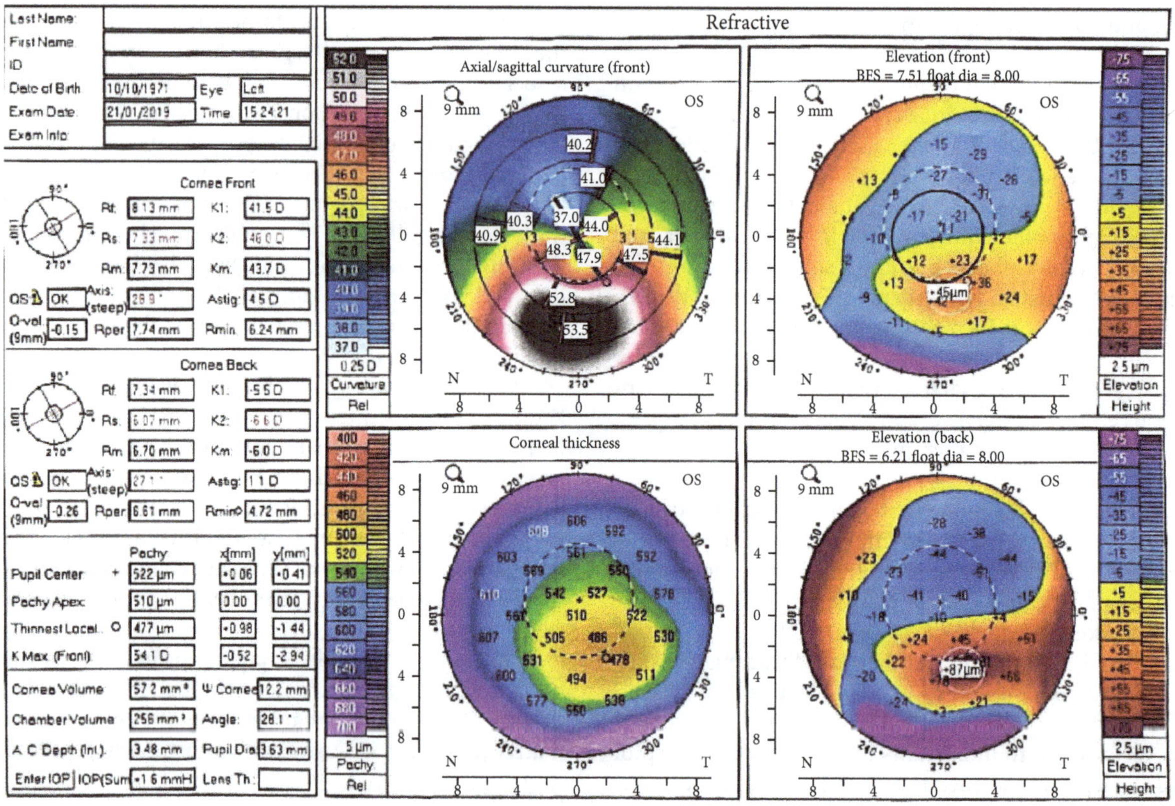

(b)

FIGURE 1: Corneal topography of the right eye with subclinical keratoconus (a) and corneal topography of the left eye showing keratoconus (b).

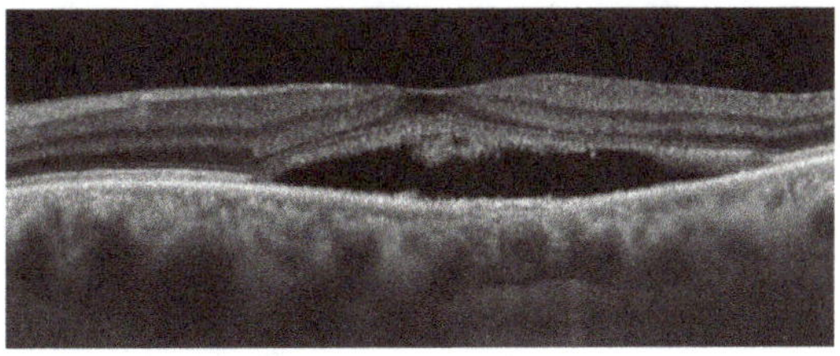

(a)

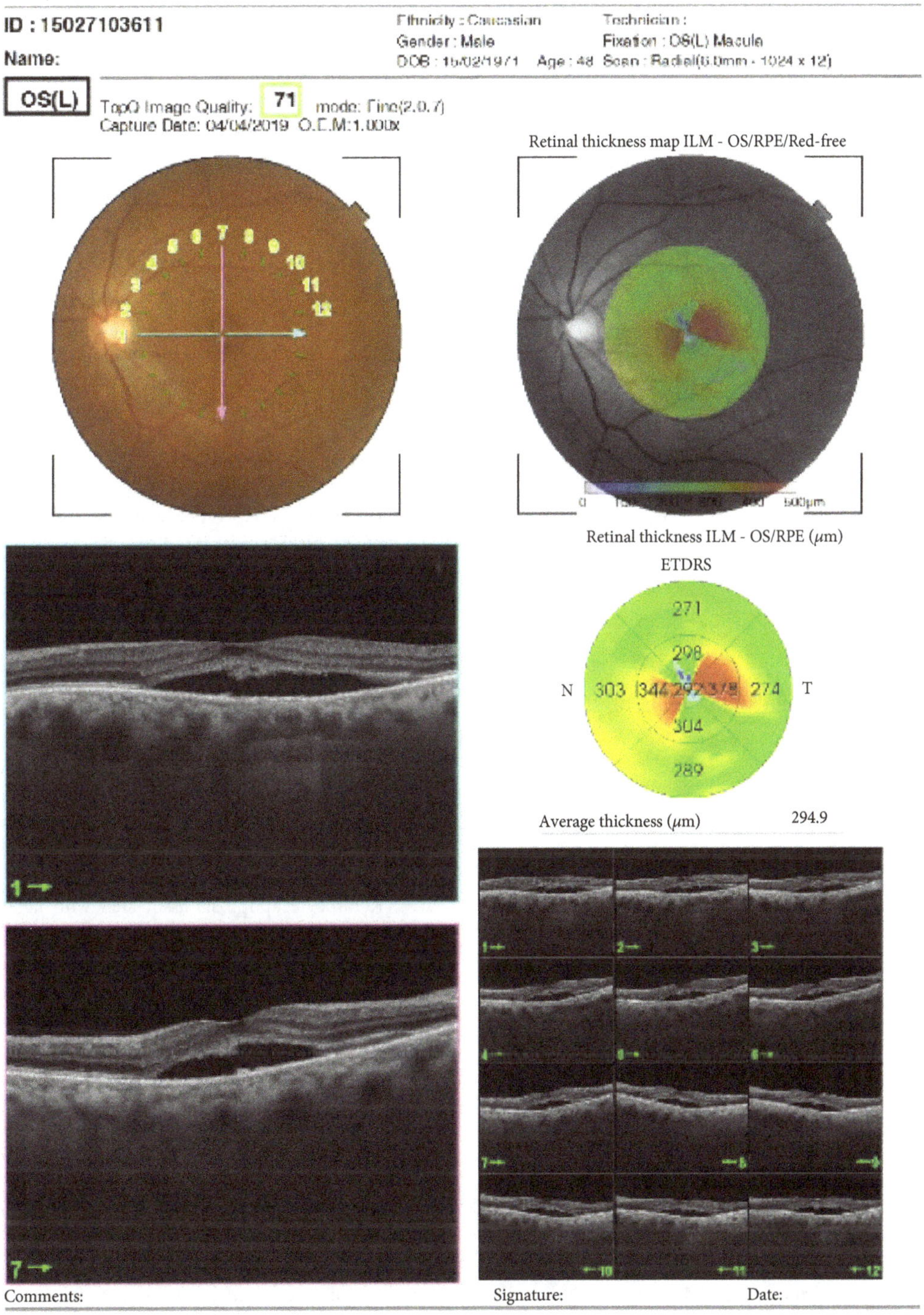

(b)

Figure 2: OCT horizontal high-resolution image (a) and retinal thickness map (b) of the left eye showing central serous chorioretinopathy.

could modify the RPE basement membrane, causing variation in the pigment epithelial integrity. These observations could explain the disturbance of the outer blood–retinal barrier [28].

Reduced expression of some proteins to RPE due to genetic disorders could explain a relationship between the two diseases, potentially reflecting a dysfunction of epithelial layers and basement membranes [29–31]. More studies are necessary to elucidate a possible connection between these diseases.

4. Conclusion

According to the literature, there is no known association between keratoconus and CSC. Genetic predisposition seems to be a plausible mechanism to explain the occurrence of both conditions on the same individual. More studies are necessary to elucidate the possible connection between these diseases.

Abbreviations

CSC: Central serous chorioretinopathy
IZ: Interdigitation zone
IOP: Intraocular pressure
IS/OS: Inner and outer
OCT: Optical coherence tomography
RPE: Retinal pigment epithelium.

Consent

The patient consented to the publication of the case in writing.

Disclosure

All authors attest that they meet the current ICMJE criteria for authorship.

References

[1] A. C. Ferdi, V. Nguyen, D. M. Gore, B. D. Allan, J. J. Rozema, and S. L. Watson, "Keratoconus Natural Progression: A Systematic Review and Meta-analysis of 11 529 Eyes," *Ophthalmology*, vol. 126, no. 7, pp. 935–945, 2019.

[2] G. L. Spaeth, H. Danesh-Meyer, I. Goldberg, and A. Kampik, *Ophthalmic Surgery: Principles and Practice E-Book: Expert Consult-Online and Print*, Elsevier Health Sciences, 2011.

[3] Y. S. Rabinowitz, "Keratoconus," *Survey of Ophthalmology*, vol. 42, no. 4, pp. 297–319, 1998.

[4] A. Gordon-Shaag, M. Millodot, and E. Shneor, "The epidemiology and etiology of keratoconus," *International Journal of Keratoconus and Ectatic Corneal Diseases*, vol. 1, no. 1, pp. 7–15, 2012.

[5] J. W. M. A. Hauser, "The genetics of keratoconus: a review," *Reproductive System & Sexual Disorders*, vol. 1, no. 2, 2012.

[6] A. Daruich, A. Matet, A. Dirani et al., "Central serous chorioretinopathy: recent findings and new physiopathology hypothesis," *Progress in Retinal and Eye Research*, vol. 48, pp. 82–118, 2015.

[7] D. R. Guyer, L. A. Yannuzzi, J. S. Slakter, J. A. Sorenson, A. Ho, and D. Orlock, "Digital indocyanine green videoangiography of central serous chorioretinopathy," *Archives of Ophthalmology*, vol. 112, no. 8, pp. 1057–1062, 1994.

[8] B. Liu, T. Deng, and J. Zhang, "Risk factors for central serous chorioretinopathy: a systematic review and meta-analysis," *Retina*, vol. 36, no. 1, pp. 9–19, 2016.

[9] T. Dada, P. Ichhpujani, and G. Spaeth, "Pearls in Glaucoma Therapy," 2011.

[10] A. A.-E. El-Khamery, A. I. Mohamed, H. E. H. Swify, and A. I. Mohamed, "Cost-effectiveness of glaucoma management with monotherapy medications in Egypt," *Journal of advanced pharmaceutical technology & research*, vol. 8, no. 1, pp. 25–28, 2017.

[11] C. P. Tătaru and V. L. Purcărea, "Antiglaucoma pharmacotherapy," *Journal of Medicine and Life*, vol. 5, no. 3, pp. 247–251, 2012.

[12] M. A. Woodward, T. S. Blachley, and J. D. Stein, "The association between sociodemographic factors, common systemic diseases, and keratoconus: an analysis of a nationwide heath care claims database," *Ophthalmology*, vol. 123, no. 3, pp. 457–465, 2016.

[13] A. Y. Nemet, S. Vinker, I. Bahar, and I. Kaiserman, "The association of keratoconus with immune disorders," *Cornea*, vol. 29, no. 11, pp. 1261–1264, 2010.

[14] F. Tréchot, K. Angioi, C. Latarche et al., "Keratoconus in inflammatory bowel disease patients: a cross-sectional study," *Journal of Crohn's and Colitis*, vol. 9, no. 12, pp. 1108–1112, 2015.

[15] J. A. Katz, "Treatment of inflammatory bowel disease with corticosteroids," *Gastroenterology Clinics of North America*, vol. 33, no. 2, pp. 171–189, 2004.

[16] T. Bourcier, V. Borderie, P. Forgez, A. Lombet, W. Rostène, and L. Laroche, "In vitro effects of dexamethasone on human corneal keratocytes," *Investigative Ophthalmology & Visual Science*, vol. 40, no. 6, pp. 1061–1070, 1999.

[17] W.-J. Kim, Y. S. Rabinowitz, D. M. Meisler, and S. E. Wilson, "Keratocyte apoptosis associated with keratoconus," *Experimental Eye Research*, vol. 69, no. 5, pp. 475–481, 1999.

[18] U. Soiberman, J. W. Foster, A. S. Jun, and S. Chakravarti, "Pathophysiology of Keratoconus: What Do We Know Today," *The open ophthalmology journal*, vol. 11, Suppl-1, M9, pp. 252–261, 2017.

[19] B. P. Nicholson, E. Atchison, A. A. Idris, and S. J. Bakri, "Central serous chorioretinopathy and glucocorticoids: an update on evidence for association," *survey of ophthalmology*, vol. 63, no. 1, pp. 1–8, 2018.

[20] S. Akkaya, "Macular and peripapillary choroidal thickness in patients with keratoconus," *Ophthalmic Surgery, Lasers and Imaging Retina*, vol. 49, no. 9, pp. 664–673, 2018.

[21] R. Gutierrez-Bonet, J. Ruiz-Medrano, P. Peña-Garcia et al., "Macular choroidal thickening in keratoconus patients: swept-source optical coherence tomography study," *Translational Vision Science & Technology*, vol. 7, no. 3, pp. 15–15, 2018.

[22] I. Maruko, T. Iida, Y. Sugano, A. Ojima, and T. Sekiryu, "Subfoveal choroidal thickness in fellow eyes of patients

with central serous chorioretinopathy," *Retina*, vol. 31, no. 8, pp. 1603–1608, 2011.

[23] S. Kuroda, Y. Ikuno, Y. Yasuno et al., "Choroidal thickness in central serous chorioretinopathy," *Retina*, vol. 33, no. 2, pp. 302–308, 2013.

[24] K. Nielsen, K. Birkenkamp-Demtro¨der, N. Ehlers, and T. F. Orntoft, "Identification of differentially expressed genes in keratoconus epithelium analyzed on microarrays," *Investigative Ophthalmology & Visual Science*, vol. 44, no. 6, pp. 2466–2476, 2003.

[25] M. L. Khaled, "In search of genetic mutations for familial keratoconus," 2019.

[26] K. Brew, D. Dinakarpandian, and H. Nagase, "Tissue inhibitors of metalloproteinases: evolution, structure and function," *Biochimica et Biophysica Acta (BBA) - Protein Structure and Molecular Enzymology*, vol. 1477, no. 1-2, pp. 267–283, 2000.

[27] J. Vranka et al., "TIMP3 expression in the human retina and choroid," *Investigative Ophthalmology and Visual Science*, vol. 37, no. 3, 1996.

[28] S. E. Jones, C. Jomary, and M. J. Neal, "Expression of TIMP3 mRNA is elevated in retinas affected by simplex retinitis pigmentosa," *FEBS Letters*, vol. 352, no. 2, pp. 171–174, 1994.

[29] K. Turksen, J. E. Aubin, J. Sodek, and V. I. Kalnins, "Localization of laminin, type IV collagen, fibronectin, and heparan sulfate proteoglycan in chick retinal pigment epithelium basement membrane during embryonic development," *Journal of Histochemistry & Cytochemistry*, vol. 33, no. 7, pp. 665–671, 2017.

[30] C. M. Eandi, L. V. del Priore, E. Bertelli, M. D. Ober, and L. A. Yannuzzi, "Central serous chorioretinopathy in patients with keratoconus," *Retina*, vol. 28, no. 1, pp. 94–96, 2008.

[31] S. Sawaguchi, B. Y. Yue, J. Sugar, and J. E. Gilboy, "Lysosomal enzyme abnormalities in keratoconus," *Archives of Ophthalmology*, vol. 107, no. 10, pp. 1507–1510, 1989.

11

A Female Case of X-Linked Retinoschisis with Macular Hole Bilaterally

A. Altun

Department of Ophthalmology, Bahcesehir University, Faculty of Medicine, Istanbul, Turkey

Correspondence should be addressed to A. Altun; aaltun06@gmail.com

Academic Editor: Maurizio Battaglia Parodi

Purpose. We aimed at reminding that X-linked retinoschisis may also be seen in female patients and share our vitreoretinal surgical experience. *Methods.* The patient underwent pars plana vitrectomy including the closure of the macular holes with inverted ILM flap technique bilaterally. Lens extractions were performed by phacoemulsification during the removal of silicone oil endotamponade. *Patient.* An 18-year-old girl with X-linked retinoschisis and large macular holes in both eyes presented to the clinic of ophthalmology. It was confirmed that the patient had RS1 mutation *Results.* Nine-month-follow-up was uneventful for retinal findings. Significant improvement in visual acuity was achieved, and macular holes were remained closed. *Conclusion.* In cases with large macular holes due to XLR, an inverted ILM flap technique might be safe and effective. Four-month-silicone-endotamponade might be sufficient.

1. Introduction

X-linked retinoschisis (XLR) is a rare macular disease that is observed in hemizygous males and homozygous females. XLR is a common cause of macular dysfunction in young men due to the allelic heterogeneity at the retinoschisis (X-linked, juvenile) locus 1 (RS1), with a prevalence of 1 in 5000 to 1 in 25,000 [1, 2]. Today, it is estimated to be very low compared to men, but the prevalence of XLR in the female population has not yet been determined. In this paper, we aimed at sharing our findings and the results of vitreoretinal surgery in an 18-year-old girl with bilateral macular hole with XLR.

2. Case Presentation

An 18-year-old female patient was admitted to our clinic with a decrease in visual acuity for 3 years. Intravitreal anti-vascular endothelial growth factor (anti-VEGF) and dexamethasone implant injections were applied 3 times to the right eye and 4 times to the left eye due to the suspicion of macular edema in different clinics. In the detailed anamnesis, the patient reported that she could see very well in childhood and did not use glasses and there was no history of trauma. There was a consanguineous marriage between mother and father (they were the children of each other's aunts).

In the ophthalmological examination, it was determined that the patient was orthophoric and eye movements were free in all directions. The patient had no refractive error. The best-corrected visual acuity (BCVA) was at the level of counting fingers from 2 meters in the right eye and 3 meters in the left eye. The cornea, anterior chamber, iris, and lens findings were within normal limits. Intraocular pressure (IOP) was 12 mm in the right eye and 13 mmHg in the left eye. In funduscopic examination, macular hole (Figures 1 and 2) was detected in both eyes, which was wider in the left eye. Optical coherence tomography (OCT) revealed macular holes as well as the presence of retinoschisis in both eyes (Figure 3). There were also spots on the retina of the patient in the peripheral region. Electroretinogram showed a decrease in b-wave amplitude bilaterally. The patient did not have any additional problems at night vision. The patient

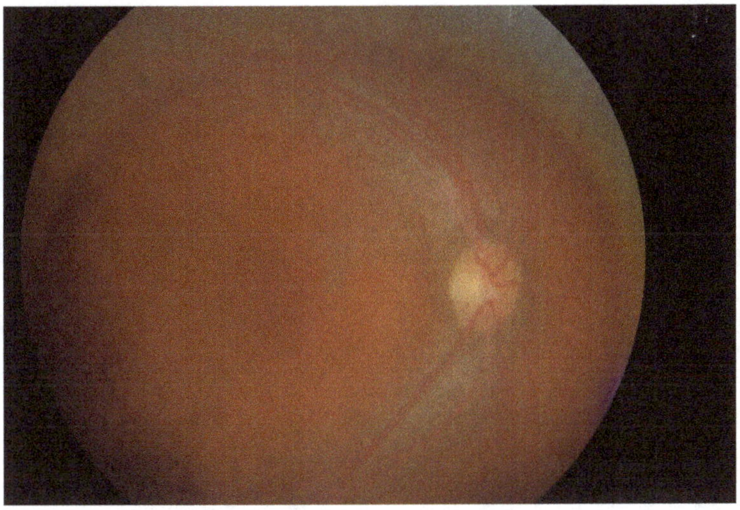

FIGURE 1: Fundus photo of the right eye.

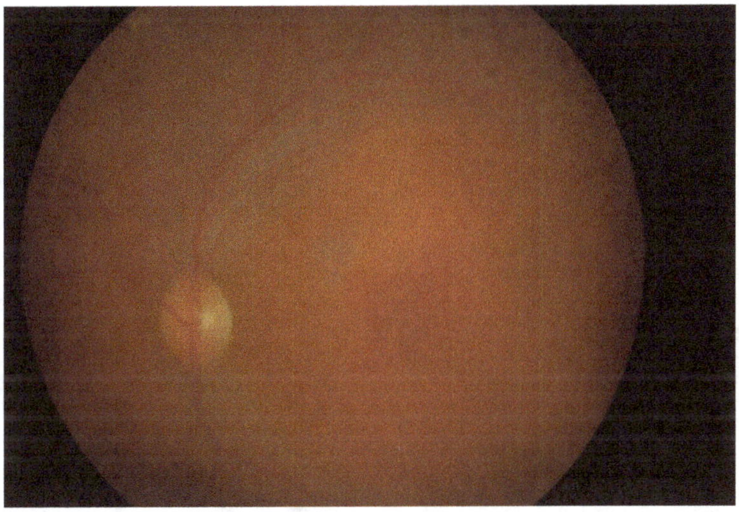

FIGURE 2: Fundus photo of the left eye.

was diagnosed as X-associated retinoschisis (XLR) due to funduscopic, OCT, and ERG findings.

3. Methods

After obtaining the informed consent, under general anesthesia, 23 gauge pars plana vitrectomy, inner limiting membrane (ILM) peeling, and the closure of macular holes were performed with an inverted ILM flap technique.

During PPV, a third-hand effect was created with the help of perfluorocarbon to stabilize the macula and prevent iatrogenic tearing during the ILM peeling phase. At the end of the operation, 1000 centistokes silicone oil endotamponade was implanted in both eyes, and the patient was kept in the prone position for 7 days in the postoperative period. Silicone endotamponade was removed after 4 months in both eyes. During the removal of silicone oil, cataract surgeries were performed with the phacoemulsification technique for lens opacification that developed post-PPV.

4. Results

During the postoperative follow-up period, no drug was needed for IOP control and always remained within normal limits. Within a month, BCVA improved to 2/10 in the right eye and 3/10 in the left eye. The patient was confirmed to have genetically RS1 mutation. During follow-up, the maculas were flat and the holes were closed. Three months later, the posterior subcapsular cataract developed in both eyes. During the removal of silicone oil in the fourth month after PPV, the patient's cataract surgeries were performed in the same sessions. At the last visit of the patient (at the 9th month after PPV), BCVA improved to 4/10 in the right eye and 6/10 in the left eye, there was no macular hole, and retina was attached in both eyes (Figure 4).

5. Discussion

XLR is one of the rare retinal diseases whose genetic cause is not yet fully understood. The association of XLR with the RS1

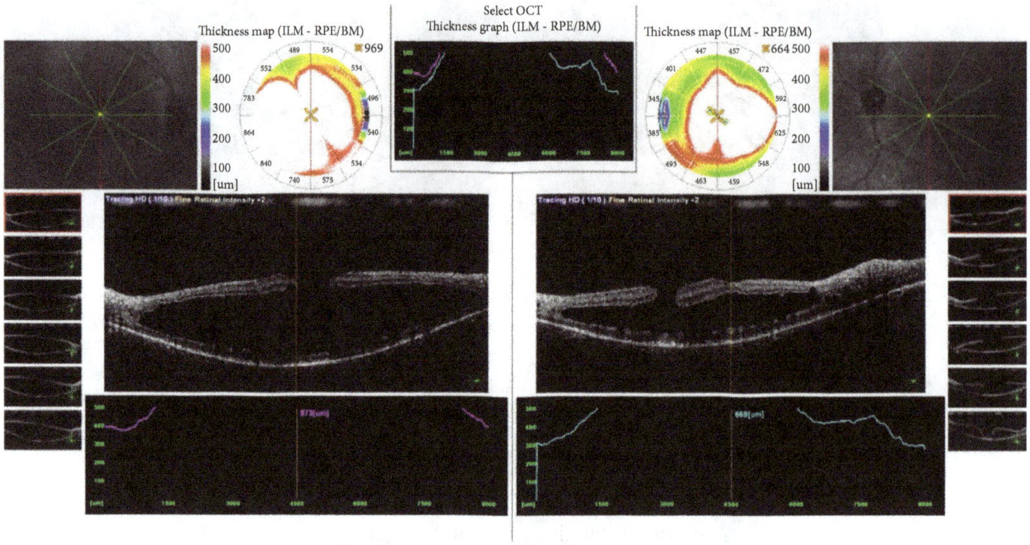

FIGURE 3: Preoperative optical coherence image of the eyes.

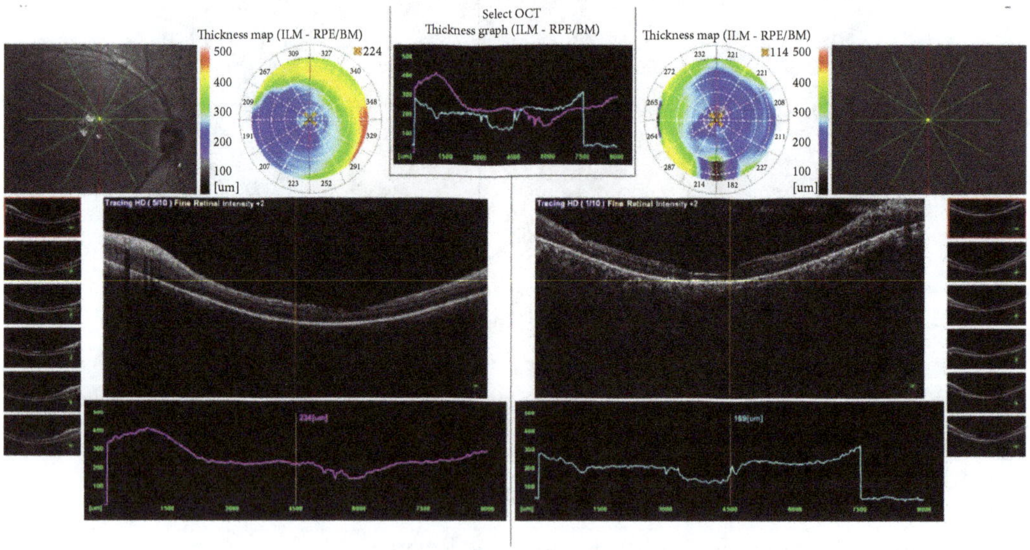

FIGURE 4: Postoperative optical coherence image of the eyes.

mutation has been previously reported in the literature [1, 2]. Our case had also RS1 mutation. Most of the cases reported in the literature have male gender [1–6]. One of the conditions that make our case special is her gender. The reason for this may be the close relative relationship between mother and father. When her detailed story was questioned, it was learned that the patient's two aunts had similar problems, but unfortunately, we did not have the chance to reach these people and confirm their eye findings.

Bilateral retinoschisis is the most frequently observed finding, as in our case. The diagnosis of XLR is made by funduscopic and OCT findings and excluding other possible causes. In XLR, retinoschisis usually affects the macula bilaterally, but only one case has been reported in the literature where only the peripheral retina is affected unilaterally [7]. In the majority of cases reported to have XLR, the macular hole is unilateral. In our case, there was a bilateral macular hole, as in the case presented by Gautam et al. [8].

Today, the pathogenesis of XLR is not fully understood [2]. Gass [3] suggested that "Muller cell cone" was a key factor in the pathogenesis of congenital XLR. The Muller cell cone is a focal point for foveal division and cyst formation in both pathologies. In XLR, the accumulation of defective retinoschisin protein in and around Muller cells causes cystic voids in multiple retinal layers. The combination of these cysts leads to the formation of larger cysts, resulting in larger glandular cavities. In the uppermost region of the schisis cavities, degeneration of the retina takes place because of tangential traction caused by elevation of the retinal tissue. Breakage of inner layers occurs and a macular hole forms.

Methods such as intravitreal dexamethasone [9] or gene therapy [10] in XLR treatment have been described in the literature. Before presenting our clinic, the patient had been injected with intravitreal anti-VEGF or dexamethasone implant in different clinics. Today, there is no evidence that anti-VEGF drugs are effective in macular edema or retinal dissociation that may develop in XLR.

We preferred a surgical treatment option for our case. We performed PPV and an inverted ILM flap technique to close the macular holes. Although the macular holes were closed in one month, we extended the silicone oil endotamponade for up to 4 months to support the separated retinal layers. During PPV, we observed that the cortical vitreous was strictly connected to the retina in both eyes. This experience reinforces the traction hypothesis of Shukla et al., Greven et al., and Shanmugam et al. [4–6] on the macula in pathophysiology. Yu et al. [11] reported that vitreoretinal traction associated with interface tight connection was found in 9% of their cases.

In the majority of cases reported to have XLR, the macular hole is unilateral. In our case, there were bilateral macular hole, as in the case presented by Yu et al. [11].

6. Conclusion

X-linked retinoschisis (XLR) can rarely be observed in females, especially in daughters of close-relative parents. Inverted ILM flap application under perfluorocarbon can be a safe technique in the surgical treatment of large macular holes in patients with XLR. In these cases, it may be sufficient for the silicone oil to remain in the eye for 4 months for endotamponade.

Additional Points

Summary Statement. In rhegmatogenous X-linked retinoschisis cases, the inverted ILM flap technique and four-month silicone tamponade might be a sufficient and efficient treatment method.

References

[1] E. H. Wood, I. Lertjirachai, B. K. Ghiam et al., "The natural history of congenital X-linked retinoschisis and conversion between phenotypes over time," *Ophthalmology Retina*, vol. 3, no. 1, pp. 77–82, 2019.

[2] H. Kondo, K. Oku, S. Katagiri et al., "Novel mutations in the RS1 gene in Japanese patients with X-linked congenital retinoschisis," *Human Genome Variation*, vol. 6, no. 1, p. 3, 2019.

[3] J. D. M. Gass, "Müller cell cone, an overlooked part of the anatomy of the fovea centralis," *Archives of Ophthalmology*, vol. 117, no. 6, pp. 821–823, 1999.

[4] D. Shukla, K. B. Naresh, A. Rajendran, and R. Kim, "Macular hole secondary to X-linked retinoschisis," *Eye*, vol. 20, no. 12, pp. 1459–1461, 2006.

[5] C. M. Greven, R. J. Moreno, and W. Tasman, "Unusual manifestations of X-linked retinoschisis," *Transactions of the American Ophthalmological Society*, vol. 88, pp. 211–225, 1990.

[6] M. P. Shanmugam and A. Nagpal, "Foveal schisis as a cause of retinal detachment secondary to macular hole in juvenile X-linked retinoschisis," *Retina*, vol. 25, no. 3, pp. 373–375, 2005.

[7] H. Oummad, M. Elkaddoumi, J. Maré, M. Lezrek, and O. Cherkaoui, "Bilateral macular retinoschisis associated with unilateral peripheral retinoschisis," *The Pan African Medical Journal*, vol. 28, p. 38, 2017.

[8] M. Gautam, H. Murthy, and N. S. Muralidhar, "Bilateral macular holes in X-linked retinoschisis: now the spectrum is wider," *Indian Journal of Ophthalmology*, vol. 59, no. 6, pp. 507–509, 2011.

[9] S. Mukhtar, S. M. Potter, and S. G. Khurshid, "Dexamethasone intravitreal implant for X-linked (juvenile) retinoschisis," *Retinal Cases & Brief Reports*, vol. 13, no. 1, pp. 18–20, 2019.

[10] C. Cukras, H. E. Wiley, B. G. Jeffrey et al., "Retinal AAV8-RS1 gene therapy for X-linked retinoschisis: initial findings from a phase I/IIa trial by intravitreal delivery," *Mol Ther*, vol. 26, no. 9, pp. 2282–2294, 2018.

[11] J. Yu, Y. Ni, P. A. Keane, C. Jiang, W. Wang, and G. Xu, "Foveomacular schisis in juvenile X-linked retinoschisis: an optical coherence tomography study," *American Journal of Ophthalmology*, vol. 149, no. 6, pp. 973–978.e2, 2010.

12

Orbital Infection by *Saksenaea vasiformis* in an Immunocompetent Host

Mingkwan Lumyongsatien,[1] Pimkwan Jaru-ampornpan,[2] Mongkol Uiprasertkul,[3] and Dinesh Selva[4]

[1]*Department of Ophthalmology, Mettapracharak Hospital, Sampran District, 52 moo2 Rhikhing, Sampran, Nakhon Pathom, Thailand 73210*
[2]*Department of Ophthalmology, Faculty of Medicine, Siriraj Hospital, Mahidol University, 2 Arun Amarin Road, Siriraj, Bangkoknoi, Bangkok, Thailand 10700*
[3]*Department of Pathology, Faculty of Medicine, Siriraj Hospital, Mahidol University, 2 Arun Amarin road, Siriraj, Bangkoknoi, Bangkok, Thailand 10700*
[4]*Department of Ophthalmology and Visual Sciences, South Australian Institute of Ophthalmology, University of Adelaide, Adelaide, South Australia, Australia*

Correspondence should be addressed to Mingkwan Lumyongsatien; mingkwan@metta.go.th

Academic Editor: Hiroshi Eguchi

Orbital mucormycosis caused by *Saksenaea vasiformis* is extremely rare. Herein, we report an immunocompetent 22-year-old Thai female who presented with two months of progressive right upper eyelid mass, associated with swelling, redness, and ptosis. She failed to improve despite multiple courses of antibiotic and steroid treatment. Computed tomography (CT) scan showed infiltration involving the upper eyelid and lacrimal gland. Fungal hyphae were revealed by histopathological study. Polymerase chain reaction (PCR) was positive for *Saksenaea vasiformis* (GenBank: accession number FR687327.1). The patient was successfully treated with surgical debridement, amphotericin B, and oral posaconazole.

1. Introduction

Saksenaea vasiformis is a fungus of the phylum Zygomycota and order *Mucorales*; it was first isolated from a soil sample in India and reported by Saksena in 1953 [1]. It is a rare zygomycosis typically associated with cutaneous and subcutaneous infection in immunocompetent hosts [2]. However, severe infections such as osteomyelitis, renal infection, rhino-orbito-cerebral infection, and disseminated forms are also documented [3, 4]. Aggressive invasion to surrounding tissues is the most usual representation of *S. vasiformis* mucormycosis.

2. Case Presentation

A 22-year-old woman with no significant medical history attended a community hospital with gradual swelling, erythematous, and ptosis of the right upper eyelid for two months. The patient had no fever, pain, or visual disturbance. She denied any previous traumatic injury or insect bite. After failure of multiple courses of treatment with dicloxacillin, tetracycline, topical steroid-antibiotic ointment, and oral steroid, she presented to Mettapracharak Eye Center. Physical examination showed the right upper eyelid swelling and ptosis with a nontender palpable firm

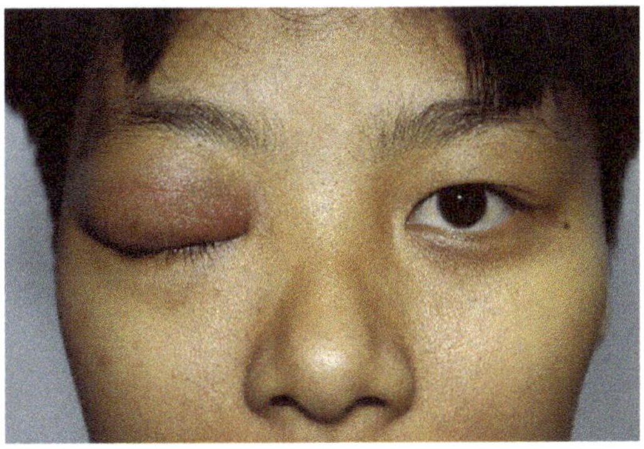

FIGURE 1: This figure shows the right upper eyelid swelling and ptosis with a palpable firm mass 20 mm in diameter.

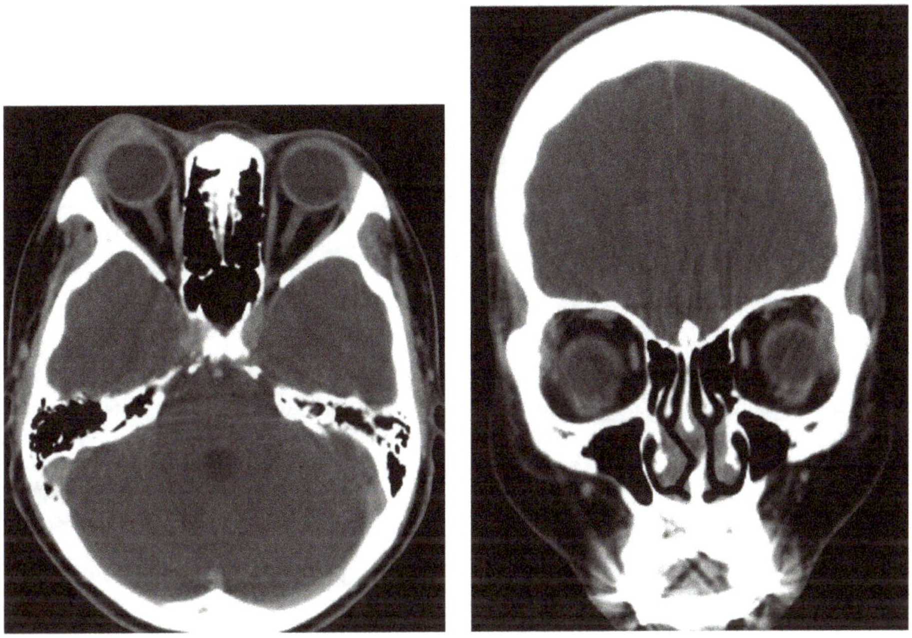

(a) (b)

FIGURE 2: (a) Computed tomography (CT) axial view. (b) Computed tomography (CT) coronal view. (a, b) An infiltrative mass at the right superolateral orbital involving the lacrimal gland and upper eyelid.

mass 20 mm in diameter (Figure 1). Best-corrected visual acuities were 20/20 bilaterally. Intraocular pressures were 28 mmHg in the right eye and 16 mmHg in the left eye. Extraocular movements were full, and there was no proptosis. Computed tomography (CT) showed an infiltrative mass at the right superolateral orbital involving the lacrimal gland and upper eyelid (Figures 2(a) and 2(b)). A biopsy was performed via a skin crease incision. A mass involving the septum and orbital fat with multiple loculated abscess was observed intraoperatively (Figure 3). Histopathology demonstrated granulomatous inflammation (Figure 4(a)) with broad nonseptate and sparsely septate hyphae with the right angle branching on periodic acid-Schiff (PAS) (Figure 4(b)) and Grocott methenamine silver (GMS) staining (Figure 4(c)) with no vascular invasion. The patient was commenced on intravenous amphotericin B 40 mg as a 24-hour infusion. Additional surgical debridement was then performed. PCR from the debrided tissue identified *Saksenaea vasiformis* with 98.33% identity (GenBank: accession number FR687327.1). There were negative cultures for bacteria and fungus. There was significant clinical improvement after one week of treatment. However, repeat biopsy on day 28 showed numerous hyphae still

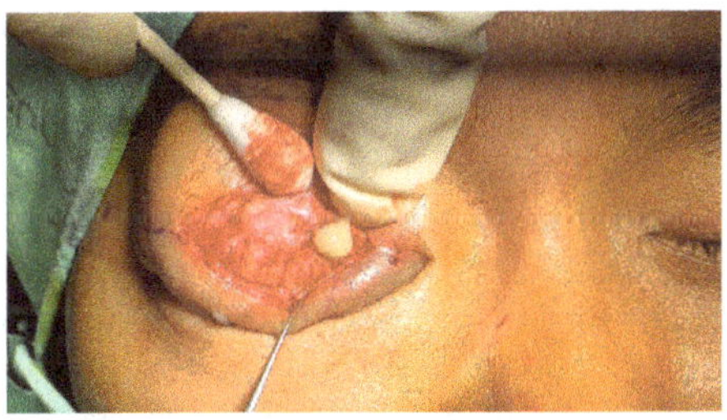

FIGURE 3: A mass involving the septum and orbital fat with multiple loculated abscesses.

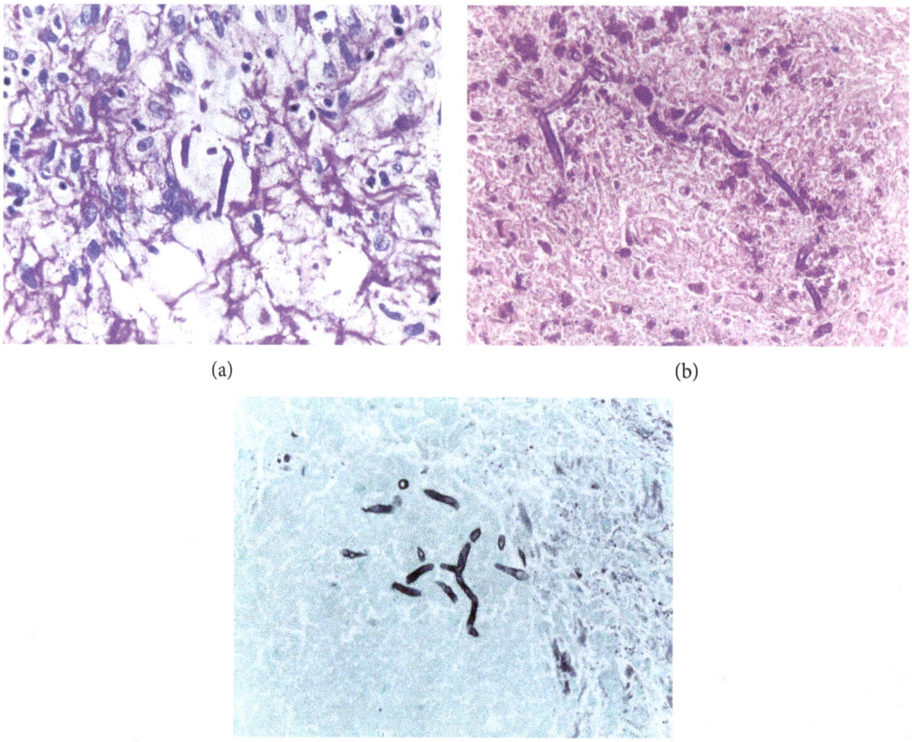

Figure 4: (a) Histopathologic section shows fungal hyphae in granulomatous inflammation background (H&E 400x). (b) Periodic acid-Schiff (PAS) (600x). (c) Grocott methenamine silver (GMS) staining (600x). (b, c) Broad nonseptate and septate hyphae with the right angle branching on PAS and GMS.

present. The patient also developed renal impairment, hypokalemia, and hypomagnesemia attributed to amphotericin B. Hence, amphotericin B was discontinued and replaced by oral posaconazole 300 mg daily for 1 month. Biopsy specimens taken at the end of treatment were negative for fungus. She underwent a levator advancement for residual ptosis. At 3-month follow-up, there was complete resolution of all symptoms and signs (Figure 5).

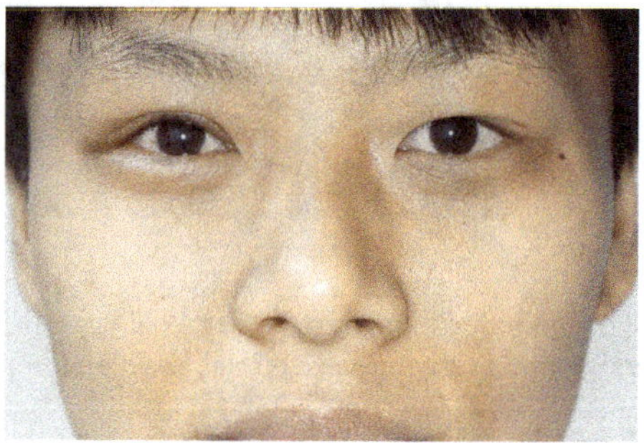

Figure 5: The patient at 3-month follow-up.

3. Discussion

The most common species of the order Mucorales that relate to mucormycosis in humans are *Rhizopus*, *Mucor*, and *Lichtheimia*. Less than 1% to 5% of the reported cases associate with *Cunninghamella*, *Apophysomyces*, *Saksenaea*, *Cokeromyces*, *Rhizomucor*, *Syncephalastrum*, and *Actinomucor* [4]. *Saksenaea vasiformis* and *Apophysomyces* are usually responsible for infections in immunocompetent hosts usually following trauma with soil contamination. However, direct inoculation via respiratory system has also been reported. The route of entry in our case remains unclear, although unnoticed minor trauma or an insect bite may be a possibility.

Saksenaea vasiformis infection was first reported in the facial wounds of a young man following an accident in 1976 [5]. Subsequently, 46 cases have been documented [6]. *S. vasiformis* orbital involvement is extremely rare with 3 published cases associated with sinusitis [3, 7, 8] and 1 individual with isolated orbital infection after aquatic exposure [2]. The prognosis for rhino-orbito-cerebral Saksenaea infection appears to be poor with 83% of mortality rate [3, 4].

Tissue specimens with mucormycosis histopathological identification are often negative cultures. In a review of 929 reported cases of mucormycosis, only 50% were found to be culture positive [9]. Identification of Saksenaea can be a challenge because it fails to sporulate in routine mycological media. Sporulation can be induced in nutrient-depleted media such as distilled water [10]. Funnel-shaped, pigmented sporangia and rhizoids are pathognomonic for *S. vasiformis* [5].

Molecular-based diagnosis such as pan-fungal polymerase chain reaction (PCR) assays enables prompt identification with high sensitivity and specificity. It may be performed on fresh tissue, paraffin-embedded specimens, cerebrospinal fluid (CSF), bronchoalveolar lavage fluid, vitreous fluid, and blood [11]. The molecular identification of fungal species in our case was achieved from fresh tissue by PCR amplification with pan-fungal primers targeted to internal transcribed spacer (ITS) of ribosomal DNA followed by direct sequencing [12]. The whole ITS1-5.8S-ITS2 region primers were synthesized by Bioneer Corporation, Korea. The Basic Local Alignment Search Tool (BLAST) program of GenBank at NCBI website was employed to search for sequence identifier.

Histopathology demonstrates multiple granulomatous inflammation with central necrosis. Fungal hyphae compatible with Mucormycetes in foci of granulomas and vascular invasion may be seen.

The treatment of *S. vasiformis* is aggressive debridement with systemic antifungal drugs. Vascular invasion and tissue necrosis in mucormycosis can lead to poor antifungal penetration. Thus, surgical debridement is critical for thorough eradication of this fungus. The timing and extent of debridement necessary for mucormycosis remains debatable. One retrospective study supported intraoperative frozen sections for margin control of infected tissues [13]. Another report used repeated biopsies to guide the duration of antifungal treatment [14]. In general, amphotericin B (AmB) is the first-line drug, and lipid formulations are significantly less nephrotoxic and provide more safety at higher doses [4, 15]. Posaconazole, a new generation triazole, can be used as an alternative to amphotericin B in the event of the toxicity [2, 4, 5].

4. Conclusions

Saksenaea vasiformis is an emerging fungal pathogen in humans that often affects immunocompetent hosts. As for the localized infection of periorbital, face, and head areas, sinus-rhino-orbito-cerebral infections are the most common associated sites, followed by cutaneous and subcutaneous infections. The clinical manifestations may be presented as granulomatous or necrotic lesions, cellulitis, or abscesses with purulent exudate and necrotic eschars. The diagnosis relies on a constellation of a high index of suspicion on lesions that fail to respond with conventional treatments or necrotic lesions related to previous trauma. Histopathological examination of the tissues is the gold standard for definite diagnosis of zygomycosis. Molecular-based diagnosis is a practical identification method for Zygomycetes species, so that appropriate treatment can be instigated based on antifungal sensitivities. Aggressive surgical debridement with systemic antifungal drugs is the treatment of choice for the disease.

Consent

The patient consented to publication of the case in writing.

References

[1] S. B. Saksena, "A new genus of the Mucorales," *Mycology*, vol. 45, no. 3, pp. 426–436, 2018.

[2] P. Reich, T. Shute, C. Lysen et al., "Saksenaea vasiformis orbital cellulitis in an immunocompetent child treated with posaconazole," *Journal of the Pediatric Infectious Diseases Society*, vol. 7, no. 3, pp. e169–e171, 2018.

[3] S. J. Taj-Aldeen, A. Falamarzi, A. AlMuzrkchi, and J. Guarro, "Rare pediatric rhino-orbital infection caused by Saksenaea vasiformis," *Infection*, vol. 40, no. 6, pp. 703–707, 2012.

[4] M. Z. R. Gomes, R. E. Lewis, and D. P. Kontoyiannis, "Mucormycosis caused by unusual mucormycetes, non-Rhizopus, -Mucor, and -Lichtheimia species," *Clinical Microbiology Reviews*, vol. 24, no. 2, pp. 411–445, 2011.

[5] W. T. Pilch, N. Kinnear, and D. B. Hennessey, "Saksenaea vasiformisinfection in an immunocompetent patient in rural Australia," *BML Case Reports*, vol. 2017, 2017.

[6] K. Samaras, A. M. Markantonatou, D. Karapiperis et al., "Saksenaea vasiformis infections: a case of an immunocompetent adult after mild injury and a literature review," *Journal de Mycologie Medicale*, vol. 29, no. 3, pp. 260–264, 2019.

[7] V. P. Baradkar, M. Mathur, S. Taklikar, M. Rathi, and S. Kumar, "Fatal rhino-orbito-cerebral infection caused by Saksenaea vasiformis in an immunocompetent individual: first case report from India," *Indian Journal of Medical Microbiology*, vol. 26, no. 4, pp. 385–387, 2008.

[8] G. Gonis and M. Starr, "Fatal rhinoorbital mucormycosis caused by Saksenaea vasiformis in an immunocompromised child," *The Pediatric Infectious Disease Journal*, vol. 16, no. 7, pp. 714–716, 1997.

[9] S. P. Hammond, R. Bialek, D. A. Milner, E. M. Petschnigg, L. R. Baden, and F. M. Marty, "Molecular methods to improve diagnosis and identification of mucormycosis," *Journal of Clinical Microbiology*, vol. 49, no. 6, pp. 2151–2153, 2011.

[10] W. Vega, M. Orellana, L. Zaror, J. Gené, and J. Guarro, "Saksenaea vasiformis infections: case report and literature review," *Mycopathologia*, vol. 162, no. 4, pp. 289–294, 2006.

[11] S. E. Kidd, S. C.-A. Chen, W. Meyer, and C. L. Halliday, "A new age in molecular diagnostics for invasive fungal disease: are we ready?," *Frontiers in Microbiology*, vol. 10, article 2903, 2020.

[12] P. Schwarz, S. Bretagne, J. C. Gantier et al., "Molecular identification of zygomycetes from culture and experimentally infected tissues," *Journal of Clinical Microbiology*, vol. 44, no. 2, pp. 340–349, 2006.

[13] C. Reed, R. Bryant, A. S. Ibrahim et al., "Combination polyene-caspofungin treatment of rhino-orbital-cerebral mucormycosis," *Clinical Infectious Diseases*, vol. 47, no. 3, pp. 364–371, 2008.

[14] D. Blanchet, E. Dannaoui, A. Fior et al., "Saksenaea vasiformis infection, French Guiana," *Emerging Infectious Diseases*, vol. 14, no. 2, pp. 342–344, 2008.

[15] B. Spellberg and A. S. Ibrahim, "Recent advances in the treatment of mucormycosis," *Current Infectious Disease Reports*, vol. 12, no. 6, pp. 423–429, 2010.

13

Simultaneous Presentation of Uveitic Disc Edema and Papilledema in an Adult

Chase A. Liaboe, Michael S. Lee, and Justin J. Y. Yamanuha

University of Minnesota, Department of Ophthalmology and Visual Neurosciences, Phillips Wangensteen Building, 9th Floor, 516 Delaware St SE, Minneapolis, MN 55455, USA

Correspondence should be addressed to Justin J. Y. Yamanuha; yamanuha@umn.edu

Academic Editor: Nicola Rosa

Purpose. To present a case of simultaneous uveitic disc edema and increased intracranial pressure (IICP) in an adult. *Methods.* Retrospective case report. *Patients.* A 29-year-old woman affected by bilateral optic disc edema from bilateral posterior uveitis complicated by IICP with papilledema. *Results.* Laboratory workup was negative for infectious and systemic inflammatory causes of uveitis. Computed Tomography scan of the chest was negative for Sarcoidosis. Magnetic Resonance Imaging of the brain and orbits revealed a partially empty sella, bilateral posterior globe flattening without optic nerve sheath enhancement, masses, white matter lesions, or meningeal enhancement. Cerebral Magnetic Resonance Venography showed narrowing of the right and left transverse sinuses without thromboses. Prednisone was initiated for the uveitis which improved the vision but caused weight gain. Neurology evaluation with a lumbar puncture in the lateral decubitus position revealed elevated opening pressure and otherwise normal cerebrospinal fluid. Ocular ultrasonography was considered but not available to measure optic nerve sheath diameter. Oral acetazolamide 1000 mg twice daily was started for papilledema as prednisone was tapered. Periocular steroid and intravitreal bevacizumab injections were used for sight threatening cystoid macular edema and choroidal neovascularization, respectively. *Discussion.* While previously described in children, we report the first known case of bilateral uveitic disc edema and papilledema in an adult. This report will discuss recommendations for evaluation of these rarely concurrent conditions and therapy for both uveitic disc edema and papilledema.

1. Introduction

Bilateral optic disc edema (ODE) can result from intermediate or posterior uveitis as well as increased intracranial pressure (IICP). Evaluation for the former typically includes optical coherence tomography (OCT), fluorescein and indocyanine green angiography, and laboratory evaluation for infectious and inflammatory causes of uveitis. The workup for possible papilledema includes brain Magnetic Resonance Imaging (MRI) for intracranial masses, hydrocephalus, meningitis, or encephalitis and Cerebral Magnetic Resonance Venography (MRV) for venous sinus thromboses. Ocular ultrasonography by a trained examiner has been shown to safely measure optic nerve sheath diameter [1] and may also be considered in the evaluation for papilledema. A lumbar puncture is also recommended to measure intracranial pressure and analyze the cerebrospinal fluid. A thorough medication history is paramount in these cases as use or tapering of corticosteroids, oral contraceptive pills, tetracycline antibiotics, or Vitamin A retinoid derivatives can cause IICP. Concurrent presentation of bilateral uveitic disc edema and papilledema has been previously reported in children [2, 3]. Treatment of uveitis with systemic corticosteroids in children has also been shown to cause IICP [4], but presentation of bilateral uveitis and papilledema before or after treatment has not been reported in adults.

2. Purpose

We present the first reported case of an adult with simultaneous bilateral uveitic disc edema and IICP which worsened with systemic corticosteroids and discuss the need for treatment of both uveitis and papilledema when present concurrently.

3. Methods and Patient

A retrospective case report of a single patient is presented herein. The University of Minnesota Institutional Review Board (IRB) exempted review for this deidentified case report.

4. Results: Case History

A 29-year-old woman without prior ocular history presented with blurry vision in the left eye (LE). Medical history was significant for viral meningitis (age 11), Hashimoto's thyroiditis, psoriasis, and treated Chlamydia (age 22). Family history was significant for systemic lupus erythematosus in her mother, but there was no family history of uveitis or other eye conditions. There was no recent travel or exposure. Systemic review revealed intermittent headaches, however was negative for other symptoms of systemic disease such as fevers, rashes, mouth sores, genital ulcers, joint pains, or night sweats.

Initial best corrected visual acuity was 20/20 in the right eye (RE) and 20/500 with pinhole in the left eye (LE). The pupils, intraocular pressure, motility, and alignment were normal. Slit lamp examination showed a quiet anterior segment in the RE and keratic precipitates with 3+ cell and flare in the LE. Dilated funduscopic exam of the RE showed 1+ vitreous cell and optic disc edema (ODE) (Figure 1).

Dilated funduscopic exam of the LE showed 3+ vitreous cell, ODE, a gray macular lesion, and peripheral white lesions (Figure 2).

Initial posterior pole fluorescein angiography (FA) in the RE showed optic nerve and small vessel hyperfluorescence (Figure 3).

Initial FA in the LE showed optic nerve and small vessel hyperfluorescence as well as a choroidal neovascular membrane (CNVM) (Figure 4). Indocyanine green (ICG) angiography was not available at the initial evaluation.

The patient received an initial diagnosis of bilateral ODE, intermediate uveitis RE, and posterior uveitis LE and was started on topical prednisolone acetate four times daily in both eyes (BE).

Laboratory evaluation was initiated for infectious and inflammatory causes of uveitis and revealed the following normal results: Lyme IgM and IgG, Toxoplasma IgM and IgG, Quantiferon, RPR, TPA-ABS, ACE, ANCA, CBC, and ESR. Computed Tomography (CT) scan of the chest showed scattered calcified lymph nodes inconsistent with Sarcoidosis. Magnetic Resonance Imaging (MRI) of the brain and orbits was performed showing the bilateral ODE and revealed bilateral posterior globe flattening, a partially empty sella, amild distension of the perioptic nerve sheaths, but no optic nerve enhancement, white matter lesions, masses, or meningeal enhancement. Magnetic Resonance Venography (MRV) of the brain demonstrated narrowing of the right and left transverse sinuses without thromboses (Figure 5).

The initial lumbar puncture (LP) revealed elevated opening pressure of 35 cm H_20 and unremarkable CSF evaluation for protein, glucose, white and red blood cells, Zoster, Syphilis, and ACE. The patient was started on oral prednisone 60 mg daily for the uveitis, but treatment for the IICP was not initiated at this time for unclear reasons. The patient subsequently developed a thirty-pound weight gain and worsening headaches when attempting to quickly taper the oral prednisone, so this medication was gradually tapered over a few months. The vitreous inflammation did decrease in the LE, but visual acuity did not improve beyond 20/250 even after an intravitreal injection of bevacizumab for the CNVM.

Three months after initial presentation, while on prednisone 20 mg daily, the patient presented to the Emergency Department for worsening headaches. An LP at this time

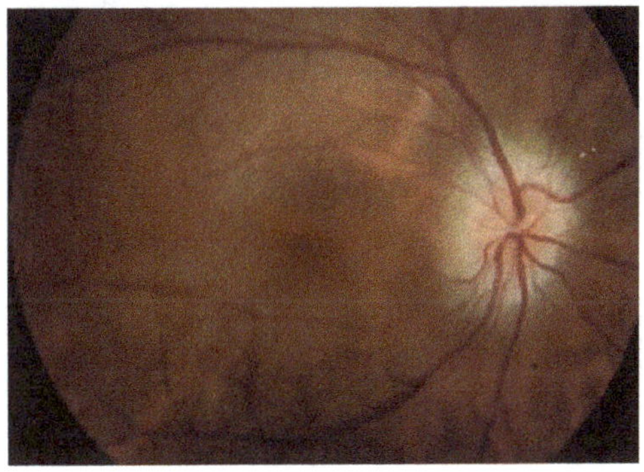

FIGURE 1: Initial fundus photo of the RE showing optic disc edema.

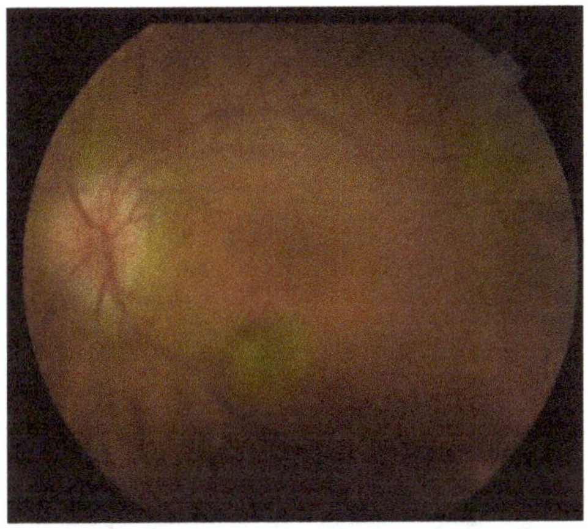

FIGURE 2: Initial fundus photo of the LE showing disc edema and a gray macular lesion.

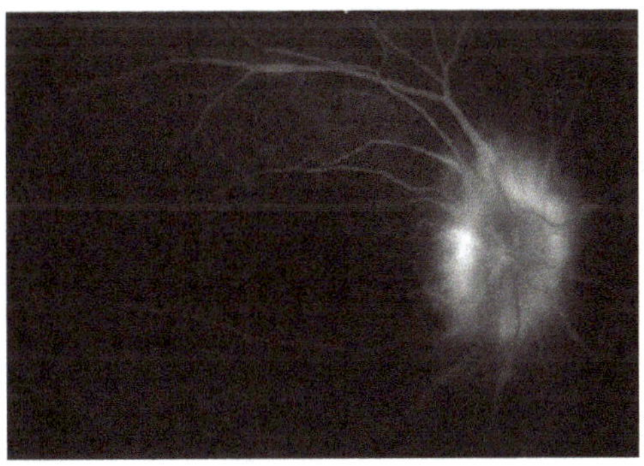

FIGURE 3: Initial FA in the RE showing optic disc and small vessel hyperfluorescence.

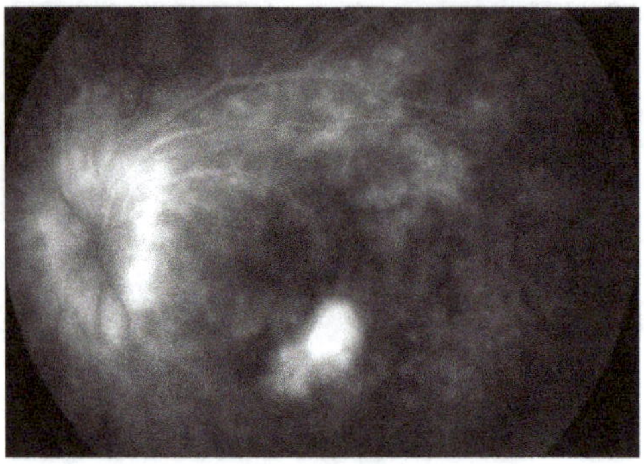

FIGURE 4: Initial FA in the LE showing optic disc and small vessel hyperfluorescence along with a CNVM.

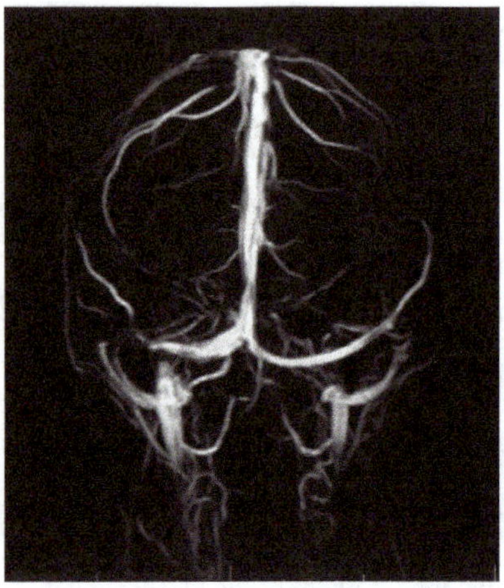

FIGURE 5: MRV showing narrowing of right and left transverse cerebral sinuses without thromboses.

showed opening pressure of 45 cm H_20. Ocular ultrasonography was not available to confirm the diagnosis of papilledema at that visit. Neurology recommended initiating oral acetazolamide 1000 mg twice daily to treat the IICP as well as the headaches and tapered the prednisone over a few weeks.

Subsequent evaluation revealed best corrected visual acuity of 20/20 RE and 20/200 with pinhole LE. Intraocular pressure was normal in BE, and an afferent pupillary defect was identified in the LE. Slit lamp examination showed a trace anterior chamber cell in the RE and 2+ anterior chamber cell and flare with keratic precipitates in the LE. Dilated funduscopic exam showed a trace anterior vitreous cell, 360 degrees of ODE, and focal retinal atrophic spots in the RE (Figure 6) and 1+ anterior vitreous cell and haze, 360 degrees of ODE, cystoid macular edema (CME), a gray macular lesion, and scattered atrophic spots throughout the periphery of the LE (Figure 7).

Widefield FA showed optic disc, small vessel, and segmental large vessel hyperfluorescence in the RE (Figure 8) and optic disc, macular, and diffuse small vessel hyperfluorescence LE (Figure 9).

Widefield ICG angiography was also performed and revealed hypocyanescent spots in the periphery of the RE (Figure 10) and a hypercyanescent spot in the macula with peripheral hypocyanescent spots in the LE (Figure 11).

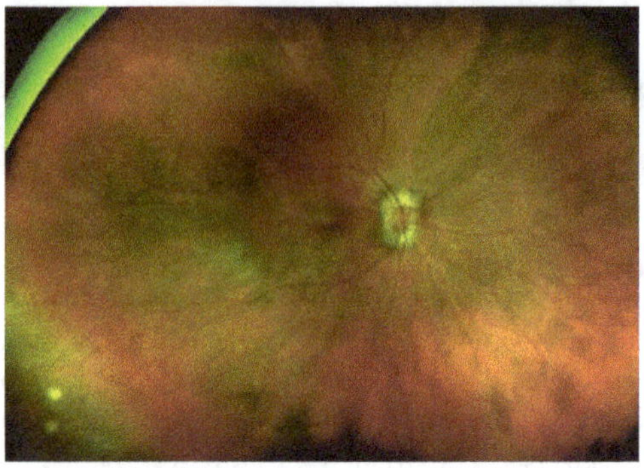

FIGURE 6: Widefield fundus photograph of the right eye showing optic disc edema and temporal atrophic spots.

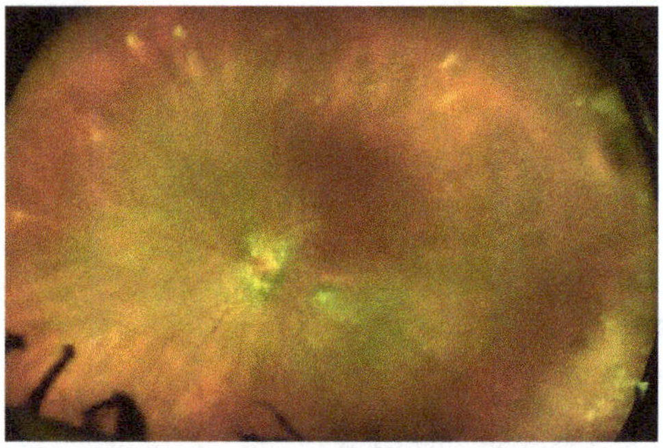

FIGURE 7: Widefield fundus photograph of the left eye showing optic disc edema, macular thickening with a gray macular lesion, and scattered atrophic peripheral spots.

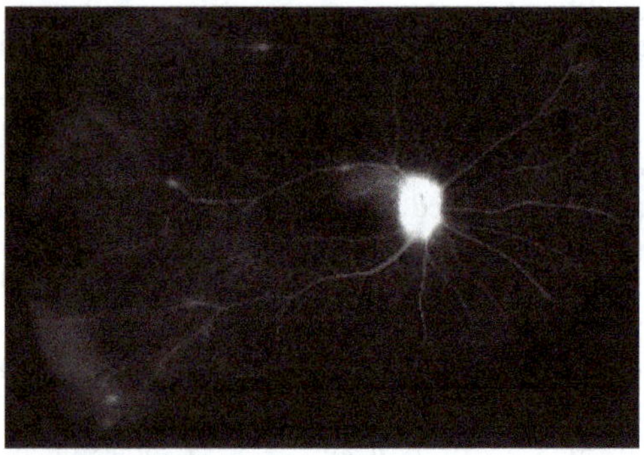

FIGURE 8: Widefield FA of the RE showing optic disc and segmental large vessel hyperfluorescence.

Automated visual field testing showed an enlarged blind spot in the RE and a superior cecocentral defect in the LE. OCT of the macula showed peripapillary nerve fiber layer thickening with normal foveal contour in the RE (Figure 12) and peripapillary nerve fiber layer thickening, diffuse CME, and a pigment epithelial detachment in the LE (Figure 13). Retinal nerve fiber layer- (RNFL-) OCT was thick in both eyes.

The patient's diagnoses were refined to bilateral ODE, multifocal choroiditis, retinal vasculitis, and CME with a CNVM LE. As corticosteroids were relatively contraindicated given prior weight gain and IICP, the patient underwent additional safety lab testing for corticosteroid sparing

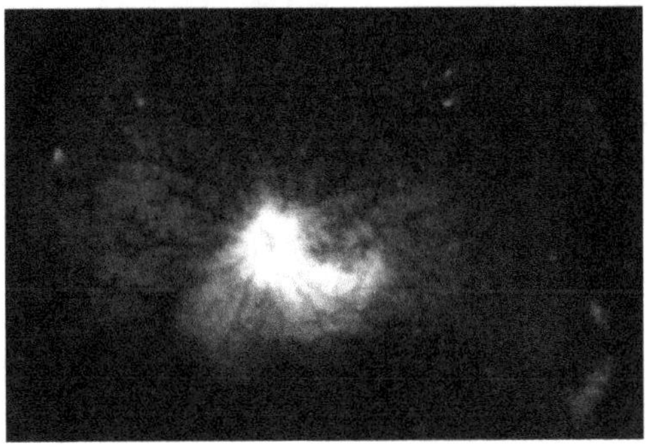

FIGURE 9: Widefield FA of the LE with disc, macular, and diffuse small vessel hyperfluorescence.

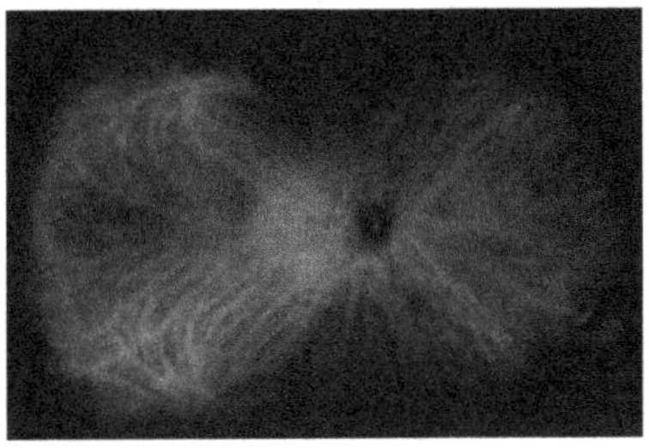

FIGURE 10: Widefield ICG showing peripheral hypocyanescent spots in the periphery of the RE.

FIGURE 11: Widefield ICG showing a hypercyanescent spot in the macula and hypocyanescent spots in the periphery of the LE.

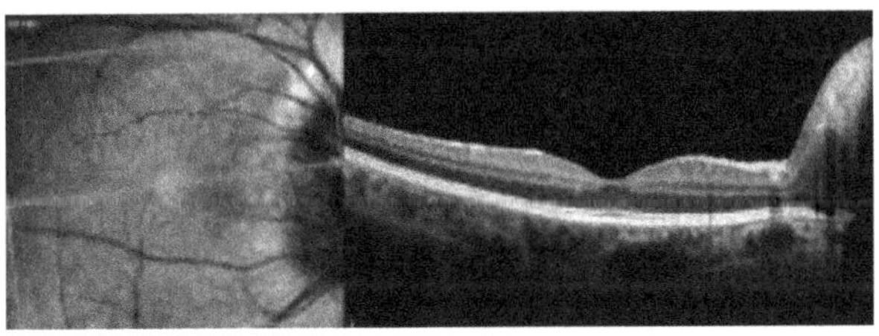

FIGURE 12: OCT of the macula showed peripapillary nerve fiber layer thickening with normal foveal contour in the RE.

immune suppression for the bilateral noninfectious uveitis. She received a periocular triamcinolone to the LE for the uveitis and CME and a second intravitreal bevacizumab injection in the LE for the inflammatory CNVM. There was improvement in acuity to 20/200 along with reduced macular edema (Figure 14).

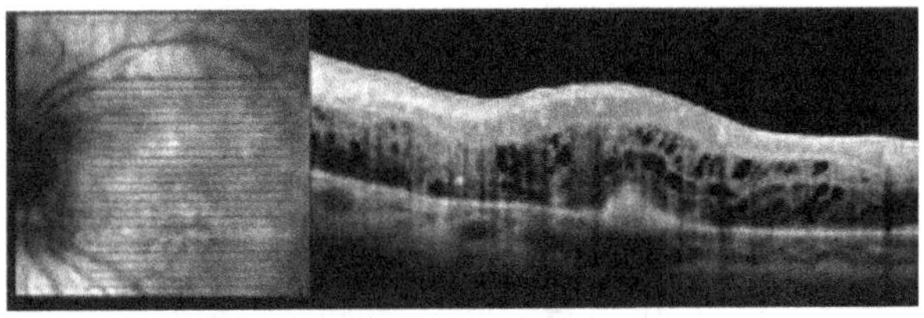

FIGURE 13: OCT of the LE with peripapillary nerve fiber layer thickening, cystoid macular edema with a focal pigment epithelial detachment.

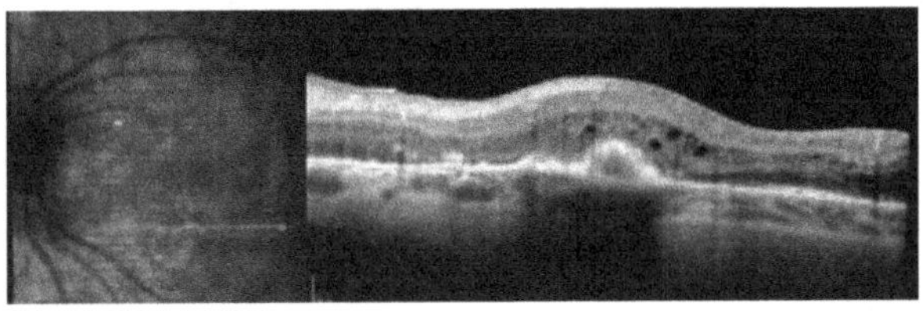

FIGURE 14: OCT of the LE three weeks after sub-Tenon's triamcinolone and intravitreal bevacizumab with improved macular edema.

Treatment for the IICP was continued with acetazolamide which was titrated up to 1250 mg twice daily with slow improvement in the bilateral ODE by RNFL. Oral corticosteroids were discouraged given the IICP. Steroid sparing immune suppressive therapy was strongly recommended given the bilateral uveitis, cystoid macular edema, and CNVM LE.

5. Discussion

Simultaneous posterior uveitis and papilledema have previously been reported by Margalit et al. who described a child with idiopathic intracranial hypertension and posterior uveitis [2] and Eken et al. who described a 16-year-old with bilateral posterior uveitis and papilledema from hydrocephalus secondary to a Chiari I malformation [3]. This is the known case of simultaneous posterior uveitis and IICP in an adult.

The evaluation of bilateral ODE, even in the presence of posterior uveitis, should include brain MRI-MRV and LP. When available, ocular ultrasonography can also be a useful noninvasive diagnostic tool for identifying optic nerve sheath distension as demonstrated by Vitiello et al. [1]. In this patient, ocular ultrasonography was not available to confirm the diagnosis of optic nerve sheath distension. Evaluation should also include visual field testing and RNFL for ODE. OCT as well as retinal fluorescein and choroidal indocyanine green angiography should be performed to assess uveitic disc edema associated with cystoid macular edema, retinal vascular inflammation, and multifocal choroiditis. Consultation with Rheumatology should be considered in such cases to evaluate for Behcet's disease, which can cause uveitic disc edema and papilledema from cerebral sinus thromboses [5]. As this patient did not have any oral or genital ulcers, she deferred the recommended Rheumatology consultation.

In this case, treatment of the uveitis with systemic corticosteroids partially improved the uveitis but caused weight gain and worsening headaches. This may have contributed to elevation of the intracranial pressure as demonstrated by higher opening pressure with the second LP. As treatment of uveitis with systemic corticosteroids has been shown to cause IICP in children [4], physicians must also be mindful of this association in adults. In this case, earlier initiation of oral acetazolamide should likely have commenced along with the systemic corticosteroids, although it is unclear if its delayed initiation will have a negative impact on the ultimate outcome. The periocular steroids for CME and intravitreal antivascular endothelial growth factor (VEGF) injections for the inflammatory CNVM were important for the acute sight threatening complications of uveitis, but the long-term focus will be on steroid sparing immune suppressive therapy in addition to therapy for the IICP.

It can be difficult to distinguish uveitic disc edema from papilledema. As such, monitoring uveitic disc edema and CME with angiography and OCT must continue, in addition to RNFL and visual field studies for papilledema as well as ocular ultrasonography if available. Treatment of uveitic disc edema should focus on reducing associated optic disc and retinal vascular leakage by angiography as well as reduction of CME and any CNVM with eye injections. Treatment of papilledema also needs to be optimized to preserve visual field and normalize retinal nerve fiber layer thickening. The ultimate goal of such multifaceted therapy is to prevent permanent vision loss as a result of optic disc and retinal atrophy. The prognosis in such cases of multifactorial optic nerve pathologies (uveitic disc edema and papilledema) as well as retinal vascular pathologies (diffuse small vessel leakage, CME, and CNVM) is unknown, but comprehensive monitoring is paramount to ensure optimal visual outcomes.

In summary, we present a case of simultaneous posterior bilateral uveitis and papilledema in an adult. Clinicians should consider neuroimaging and CSF analysis in such scenarios in addition to OCT and retinal angiography and ocular ultrasonography to monitor treatment of both uveitic disc edema and papilledema.

Acknowledgments

Publication fees, if applicable, will be furnished by the University of Minnesota.

References

[1] L. Vitiello, M. De Bernardo, P. Cornetta, and N. Rosa, "Bedside ocular ultrasound evaluation of pediatric optic neuritis," *The Journal of Emergency Medicine*, vol. 57, no. 6, pp. 883-884, 2019.

[2] E. Margalit, J. U. Sung, D. V. Do, K. Yohay, and Q. D. Nguyen, "Panuveitis in association with pseudotumor cerebri," *Journal of Child Neurology*, vol. 20, no. 3, pp. 234–236, 2016.

[3] V. Eken, F. Nilufer Yalcindag, F. Batioglu, and C. T. Isikay, "A case of bilateral uveitis and optic disc swelling with Chiari I malformation," *Saudi J Ophthalmol*, vol. 26, no. 3, pp. 335–337, 2012.

[4] D. Curragh and E. McLoone, "Pseudotumour cerebri syndrome in two children on systemic steroid therapy for uveitis," *Ocular Immunology and Inflammation*, vol. 26, no. 2, pp. 295–297, 2016.

[5] J. Shi, X. Huang, G. Li et al., "Cerebral venous sinus thrombosis in Behçet's disease: a retrospective case-control study," *Clinical Rheumatology*, vol. 37, no. 1, pp. 51–57, 2018.

14

Evolution of Lightning Maculopathy: Presentation of Two Clinical Cases and Brief Review of the Literature

Simanta Khadka,[1] **Raghunandan Byanju**,[1] **Sangita Pradhan**,[1] **Suchan Poon**,[1] **and Rinkal Suwal**[2]

[1]*Bharatpur Eye Hospital, Bharatpur, Chitwan, Nepal*
[2]*BP Eye Foundation, Hospital for Children, Eye, ENT, and Rehabilitation Services (CHEERS), Madhyapur Thimi, Bhaktapur, Nepal*

Correspondence should be addressed to Simanta Khadka; simantakhadka@gmail.com

Academic Editor: Sandra M. Johnson

Lightning is a naturally occurring atmospheric phenomenon. Though uncommon, it is a potentially devastating and underreported natural calamity. Lightning accounts for the second leading cause of weather-related death in most parts of the world. Among the survivors of lightning injury, more than half of the victims may suffer from some form of ophthalmic injury. The lightning-associated ocular injury varies from a range of anterior segment to posterior segment pathologies. We report on two clinical cases of ocular injuries among the survivors of lightning injury. Anatomical involvement is seen at different levels with presentation as uveitis, pupillary abnormality, maculopathy, and later development of lenticular opacification. Optical coherence tomography (OCT), a noninvasive diagnostic tool, is particularly useful in the evaluation of lighting maculopathy as well as to monitor its progression through the course of time. Visual prognosis depends upon the structures of the eyes affected in the injury. The presence of irreversible retinal damage as well as optic nerve damage often result in poor visual outcome in the absence of significant anterior segment pathology. This report highlights the evolution of maculopathy through the course of time and signifies the importance of long-term follow-up postlightning injury.

1. Introduction

Lightning is a naturally occurring atmospheric phenomenon. It is estimated that the earth is hit by lightning more than 100 times in each second, and around 50,000 thunderstorms occur every day, resulting in fire, injury, and even loss of life or properties [1]. The odds of being struck by lightning are about 1 in 960,000; however, almost 9 out of 10 victims may escape death [2]. Electrocution or electrofulguration is the commonest mode of injuries due to lightning strike accounting for high morbidity (75%) and mortality (20-30%) [3–5]. The most common cause of death is attributed to ventricular fibrillation or asystolic cardiac arrest [6].

Among the survivors of lightning injury, more than half of the victims suffer from some form of ophthalmic injury [7]. Numerous literatures have reported the spectra of lightning strike-associated ocular injuries [8–18]. The ocular injuries can vary with a range of anterior segment pathologies [16], consisting of thermal keratopathy, hyphema, uveitis, and cataract to posterior segment pathologies, which constitute of vitreous and retinal hemorrhage, cystoid macular edema, retinal detachment, retinal vascular occlusion, chorioretinal rupture, macular hole, and lightning maculopathy [9, 16, 19]. Neurological injuries, namely, optic neuropathy, papillitis, anisocoria, cranial nerve palsies, nystagmus, abnormal pupillary reflex, and Horner syndrome have also been reported in few instances [16, 19].

Here, we report on two cases of ocular injuries among the survivors of lightning injury. Anatomical involvement is seen at different levels with presentation as uveitis, pupillary abnormality, maculopathy, and later development of lenticular opacification. We describe the evolution of maculopathy demonstrated by optical coherence tomography (OCT) and include a brief review of the literature.

2. Case Description

2.1. Case 1. A 37-year-old male with unremarkable medical history presented with bilateral diminution of vision. The symptoms began three days prior to presentation when he was sleeping on a floor of a rural house (cemented floor, brick walls, and galvanized zinc roof). He recounted being woken briefly by a sudden appearance of a bright flash from a nearby lightning (approximately six meters away) during the rainy season of July 2018, following which he had loss of consciousness lasting for approximately 45 minutes. After regaining consciousness, he noticed blurring of vision in both eyes (BE), which improved initially but worsened afterward for which he sought ophthalmic consultation. He also noticed decreased hearing in the left side. On initial evaluation, his best-corrected visual acuity (BCVA) was 6/18 in the right eye (RE) and 6/60 in the left eye (LE). His ocular movement was preserved. The eyelids, ocular adnexa, and pupils were symmetrical, but there was relative afferent pupillary defect in LE. The rest of his anterior segment evaluation was within normal limits including absence of lenticular opacification but there was presence of 1+ anterior chamber (AC) cells in LE. Dilated fundus evaluation revealed a bilateral dull foveal reflex simulating a macular hole- (MH-) like appearance in BE (Figure 1). However, the Watzke-Allen test result was negative. The intraocular pressure (IOP) was 14 mmHg in RE and 16 mmHg in LE. Spectral-domain optical coherence tomography (SD-OCT) (Topcon 3D OCT, 2000 series, Japan) demonstrated evidence of intraretinal cystoid abnormalities prominent in RE, subfoveal outer retinal hyporeflective space suggestive of foveal cyst in LE, and increased retinal pigment epithelium (RPE) hypereflectivity in BE (Figure 2). He was treated with topical steroid and cycloplegic agent in BE.

He then presented four weeks later with slight improvement in BCVA of 6/12 in RE, but the vision in LE was static. The SD-OCT showed intraretinal cystoid changes in the middle retinal layers which was exaggerated compared to previous scan in RE (Figure 3(a)), and persistent foveal cyst appeared as hyporeflective lucency in the outer retinal layer just anterior to retinal pigment epithelium in LE (Figure 3(b)). He was then continued on topical steroid and cycloplegic agent for four more weeks.

After two months of injury, his BCVA improved to 6/9 in RE only and 6/60 in LE. Fundus examination revealed an interval development of central macular thickening, and the SD-OCT confirmed intraretinal cystoid changes with disruption of the subfoveal ellipsoid zone in RE. Similarly, the foveal cyst was continual in LE (Figure 4). He was then prescribed topical nonsteroidal anti-inflammatory drugs in BE. He pursued his profession as a cook overseas and committed to seek medical advice in case of need.

He followed up with us at an interval of one and half-year following the injury upon his arrival. The documented BCVA was 6/9 RE and 6/60 LE. A mild cortical and posterior subcapsular cataract was evident on slit-lamp examination. Fundus examination showed dull foveal reflex (Figure 5). The Watzke-Allen test was negative, but he still complained of mild distortion in the Amsler grid test of LE. OCT affirmed the restoration of foveal contour in RE (Figure 6(a)). Nonetheless, there was still presence of few intraretinal cystoid abnormalities in LE. The previous hyporeflective foveal cyst was absent, and further loss of the outer retinal layers was evident in the macula (Figure 6(b)).

His continual follow-up with us at the passage of two years postlightning injury (July 2020) revealed a BCVA of 6/9 RE and 6/60 LE. Early anterior and posterior subcapsular lenticular opacification was present during slit-lamp examination (Figure 7) and a dull foveal reflex in dilated fundus examination (Figure 8). Automated Humphrey 24–2 Swedish Interactive Threshold Algorithm (SITA) standard visual field analysis revealed mild deficit extending from the blind spot in the left eye. OCT revealed normal restoration of foveal anatomy in RE (Figure 9(a)), whereas the intraretinal cystoid abnormality was almost absent but the nasal retina was grossly atrophic in LE (Figure 9(b)).

2.2. Case 2. A 42-year-old male with no ocular and medical history was struck by lightning (June 2019) while on his way back home resulting in a loss of consciousness. Upon arousal after 20 minutes, he complained of pain and swelling of the right side of his face. He was then brought to the emergency department of a general hospital where the primary management of his condition was done, and the neuroimaging revealed no abnormality. He was then referred to us for the complaint of BE blurring of vision associated with pain and photophobia after two days. Upon evaluation, the BCVA was 6/24 in RE and 6/18 in LE. The ocular motility was full in all cardinal gazes, and no pupillary abnormality was noted bilaterally. Anterior segment examination showed mild conjunctival congestion in BE with presence of 2+ AC cells in RE and 1+ AC cells in LE. Dilated fundus examination revealed bilateral dull foveal reflex and bilateral central yellow-white lesion surrounded by orange-brown pigmentation in the macular region (Figure 10). SD-OCT did not divulge any significant abnormality except for slight blunting of inner retinal layers more prominent in right (Figures 11(a) and 11(b)). He was treated with topical steroid and cycloplegic agent for traumatic iritis.

Three weeks after the injury, the BCVA was similar to the vision at presentation, but the patient complained of marked distortion. Upon examination, the iritis has quietened. The Watzke-Allen test was negative, but the distortion of the lines in Amsler grid was more pronounced. OCT showed an increase in central macular thickness with loss of foveal contour, intraretinal cystoid abnormalities in the middle retinal layers, and disruption of ellipsoid zone. The changes were more marked in RE compared to LE (Figures 11(c) and 11(d)). The patient was continued on topical steroid. On follow-up evaluation at five weeks postinjury, the BCVA had declined to 6/60 RE and 6/24 LE. Fundus examination showed interval development of macular edema BE, similarly OCT confirmed the increment in cystoid abnormalities more in the right (Figures 11(e) and 11(f)).

At the end of two months, the BCVA was restored as of baseline to 6/24 in RE, whereas it improved to 6/12 in LE.

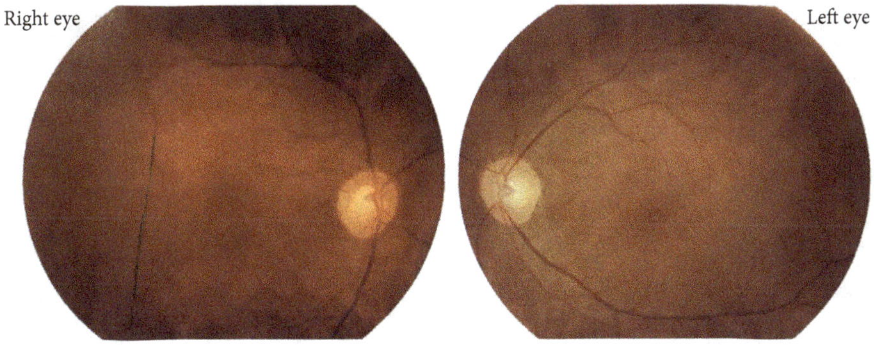

FIGURE 1: Fundus photograph at the time of presentation. Presence of bilateral dull foveal reflex and central yellow-white lesion surrounded by orange-brown pigmentation is shown in the macula. The lesion is prominent in the left eye.

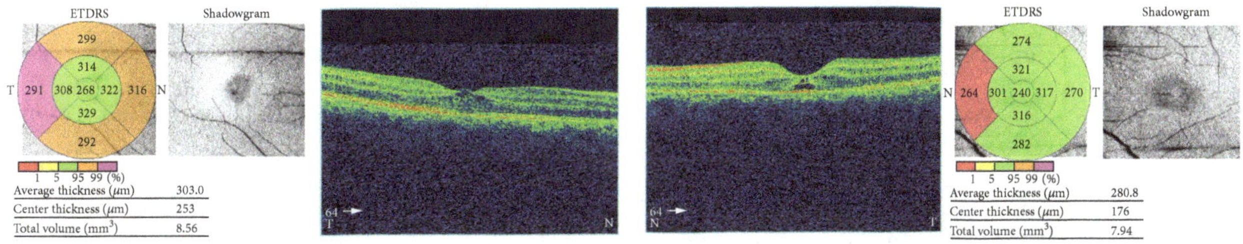

(a) (b)

FIGURE 2: Spectral-domain optical coherence tomography (SD-OCT) at presentation. (a) Right eye with few intraretinal cystoid changes. (b) Left eye with a foveal cyst.

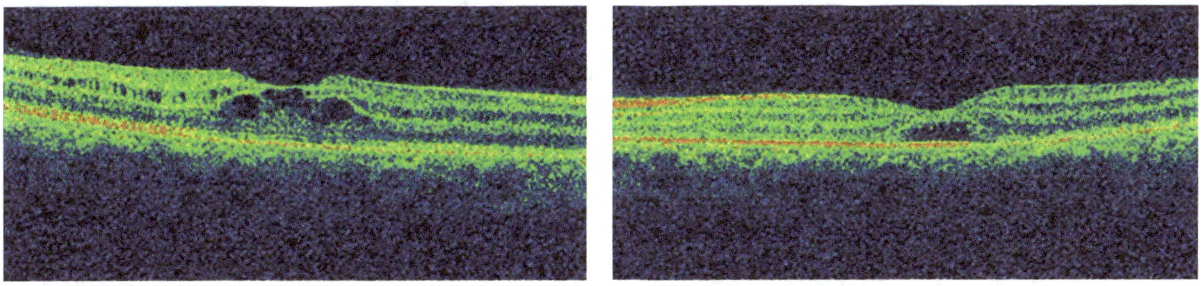

(a) (b)

FIGURE 3: SD-OCT at four weeks following lightning injury. (a) Right eye with intraretinal cystoid changes. (b) Left eye with a foveal cyst. The cyst has increased fluid volume compared to OCT at presentation.

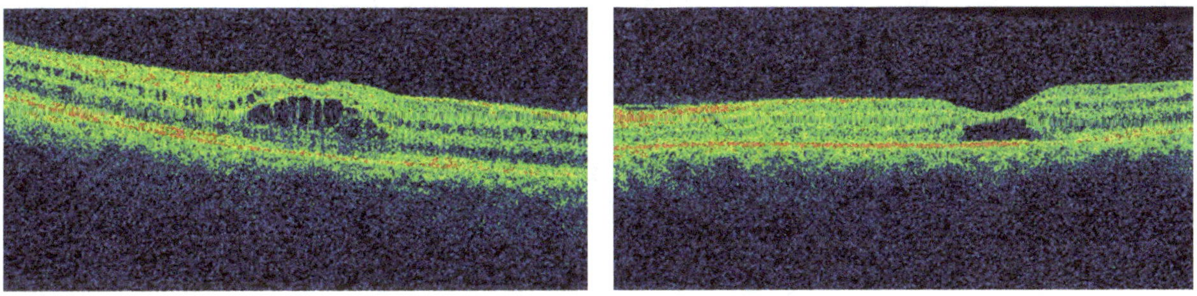

(a) (b)

FIGURE 4: SD-OCT at two months following injury. (a) Right eye with interval development of intraretinal cystoid abnormalities. (b) Left eye with persistent foveal cyst.

The OCT of RE was analogous to the previous finding, but increment in central macular thickness was noted. There was slight restoration of foveal anatomy but still presence of subfoveal cystic changes in LE (Figures 11(g) and 11(h)). He was advised to for topical nonsteroidal anti-inflammatory drugs BE. Serial OCT scans were obtained during his follow-

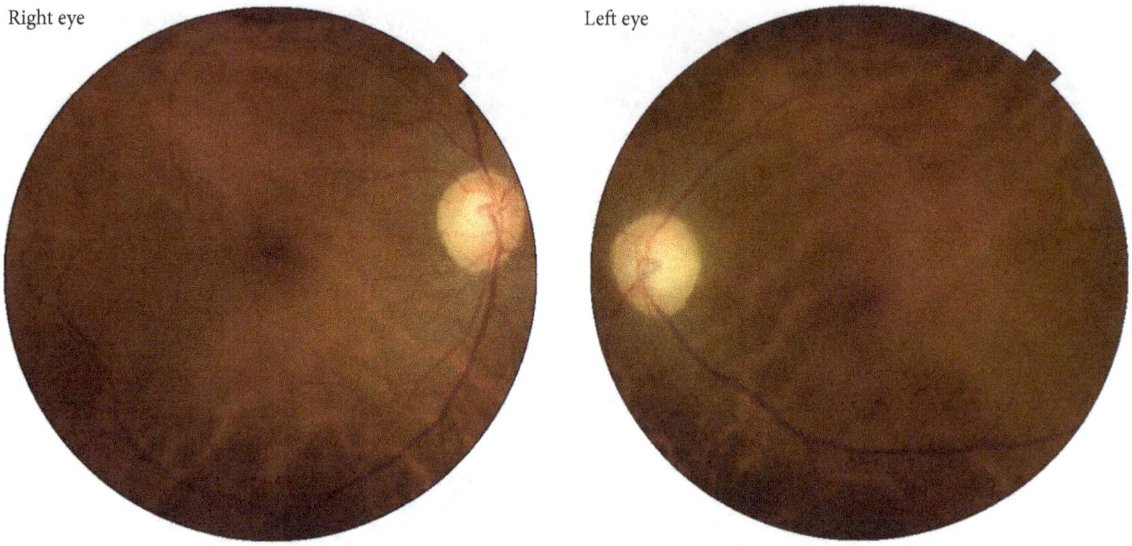

FIGURE 5: Fundus photo at the end of one and half-year following the injury.

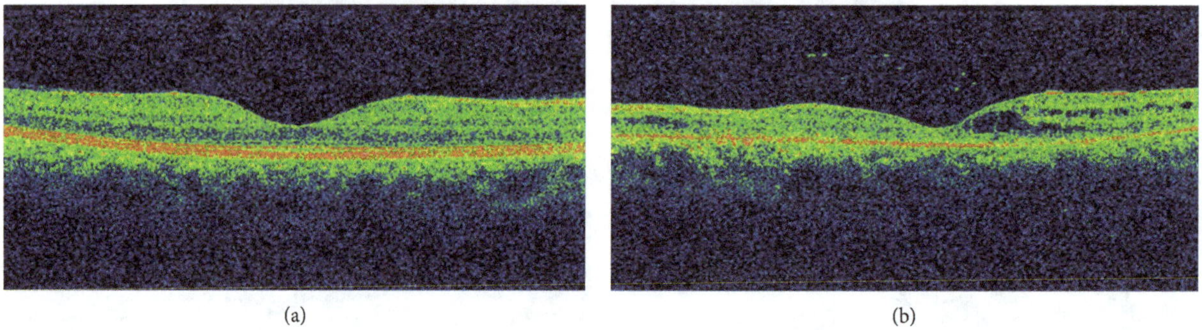

FIGURE 6: SD-OCT at one and half-year follow-up. (a) Right eye with near normal restoration of foveal anatomy. (b) Left eye showing few cystoid abnormalities but atrophy of the nasal retina.

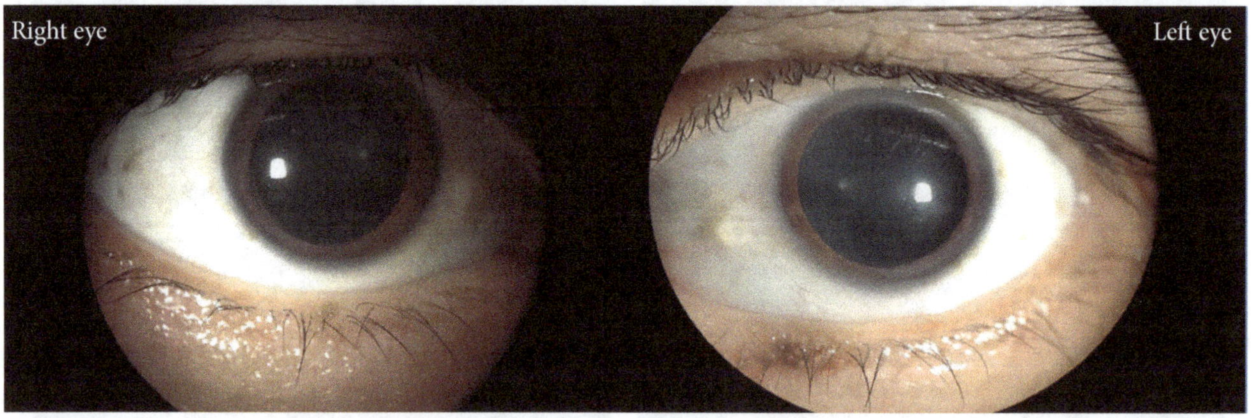

FIGURE 7: Anterior segment diffuse photography at the end of two years follow-up. Anterior subcapsular opacification is visible in the photography, which is more prominent in the right eye compared to the left.

up over the next two months. By the end of four months, the BCVA in RE was 6/24 and 6/12 in LE. Development of early posterior subcapsular cataract was evident during slit lamp examination. OCT demonstrated decreased intraretinal cystic changes in BE (Figures 11(i) and 11(j)).

Five months after the event, the BCVA RE improved to 6/18 RE and was static to 6/12 LE. Dilated fundus examination revealed no other findings except for dull foveal reflex. Repeated OCT scan established interval restoration of foveal anatomy in RE. The outer layers of the retina could be

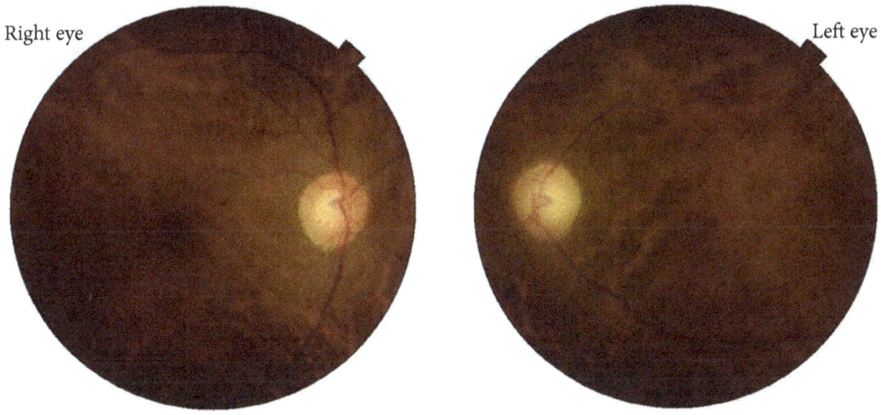

FIGURE 8: Fundus photo at the end of two years follow-up showing dull foveal reflex in both eyes.

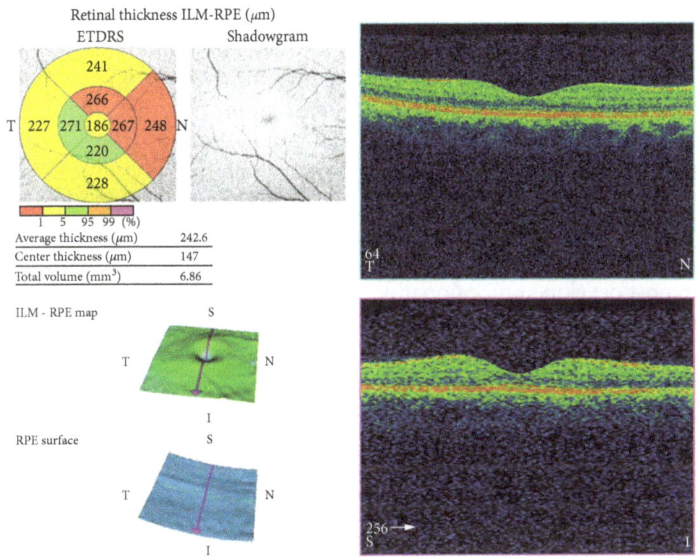

(a)

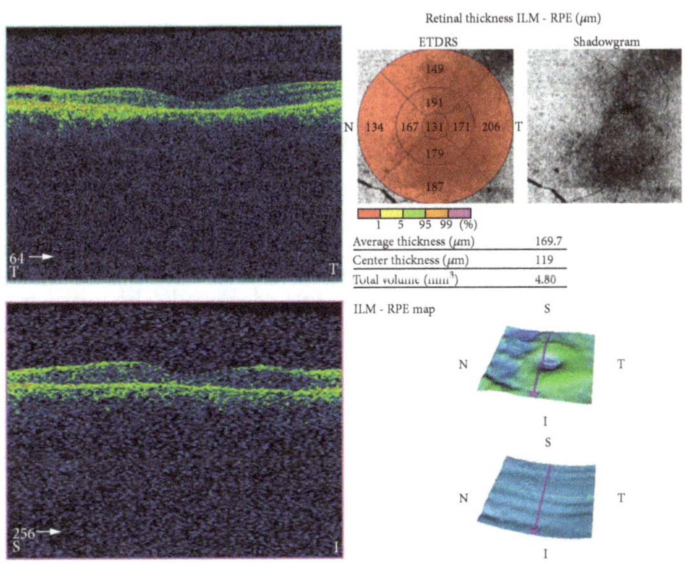

(b)

FIGURE 9: OCT at the end of two years follow-up. (a) Right eye with restoration of foveal anatomy. (b) Left eye with gross retinal atrophy.

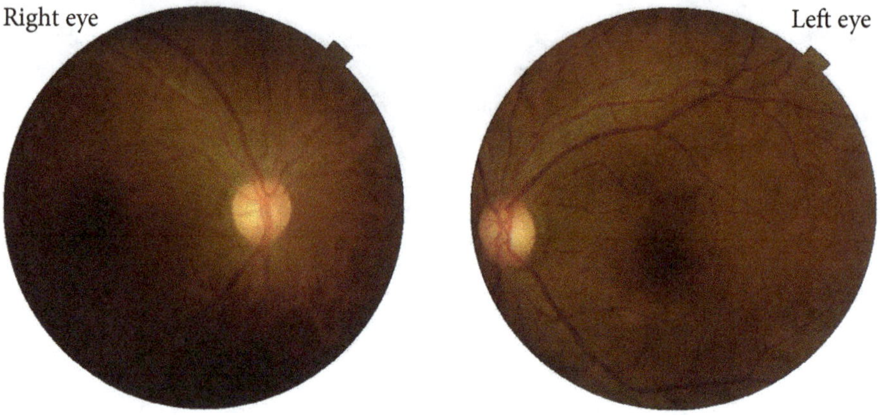

FIGURE 10: Fundus photography at presentation showing macular lesion simulating macular hole. Bilateral central yellow-white lesion surrounded by orange-brown pigmentation in the macular region is visualized.

distinguished, and there was resolution of intraretinal cystic abnormalities, but the foveal contour was not restored completely (Figure 11(k)). Similarly, in LE, there was persistent cystic space with restoration of outer layers of the retina (Figure 11(l)). The patient lost for follow-up afterward.

3. Discussion

The patients discussed in our report developed maculopathy induced by lightning injury, which resembled MH in clinical appearance. This simulation is due to macular edema and cystic changes in the retina [9]. To the best of our knowledge, this could be the first case to report the evolution and sequelae of macular changes associated with lightning during a period of two years. Similarly, the data of the second patient was available for only up to five months following the injury, and then we lost the follow-up. In both cases, the documented anterior segment pathology of cataract was evident, and there was gradual progression in the opacification. Afferent pupillary defect was elicited from the time of presentation and persisted until the last follow-up in the first case. The injuries reported in our patients signify a multitude of ocular pathologies in lightning-induced injury to the eye.

Lightning accounts for the second leading cause of weather-related death in most parts of the world. Though uncommon, it is a potentially devastating and under reported natural calamity as it does not cause a mass casualty [20]. The distribution and frequency of lightning vary on different geographical locations and meteorological distribution across the globe [21]. Nepal, the Himalayan nation, is very much more prone to lightning activity which is favored by the surface temperature, atmospheric moisture, elevation, and the topography of this region [22].

The first documented report of lightning-induced ocular injury dates to 1722 by St Yves [23]. The possible mechanism of injury to the tissues by lightning may occur by several ways: direct strike, side flash or spray, or ground strike [16]. Direct strike occurs when the victim comes in direct contact with lightning, which is believed to be the most damaging mode of injury. The transmission can occur by touching the direct path of the current such as a pole or tree. Side splash, side flash, or spray injury can result when lightning jumps from the primary contact point to the victim [24]. If the lightning impacts the ground first and then spreads to a victim, a ground strike or stride injury can occur [25]. The injury reported in both of our patients is due to the ground strike current. The affection of hearing and ocular injury in the first case also supports the evidence of ground strike [8].

The power of lightning is estimated to be between 10,000 and 200,000 amperes of current, with an estimated voltage ranging from 20 million to 1 billion volts [26]. The extent of tissue destruction depends upon several variables, including the voltage, amperage, resistance, pathway, and duration of current flow [27]. When the eye is considered as a component of an electric circuit, the melanin granules of the RPE [28] and the uvea act as a main obstacle for the flow of the current [9]. The mechanism for tissue damage following lightning injury is attributed to direct electrolysis, resistance-induced heat, or mechanical disruption by the associated shock wave [11]. Secondary damage may also result from tissue edema, ischemia, or reperfusion injury [16].

The high melanin content of macula makes it highly sensitive to thermal damage. The resistance offered by melanin within the pigment epithelium of retina leads to heat production. Additionally, cylindrical shockwave produced by lightning can also lead to mechanical injury of the RPE. Localized inflammation could contribute to RPE dysfunction and retinal vascular incompetence resulting in decreased fluid transport across the retina and development of intraretinal edema [9]. The initial macular lesion with resemblance to Berlin's edema seen early after the lightning strike may be replaced or evolve into lesion later described as a intraretinal cyst or lesion simulating MH [19]. Negative Watzke-Allen test results, lack of posterior vitreous detachment, and operculum support the diagnosis of lightning maculopathy, which is a predominant feature of full-thickness MH [9, 14]. Macular cystic changes and full-thickness MH due to lightning need to be differentiated in the early stage as the management approach in this condition is completely different. Maculopathy with cystic change may spontaneously resolve with observation only, but for full-thickness MH, surgical intervention may be required [14]. However,

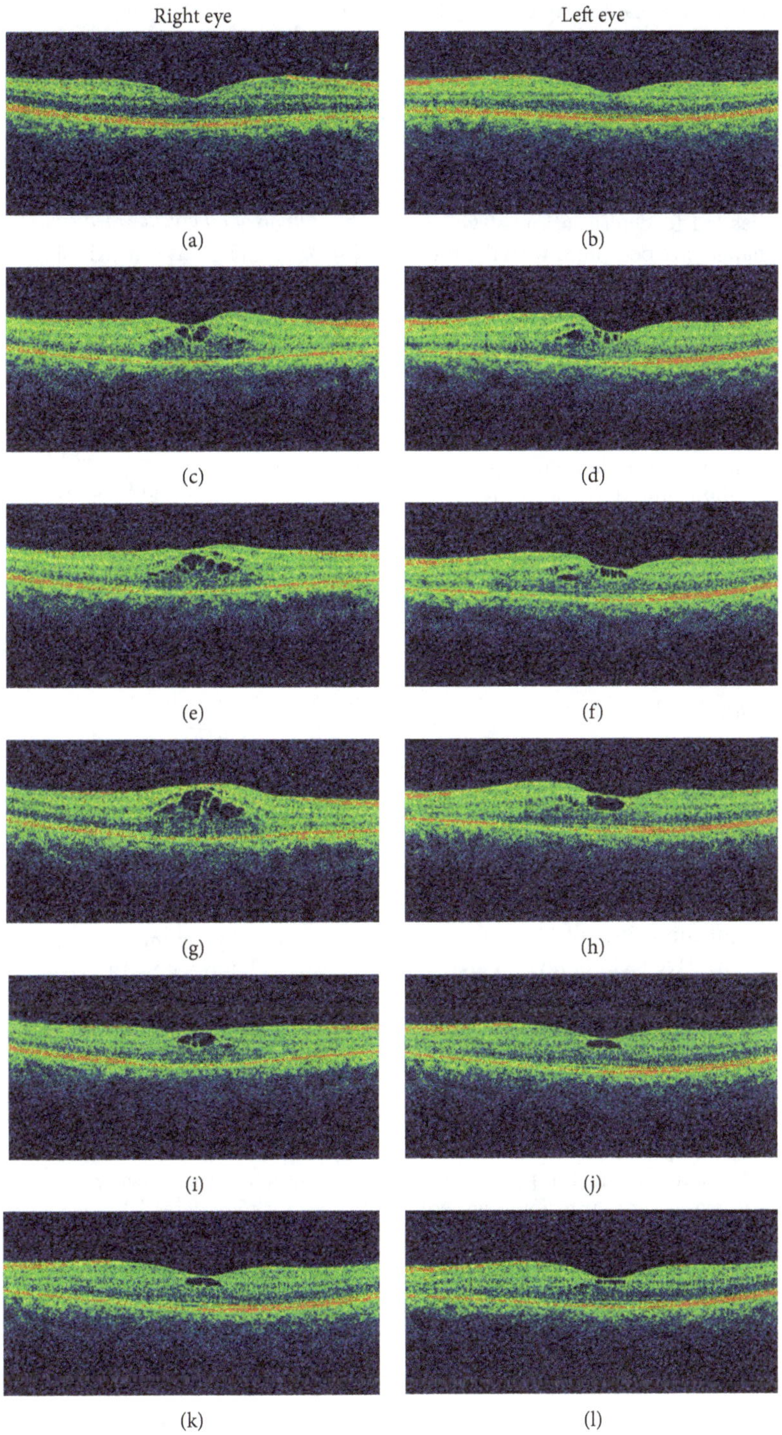

Figure 11: (a)–(l) Serial OCT scans showing the evolution of maculopathy obtained at the time of presentation to the last follow-up visit at the end of five months postinjury. (a, b) OCT at presentation showing normal appearance. (c, d) OCT at three weeks of injury with development of intraretinal cystoid abnormalities. (e, f) Five weeks following injury showing increment in cystoid changes. (g, h) Interval increment in macular thickness as well as cystoid pockets more marked in the right at the end of two months. (i, j) Four months interval with decreased cystoid changes in both eyes. (k, l) OCT at the end of last follow-up visit at five months showing resolution of cystoid spaces and restoration of fovea in the right; however, presence of foveal cyst in the left was evident.

lightning-induced MH may undergo spontaneous closure in a few instances [19]. OCT is helpful for delineating the difference in identification of MH and lightning-induced maculopathy. [14] The OCT appearance of the macular lesion shares a common appearance with solar retinopathy, [29] and welder's maculopathy [28] among other pathologies of photic maculopathy which is essentially due to a photochemical reaction. Hence, meticulous inquiry of the previous exposure of these factors needs to be excluded.

We were able to document the evolution of macular changes with the help of OCT. The change of macular lesions over the period of time also helps in predicting the prognosis [30, 31]. Apart from the solitary cystic changes in the macula previously reported through OCT, [32] we were able to demonstrate the delayed onset intraretinal cystic changes [33]. The eventual atrophy of the fovea due to obliteration of the nasal photoreceptor layer has led to deterioration of vision in the first case, and these changes are persistent with the previous report on evolution of lightning maculopathy [14, 31].

The inflammatory changes in the uveal tissues are also of frequent occurrence [15]. The iritis might appear within days to weeks following injury, but these are transitory and generally mild to moderate in severity [34]. The pigmented portion of iris also gets heated up during resistance to the flow of the current which can induce denaturation of lenticular proteins and opacification [35]. The lightning strike leads to both anterior and posterior coarse subcapsular opacities. These opacities can often impair vision significantly and necessitate surgical removal [33]. The cataract in our patients was not visually significant, and we proceeded with observation. Similarly, neural injury can occur by several mechanisms. Myelin injury occurs due to resistance for the current flow, coagulation factor abnormalities, and consequential damage to the vascular supply [36].

4. Conclusion

The unpredictability of the flow of electric current through a human body results in different modalities of presentations of ocular injury. OCT, a non-invasive technology, is particularly useful in the evaluation of lighting induced maculopathy as well as its evolution through the course of time. Though observation alone may suffice, visual prognosis in lightning induced maculopathy depends upon the degree of involvement of ocular structures. The presence of irreversible retinal damage in terms of retinal atrophy as well as optic nerve damage are the major determinant factors for poor visual outcome in the absence of significant anterior segment pathology. This report signifies the importance of long term follow-up post lightning injury. Though no definite conclusions can be made, we believe that the findings from these two cases will contribute to the pool of knowledge in understanding the evolution of lightning maculopathy.

Acknowledgments

The authors would like to thank Mr Ram Janaki Pandey, Optometrist, Bharatpur Eye Hospital, for obtaining the OCT scans and fundus photography.

References

[1] U. Okafor, "Lightning injuries and acute renal failure: a review," *Renal Failure*, vol. 27, no. 2, pp. 129–134, 2005.

[2] R. J. Vavrek, R. Kithil, R. Holle, J. Allsopp, and M. A. Cooper, "The science of thunder," *Earth Science*, vol. 22, no. 3, pp. 5–9, 2006.

[3] O. Alyan, O. Ozdemir, O. Tufekcioglu, B. Geyik, D. Aras, and D. Demirkan, "Myocardial injury due to lightning strike: a case report," *Angiology*, vol. 57, no. 2, pp. 219–223, 2006.

[4] M. A. Cooper, "Lightning injuries: prognostic signs for death," *Annals of Emergency Medicine*, vol. 9, no. 3, pp. 134–138, 1980.

[5] S. R. Craig, "When lightning strikes: pathophysiology and treatment of lightning injuries," *Postgraduate Medicine*, vol. 79, no. 4, pp. 109–124, 1986.

[6] R. Edlich, H.-M. A. Farinholt, K. L. Winters, L. Britt, and W. B. Long III, "Modern concepts of treatment and prevention of electrical burns," *Journal of Long-Term Effects of Medical Implants*, vol. 15, no. 5, pp. 511–532, 2005.

[7] J. Edelstein, W. Peters, and R. Cartotto, "Lightning injury: a review and case presentations," *Canadian Journal of Plastic Surgery*, vol. 2, no. 4, pp. 164–168, 1994.

[8] K. A. Rao, L. G. Rao, A. N. Kamath, and V. Jain, "Bilateral macular hole secondary to remote lightning strike," *Indian Journal of Ophthalmology*, vol. 57, no. 6, pp. 470–472, 2009.

[9] J. T. Handa and G. J. Jaffe, "Lightning maculopathy," *Retina*, vol. 14, no. 2, pp. 169–172, 1994.

[10] R. V. Campo and R. S. Lewis, "Lightning-induced macular hole," *American Journal of Ophthalmology*, vol. 97, no. 6, pp. 792–794, 1984.

[11] W.-D. A. Lagrèze, T. G. Bömer, and L. P. Aiello, "Lightning-induced ocular injury," *Archives of Ophthalmology*, vol. 113, no. 8, pp. 1076-1077, 1995.

[12] A. Espaillat, R. Janigian Jr., and K. To, "Cataracts, bilateral macular holes, and rhegmatogenous retinal detachment induced by lightning," *American Journal of Ophthalmology*, vol. 127, no. 2, pp. 216-217, 1999.

[13] E. Pradhan, A. Khatri, A. A. Ahmed et al., "Lightning injury to eye: brief review of the literature and case Series," *Clinical Ophthalmology*, vol. Volume 14, pp. 597–607, 2020.

[14] S. J. Moon, J. E. Kim, and D. P. Han, "Lightning-induced maculopathy," *Retina*, vol. 25, no. 3, pp. 380–382, 2005.

[15] J. E. Toquica and H. F. Gomez, "Ocular injuries caused by lightning strikes: review of the literature and presentation of two clinical cases," *Vision Pan-America, The Pan-American Journal of Ophthalmology*, vol. 15, no. 3, pp. 84–86, 2016.

[16] M. E. Norman, D. Albertson, and B. R. Younge, "Ophthalmic manifestations of lightning strike," *Survey of Ophthalmology*, vol. 46, no. 1, pp. 19–24, 2001.

[17] P. S. Dhillon and M. Gupta, "Ophthalmic manifestations post-lightning strike," *Case Reports*, vol. 2015, article bcr2014207594, 2015.

[18] R. Shrestha, R. K. Shah, and P. Joshi, "Lightning Maculopathy: a case report," *Nepal Medical Journal*, vol. 2, no. 1, pp. 98–101, 2019.

[19] M. S. Lee, K. B. Gunton, D. H. Fischer, and A. J. Brucker, "Ocular manifestations of remote lightning strike," *Retina*, vol. 22, no. 6, pp. 808–810, 2002.

[20] A. E. Ritenour, M. J. Morton, J. G. McManus, D. J. Barillo, and L. C. Cancio, "Lightning injury: a review," *Burns*, vol. 34, no. 5, pp. 585–594, 2008.

[21] H. J. Christian, R. J. Blakeslee, D. J. Boccippio et al., "Global frequency and distribution of lightning as observed from space by the Optical Transient Detector," *Journal of Geophysical*

Research: Atmospheres, vol. 108, no. D1, pp. ACL 4-1–ACL 4-15, 2003.

[22] K. Saha, N. P. Damase, T. Banik et al., "Satellite-based observation of lightning climatology over Nepal," *Journal of Earth System Science*, vol. 128, no. 8, p. 221, 2019.

[23] C. Saint Yves, "Les causes accidentelles qui peuvent blesser la vuë," in *Nouveau Traité des Maladies des Yeux, les Remedes qui y Conviennent, & les Operations de Chirurgie que Leurs Guérisons Exigent*, vol. 1722, pp. 368–370, Pierre-Augustin Le Mercier, Paris, France, 1722.

[24] C. Tribble, J. Persing, R. Morgan, J. Kenney, and R. Edlich, "Lightning injuries," *Comprehensive Therapy*, vol. 11, no. 2, pp. 32–40, 1985.

[25] T. D. Epperly and J. R. Stewart, "The physical effects of lightning injury," *Journal of Family Practice*, vol. 29, no. 3, pp. 267–273, 1989.

[26] S. Jain and V. Bandi, "Electrical and lightning injuries," *Critical Care Clinics*, vol. 15, no. 2, pp. 319–331, 1999.

[27] R. C. Lee, "Injury by electrical forces: pathophysiology, manifestations, and therapy," *Current Problems in Surgery*, vol. 34, no. 9, pp. 677–764, 1997.

[28] R. S. Lucas, C. A. Harper, M. F. McCombe, M. A. Mainster, D. H. Sliney, and E. Zamir, "Optical coherence tomography findings in Welder's maculopathy," *Retinal Cases & Brief Reports*, vol. 1, no. 3, pp. 169–171, 2007.

[29] A. Jain, R. U. Desai, R. A. Charalel, P. Quiram, L. Yannuzzi, and D. Sarraf, "Solar RETINOPATHY," *Retina*, vol. 29, no. 9, pp. 1340–1345, 2009.

[30] T. Y. A. Liu, C. See, E. Singman, and I. C. Han, "Delayed onset of intraretinal cystoid abnormalities in lightning retinopathy," *JAMA Ophthalmology*, vol. 134, no. 7, pp. 840–842, 2016.

[31] B. Armstrong, C. Fecarotta, A. C. Ho, and D. E. Baskin, "Evolution of severe lightning maculopathy visualized with spectral domain optical coherence tomography," *Ophthalmic Surgery, Lasers, and Imaging*, vol. 41, no. 6, pp. S70–S73, 2010.

[32] P. J. Rivas-Aguiño, R. A. Garcia, and J. F. Arevalo, "Bilateral macular cyst after lightning visualized with optical coherence tomography," *Clinical & Experimental Ophthalmology*, vol. 34, no. 9, pp. 893-894, 2006.

[33] S. Cazabon and T. R. Dabbs, "Lightning-induced cataract," *Eye*, vol. 14, no. 6, pp. 903-904, 2000.

[34] H. Lakosha, F. Tremblay, and I. De Becker, "High-voltage electrical trauma to the eye," *Canadian Journal of Ophthalmology*, vol. 44, no. 5, pp. 605-606, 2009.

[35] C. Hanna and F. T. Fraunfelder, "Electric cataracts: II. Ultrastructural lens changes," *Archives of Ophthalmology*, vol. 87, no. 2, pp. 184–191, 1972.

[36] J. Koller and J. Orsagh, "Delayed neurological sequelae of high-tension electrical burns," *Burns*, vol. 15, no. 3, pp. 175–178, 1989.

15

Binocular Diplopia: A Possible Adverse Effect of Fluoroquinolone Therapy

Mariama Touray,[1] Victoria Ando,[1] Erwin Samutelela,[2] and Jean-Philippe Zuber[1]

[1]Etablissements Hospitaliers du Nord Vaudois, Internal Medicine, Saint-Loup Hospital, Pompaples, Switzerland
[2]Jules-Gonin Ophthalmic Hospital, Lausanne, Switzerland

Correspondence should be addressed to Mariama Touray; mariama.touray@bluewin.ch

Academic Editor: Huban Atilla

The adverse effects of fluoroquinolones are yet to be fully elucidated. We present an interesting case of a 41-year-old male with binocular diplopia most likely induced by the use of a fluoroquinolone antibiotic.

1. Introduction

Fluoroquinolones are widely used antibiotics with proven safety and efficacy (1, 2). However, adverse effects unique to this class of antibiotic, particularly tendinopathies, have been described. The mechanism underlying this adverse effect is not yet clear. This report presents a case of diplopia likely secondary to fluoroquinolone use.

2. Case Presentation

A previously healthy 41-year-old male, with no known cardiovascular risk factors, attended the emergency department with painless horizontal binocular diplopia which had started 12 hours earlier. Three days prior to the onset of symptoms, the patient had been started on ciprofloxacin for a complicated urinary tract infection. The neuroophthalmologic examination was remarkable for the presence of horizontal binocular diplopia on leftward gaze. Visual acuity was 20/16 oculus uterque (OU) without correction. Intraocular tension was 12 mmHg OU. Slit lamp examination and fundoscopy were within normal limits OU. On the Hess-Weiss testing, we identified diminished function of the left *lateral rectus muscle* and an associated increased compensatory function of the right *medial rectus muscle*, confirming a paresis of the left *lateral rectus muscle* (Figure 1). The rest of the physical examination was unremarkable.

Blood tests revealed a slightly increased CRP without leukocytosis. TSH was normal. Cerebral imaging (MRI and CT-angiography) and orbital MRI results were within normal limits. Analysis of cerebrospinal fluid was normal. Serology tests (HIV, syphilis, Lyme disease, and TBE) were negative. Taken together, we concluded on a probable fluoroquinolone-induced unilateral tendinopathy of the left abducens muscle. Ciprofloxacin was stopped and replaced by coamoxicillin. The patient reported progressive regression of diplopia after withdrawal of ciprofloxacin. At a follow-up consultation one week after ciprofloxacin withdrawal, the patient's symptoms had fully resolved. Three months later, the Hess-Weiss testing showed a complete recovery (Figure 2).

3. Discussion

Possible tendinitis of extraocular muscles due to fluoroquinolones has already been described in one 2009 database study (3). The study collected data on 171 patients who were enrolled in a national registry for pharmacological surveillance due to suspected fluoroquinolone-induced diplopia (3). Adverse events were noted at a median time of 9.6 days from the beginning of antibiotics, although time to onset

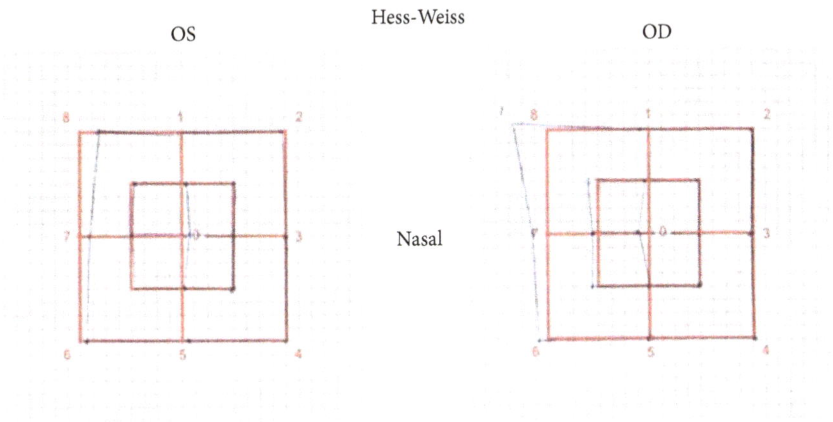

Figure 1: The Hess-Weiss test at presentation. Abbreviations: OS, oculus sinister, left eye; OD, oculus dexter, right eye.

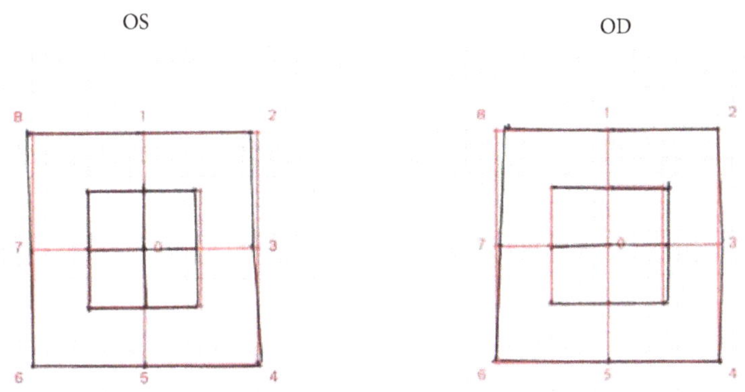

Figure 2: The Hess-Weiss test after ciprofloxacin cessation. Abbreviations: OS, oculus sinister, left eye; OD, oculus dexter, right eye.

ranged from 1 day to 5 months (3). Mean age at presentation was 51 years (3). Concomitant tendinopathy was found in 10% of patients (3).

Some risk factors are known to increase the occurrence of quinolone-induced tendinopathy, such as older age, chronic renal failure, concomitant steroid treatment, and systemic disease (4, 5). In the 2009 database study, a minority (29%) were 60 years or older, and 2% were on systemic steroids (3).

To our knowledge, only one other case report on this subject has been described in France (6) with a very similar clinical presentation to ours. The patient, a 58-year-old male with no known cardiovascular risk factors, had binocular diplopia due to paresis of the left abducens muscle arising during treatment with ofloxacin (6). The patient's diplopia reoccurred with the reintroduction of ofloxacin for a later infection, underscoring the correlation between diplopia and quinolone use (6).

Here, we present the case of a 41-year-old healthy male who presented with binocular diplopia 72 hours after introduction of fluoroquinolone therapy. Symptoms regressed rapidly after withdrawal of the culprit antibiotic, with complete remission noted at a follow-up consultation one week later.

4. Conclusion

The present case study demonstrates a correlation between the onset of diplopia after the initiation of fluoroquinolone therapy, and regression of the symptom upon withdrawal of this agent. However, fluoroquinolone-induced diplopia remains a diagnosis of exclusion. We encourage clinicians to consider discontinuing use of this antibiotic class when facing this possible diagnosis. The mechanism underlying the development of tendinopathies secondary to fluoroquinolone use is yet to be elucidated.

Abbreviations

OU: Oculus uterque, both eyes
OS: Oculus sinister, left eye
OD: Oculus dexter, right eye

Acknowledgments

We would like to express our gratitude to Ms. Karen McWilliams, technical writer, for editing our manuscript.

References

[1] L. Mandell and G. Tillotson, "Safety of fluoroquinolones: an update," *Canadian Journal of Infectious Diseases*, vol. 13, no. 1, pp. 54–61, 2002.

[2] D. C. Hooper and J. S. Wolfson, "Fluoroquinolone antimicrobial agents," *The New England Journal of Medicine*, vol. 324, no. 6, pp. 384–394, 1991.

[3] F. W. Fraunfelder and F. T. Fraunfelder, "Diplopia and fluoroquinolones," *Ophthalmology*, vol. 116, no. 9, pp. 1814–1817, 2009.

[4] G. K. Kim, "The risk of fluoroquinolone-induced tendinopathy and tendon Rupture: What Does The Clinician Need To Know?," *The Journal of clinical and aesthetic dermatology*, vol. 3, no. 4, pp. 49–54, 2010.

[5] C. Yu and B. Giuffre, "Achilles tendinopathy after treatment with fluoroquinolone," *Australasian Radiology*, vol. 49, no. 5, pp. 407–410, 2005.

[6] S. Lemercier and J. F. Pinel, *Diplopie et quinolones : cas clinique*, Journées de Neurologie de Langue Française, Paris, 2011.

16

Posner-Schlossman Syndrome in Common Variable Immunodeficiency

Madiha Huq,[1] **Neha Sanan**,[2] **Phuong Daniels**,[3] **and Robert Hostoffer**[4]

[1]*University Hospitals Parma Medical Center, Cleveland, Ohio, USA*
[2]*University Hospitals, Cleveland Medical Center, Cleveland, Ohio, USA*
[3]*Lake Erie College of Osteopathic Medicine, Erie, Pennsylvania, USA*
[4]*Allergy/Immunology Associates Inc., Mayfield Heights, Ohio, USA*

Correspondence should be addressed to Madiha Huq; madiha.huq@uhhospitals.org

Academic Editor: Stephen G. Schwartz

Introduction. Posner-Schlossman syndrome (PSS) is a rare glaucomatocyclitic crisis with clinical features including recurrent episodes of unilateral elevated intraocular pressure. Autoimmune and infectious causes have been proposed as potential etiologies of PSS. We report the first case of PSS in the setting of common variable immunodeficiency (CVID). *Case Report.* A sixty-two-year-old Caucasian female with a medical history of CVID and ulcerative colitis presented to the emergency room with complaints of acute right-sided vision changes. She reported image distortion, blurriness, and loss of central vision. Physical exam was significant for mildly injected right conjunctiva, visual acuity of 20/70 in right eye, and 20/25 in left eye. The right intraocular pressure was measured at 34 mmHg and left at 12 mmHg. The gonioscopy and dilated fundus examination were unremarkable. Cup to disc ratio was within normal limits, and no afferent pupillary defects were recorded. The patient was acutely treated with three rounds of dorzolamide/timolol and 0.2% brimonidine which decreased the right eye intraocular pressure to 24 mmHg. On follow-up exam with an ophthalmologist, anterior uveitis including an elevated pressure of 41 mmHg on the right and 18 mmHg on the left eye was noted and a PSS diagnosis was confirmed. *Conclusion.* PSS remains a rare condition with uncertain etiology and no associated systemic conditions. PSS has been postulated to be linked to autoimmune conditions. CVID is associated with many autoimmune disorders including Sjogren's, rheumatoid arthritis, and colitis. There have been a few reported CVID-associated ocular diseases including granulomatous uveitis and conjunctivitis, chronic anterior uveitis, and birdshot retinopathy. We describe the first case of PSS in a patient with CVID.

1. Introduction

Posner-Schlossman syndrome (PSS), a glaucomatocyclitic crisis with unknown etiology, was first reported in 1948. Common clinical features include recurrent episodes of unilateral markedly elevated intraocular pressure (IOP) that is associated with mild anterior uveitis. Each attack can last a few hours to a month and usually affects middle-aged adults [1, 2]. PSS typically presents with mild discomfort, halos around lights, blurring of vision, and occasional injection in one eye [2]. Ocular autoimmune disease is a rare finding with common variable immunodeficiency (CVID), and its manifestations are not commonly recorded or reported. This case report of an ocular disease with CVID forms a touchstone for the potential of other reported cases in the future and in creating a true association between the two disorders. Although the cause is largely unknown, autoimmune and infectious diseases have previously been proposed as potential etiologies of PSS [3]. In this report, we present the first case of PSS in the setting of CVID.

2. Case Report

A sixty-two-year-old Caucasian female presented to the emergency room with complaints of acute right-sided vision changes for the past 12 hours. She reported image distortion, blurriness, and loss of central vision with "flashing lights." She also experienced mild injection of her right conjunctiva and stated that she has experienced episodic blurry vision accompanied by headaches for the past several months.

Significant medical histories included CVID and ulcerative colitis. Her initial immunologic evaluation revealed a low IgG level at 223 mg/dL, normal IgA, and IgM values. The patient was placed on daily sulfamethoxazole-trimethoprim prophylaxis in the setting of recurrent upper respiratory tract infections including sinusitis and bronchitis. The patient failed the prophylactic antibiotic therapy as she continued to have recurrent, persistent sinusitis. The patient was eventually placed on immunoglobulin therapy, and her infections subsided. In addition, the patient has notably complained of intermittent blurry vision in the right eye for several years. Acutely, the patient displayed worsened right eye vision distortion and was evaluated in the emergency room.

In the emergency room, the physical exam was significant for mildly injected right conjunctiva and visual acuity of 20/70 in the right eye and 20/25 in the left eye. The right intraocular pressure (IOP) was measured at 34 mmHg and 12 mmHg in the left. Color vision was intact bilaterally with reactive and equal pupils. No signs of trauma, photophobia, eye drainage, or hyphema were noted. Extraocular eye movements were intact, and no other focal deficits were noted on neurological exam.

The ophthalmology slit lamp examination showed 4-5 trace cells in anterior chamber of right eye confirming anterior chamber uveitis. There were no keratic precipitates, and the iris appeared normal on direct illumination bilaterally. The left eye exam did not show any cells in the anterior chamber or evidence of corneal edema. Gonioscopy and dilated fundus examination were unremarkable. Cup to disc ratio was within normal limits, and no afferent pupillary defects were noted.

The patient was acutely treated with three rounds of dorzolamide/timolol and 0.2% brimonidine with a subsequent decrease in the right eye's IOP to 24 mmHg. She was discharged with brimonidine 0.2% and dorzolamide/timolol two times a day in the right eye. After four days of the initial presentation, a follow-up IOP revealed 41 mmHg of the right and 18 mmHg of the left eye. There was poor foveal reflex in the right eye, and 0-1 cells were noted in the anterior chamber. The patient was diagnosed with Posner-Schlossman syndrome given the clinical findings of elevated right unilateral ocular pressure and anterior segment inflammation with right blurry vision.

3. Discussion

PSS typically affects males between the ages of 20 and 50, but advanced ages and female gender have also been reported. Primary open angle glaucoma has been recorded with recurrent attacks of PSS, and treatment is aimed at reducing intraocular pressure and inflammation during and in between episodes [4]. Other studies have proposed initiation of treatment with confirmed optic disc or nerve changes such as ischemic or glaucomatous change; however, this still remains as an ongoing debate. With recurrent attacks as in our case report, the patient was treated as this may have eventually led to optic disc and nerve compromise if left untreated [5, 6].

PSS remains a rare condition with uncertain etiology and no associated systemic conditions. It has been proposed to be linked to autoimmune conditions [7]. A study performed in Japan involving 22 patients with PSS showed HLA-Bw54 positive in nine (approximately 41%) patients implicating a possible CD8 T-cell immunogenic role [8].

Symptoms have been noted to resolve within days to weeks with initial attacks gone unnoticed. In our case, the patient has reported episodic blurry vision in the past during primary care visits. Drug-induced uveitis was initially ruled out since this would cause a bilateral uveitis presentation. Similarly, one case of bilateral uveitis has been reported as a result of IVIG [9], but our patient presents with unilateral findings making IVIG-induced uveitis unlikely. Therefore, these episodes are consistent with the clinical course of PSS. Reoccurrence is expected, but the intervals in between each occurrence have been noted to increase with time.

CVID is a common heterogenetic immunodeficiency found in adulthood [1]. It is associated with many autoimmune disorders including Sjogren's rheumatoid arthritis and colitis. We feel that this ocular disorder represents a rare association in the spectrum of CVID. Some of which have been reported include granulomatous uveitis and conjunctivitis, chronic anterior uveitis, and birdshot retinopathy [10–12]. We predict this ocular manifestation stems from central T-cell regulatory activity with undetermined cell or immune regulatory process. We feel that PSS is of the same nature, and it represents another ocular manifestation in CVID.

Even though this case involving PSS and CVID may sound coincidental, this opinion may be more frequent in other CVID patients seeking ophthalmic evaluations. CVID may set a stage of immunity dysregulation for the manifestation of many autoimmunity disorders including PSS. We describe the first case of PSS in a patient with CVID and hope that the start of this report will lead to other reports bringing a coincidence into an association between PSS and CVID.

Abbreviations

PSS: Posner-Schlossman syndrome
CVID: Common variable immunodeficiency
OCT: Optical coherence tomography
IOP: Intraocular pressure.

Authors' Contributions

Madiha Huq DO, Neha Sanan DO, Phuong Daniels DPT, and Robert Hostoffer DO contributed to the conception and design of the study, data generation, analysis and interpretation of the data, preparation, and clinical revision of the manuscript.

References

[1] A. Posner and A. Schlossman, "Syndrome of unilateral recurrent attacks of glaucoma with cyclitic symptoms," *Archives of Ophthalmology*, vol. 39, no. 4, pp. 517–535, 1948.

[2] R. Megaw and P. K. Agarwal, "Posner-Schlossman syndrome," *Survey of Ophthalmology*, vol. 62, no. 3, pp. 277–285, 2017.

[3] J. Harrington, "Posner-Schlossman syndrome: a case report," *Journal of the American Optometric Association*, vol. 70, no. 11, pp. 715–723, 1999.

[4] M. Yanoff and J. S. Duker, *Ophthalmology*, Elsevier, Edinburgh, 5th edition, 2019.

[5] T.-H. Kim, J. L. Kim, and C. Kee, "Optic disc atrophy in patient with Posner-Schlossman syndrome," *Korean Journal of Ophthalmology*, vol. 26, no. 6, pp. 473–477, 2012.

[6] T. A. Shazly, M. Aljajeh, and M. A. Latina, "Posner-Schlossman glaucomatocyclitic crisis," *Seminars in Ophthalmology*, vol. 26, no. 4-5, pp. 282–284, 2011.

[7] J. Lippert, M. Falgiani, and L. Ganti, "Posner-Schlossman syndrome," *Cureus*, vol. 12, no. 1, pp. 65–84, 2020.

[8] R. J. Green, "Posner-Schlossman syndrome (glaucomatocyclitic crisis)," *Clinical & Experimental Optometry*, vol. 90, no. 1, pp. 53–56, 2007.

[9] E. D. Kocak, B. Z. Wang, and A. J. Hall, "Bilateral uveitis following intravenous immunoglobulin administration," *American Journal of Ophthalmology Case Reports*, vol. 6, no. 6, pp. 74–76, 2017.

[10] J. Oh, A. Marks, K. Wessell et al., "Common variable immunodeficiency associated with birdshot-like chorioretinopathy," *Annals of Allergy, Asthma & Immunology*, vol. 112, no. 5, pp. 472–474, 2014.

[11] S. Carter, K. Xie, D. Knight, D. Minkcler, and S. Kedhar, "Granulomatous uveitis and conjunctivitis due to common variable immune deficiency: a case report," *Ocular Immunology and Inflammation*, vol. 27, no. 7, pp. 1124–1126, 2018.

[12] E. Z. Oltra, C. Morris, A. D. Birnbaum, H. H. Tessler, and D. A. Goldstein, "Chronic anterior uveitis in common variable immunodeficiency," *Ocular Immunology and Inflammation*, vol. 19, no. 6, pp. 448-449, 2011.

17

Vogt-Koyanagi-Harada Disease: A Case Series in a Tertiary Eye Center

Pranav Shrestha,[1] **Sadhana Sharma**,[1] **and Ranju Kharel**[2]

[1]*Mechi Eye Hospital, Jhapa 57200, Nepal*
[2]*Department of Uveitis, B. P. Koirala Lions Center for Ophthalmic Studies (BPKLCOS), Institute of Medicine, Maharajgunj, Kathmandu 44600, Nepal*

Correspondence should be addressed to Sadhana Sharma; ssadnaa@gmail.com

Academic Editor: Nicola Rosa

Purpose. To study the clinical spectrum of Vogt-Koyanagi-Harada (VKH) disease in a tertiary eye center in Nepal. *Methods.* Baseline demographic details and clinical features of six patients diagnosed as VKH in a tertiary eye center were retrospectively reviewed. Examinations included best corrected visual acuity, intraocular pressure, and slit lamp examination of anterior and posterior segments. Baseline blood investigations, chest X-ray, fundus photography, and fundus fluorescent angiography (FFA) were performed on all the patients. *Results.* The mean age at presentation was 46 ± 8.43 years with female predominance (83.3%). The disease was complete in 16.7%, incomplete in 16.7%, and probable in 66.7% of the patients. Most cases presented in acute uveitis stage (66.7%). The most common finding in acute cases was serous retinal detachment (66.7%), followed by disc edema (58.3%), whereas in chronic cases, depigmented fundus was the most common. All cases had bilateral presentation. *Conclusion.* VKH is an important cause of bilateral loss of vision and has a good visual prognosis if aggressive treatment is initiated during the early stages.

1. Introduction

Vogt-Koyanagi-Harada (VKH) is a severe, bilateral, granulomatous panuveitis associated with extraocular manifestations. It is a cell-mediated autoimmune disorder affecting the pigmented tissues leading to amplification of inflammatory cascade against the melanocytes [1, 2]. It is more common in the adult population and has a predilection for female gender. HLA-DQ4 carriers had a higher risk of VKH, and HLA-DQ1 seemed to be protective [3]. Most of the cases are bilateral; however, in rare cases, a unilateral presentation or delayed involvement of the other eye can also occur [4, 5].

Patients may present with varied ocular manifestations like iridocyclitis, diffuse choroidal thickening, and hyperemia of the optic disc. Headache and meningismus are the main neurological manifestations, while auditory and integumentary changes may present with tinnitus and hearing loss and alopecia, poliosis, and vitiligo, respectively [6].

The four distinct phases of VKH are as follows: prodromal, acute uveitic, convalescent, and chronic recurrent. Low-grade nongranulomatous anterior uveitis along with diffuse choroiditis and exudative retinal detachment (RD) is seen in acute phases, while in chronic recurrent phases, patients present with recurrent granulomatous anterior uveitis [1]. As the frequency of ocular inflammatory attacks increases, the occurrence of ocular complications increases and is associated with worse visual prognosis.

The first international workshop defined VKH as bilateral uveitis without a history of trauma or ocular surgery [2] and classified VKH disease as (a) complete VKH with ocular, neurological, or auditory and integumentary involvement; (b) incomplete VKH with ocular and either neurological/auditory or integumentary involvement; and (c) probable VKH without extraocular manifestation [4, 5, 7, 8].

Treatment regimens include corticosteroids (intravenous, oral, and regional) and immunomodulators. Improper and inadequate treatment during the acute stage can lead to chronic recurrent VKH disease. High-dose systemic

Table 1: Diagnostic criteria of VKH.

No history of penetrating ocular trauma or surgery preceding the initial onset of uveitis	
No clinical or laboratory evidence suggestive of other ocular disease entities	
Bilateral ocular involvement	
Early manifestations	Late manifestations
Evidence of a diffuse choroiditis (with or without anterior uveitis, vitreous inflammatory reaction, or optic disc hyperemia) Focal areas of subretinal fluid or bullous serous retinal detachments	History suggestive of prior presence of findings Ocular depigmentation; sunset glow fundus or Sugiura's signs
Equivocal fundus findings: Focal areas of delay in choroidal perfusion, multifocal areas of pinpoint leakage, large placoid areas of hyperfluorescence, pooling within subretinal fluid, and optic nerve staining Diffuse choroidal thickening	Other ocular signs: (a) Nummular chorioretinal depigmented scars (b) Retinal pigment epithelium clumping and/or migration (c) Recurrent or chronic anterior uveitis
Neurological/auditory findings (may have resolved by time of examination); meningismus, tinnitus, or cerebrospinal fluid pleocytosis	
Integumentary finding (not preceding onset of central nervous system or ocular disease), alopecia, or poliosis, or vitiligo	

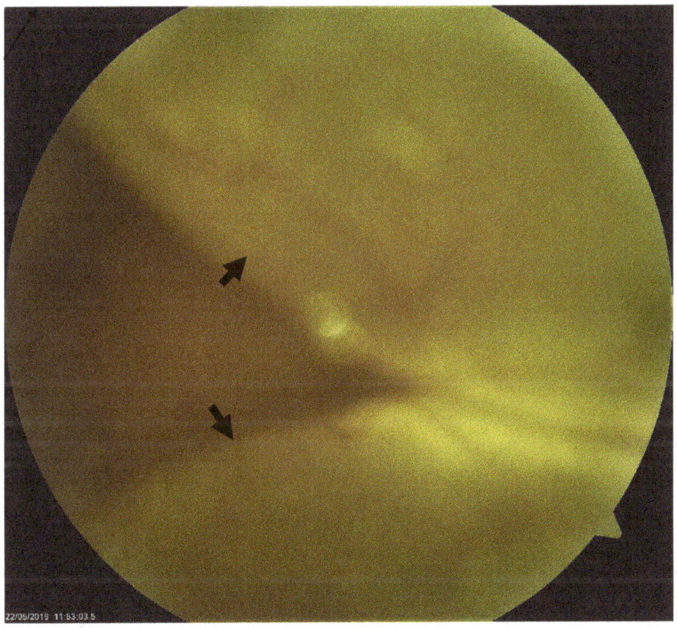

Figure 1: A VKH patient presenting in acute uveitic phase with bullous exudative retinal detachment (black arrows).

corticosteroids initiated during the early acute uveitis stage followed by slow tapering is required to suppress the inflammation. Addition of immunomodulatory agents along with steroids can improve the visual outcome and can also decrease the risk of cutaneous involvement [1].

We present a series of 6 cases of VKH presenting to a tertiary eye center in Nepal over a period of one year.

2. Methods

This is a retrospective review of medical records of VKH patients presenting to our uveitis clinic from 2015 to 2017 with a follow-up of 1-3 years. Informed consent was obtained from all the patients, and the study adhered to the Declaration of Helsinki. All patients provided a detailed history and underwent ocular examination including visual acuity (VA), intraocular pressure (IOP), and slit lamp evaluation including fundus evaluation using 90D aspheric lens and indirect ophthalmoscopy using 20D aspheric lens. Ultrasound B scan was done when required, and patients were required to undergo fundus photography at various stages of treatment depending upon the visibility of the posterior segment. All the patients were subjected to chest X-ray and baseline blood investigation including complete blood count (CBC), erythrocyte sedimentation rate (ESR), C reactive protein (CRP), uric acid, random blood sugar (BSR), serology for HBsAg, HCV, HIV, and syphilis.

The diagnosis of VKH is made by the criteria as summarized in Table 1.

Due to the wide range of presentation, the disease is categorized as follows: probable or ocular VKH if all the ocular criteria mentioned in Table 1 are met, incomplete VKH if

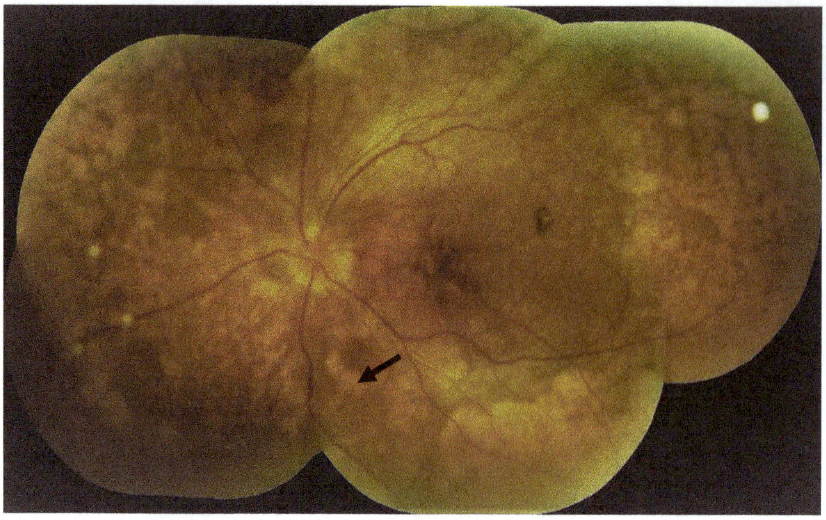

Figure 2: A VKH patient presenting in chronic stage with sunset glow fundus, multiple nummular chorioretinal depigmented scars, and pigmentary changes.

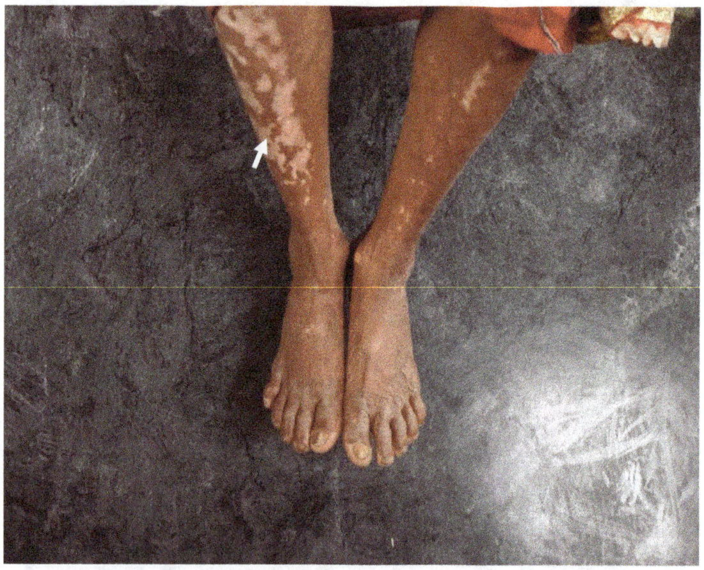

Figure 3: A VKH patient with extraocular manifestation (vitiligo).

along with ocular criteria there is presence of integumentary or neurological criteria, and complete VKH if both integumentary and neurological criteria are present.

After preliminary diagnosis of VKH was made, the patients were referred for consultation with a neurophysician, otorhinolaryngologist, and dermatologist. Depending on their expertise, further investigation like CSF examination was done solely on their discretion.

3. Results

A total of 12 eyes of six patients of different ethnicities were evaluated. Among them, 5 (83.3%) were female. The mean age at presentation was 46 ± 8.43 years (range 30–54 years). Four out of six patients (66.7%) presented in acute uveitis phase (Figure 1), while one (16.7%) patient each presented in convalescent phase and chronic recurrent phase. Among the six cases, four (66.7%) were probable VKH, one (16.7%) was incomplete, and one (16.67%) was complete.

The most common presenting symptom was diminution of vision in 91.7% (11 out of 12 eyes) and photophobia in 58.3% (7 out of 12 eyes). Majority of the eyes (58.3%; 7 out of 12) presented in the acute uveitis stage. Posterior segment findings included disc edema in 58.3% (7 out 12 eyes), exudative retinal detachment in 66.7% (8 out of 12 eyes), and choroiditis in 33.3% (4 out of 12 eyes). During the study duration, 6 eyes (50%) developed hypopigmented fundus with sunset glow appearance (Figure 2). Extraocular manifestation was present in two cases. Integumentary findings (vitiligo) (Figure 3) were present in both the cases, and one case also had neurological (headache) and auditory (tinnitus) findings.

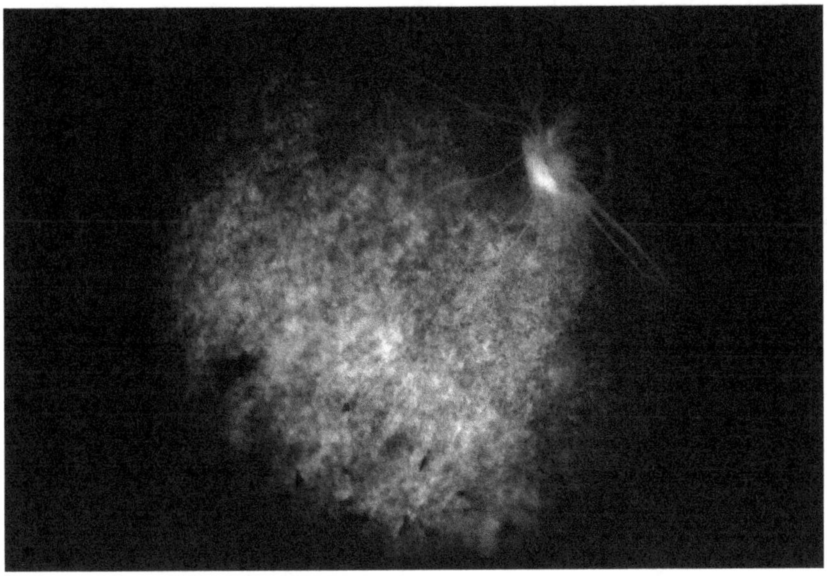

Figure 4: FFA showing multiple pinpoint hyperfluorescence in arteriovenous phase of the angiogram.

Table 2: Clinical characteristics and management of the cases of VKH.

Case no.	Sex	Age (years)	Stage of presentation	Extraocular manifestation	Presenting VA	Final VA	Medical treatment	Surgical treatment
1	F	54	Acute uveitis	None	HM and HM	6/12 and 6/18	IV steroid, azathioprine	Cataract surgery
2	F	47	Acute uveitis	None	3/60 and 6/18	6/18 and 6/12	Oral steroid, methotrexate	Cataract surgery
3	M	30	Acute uveitis	None	HM and 1/60	6/6 and 6/9	IV steroid, azathioprine, ATT	
4	F	49	Acute uveitis	Integumentary	6/12 and 6/24	6/12 and 6/24	Oral steroid	
5	F	51	Chronic recurrent	None	6/9 and 6/12	6/18 and 6/18	Oral steroid, methotrexate, ATT	
6	F	45	Convalescent	Neurological, integumentary, and auditory	6/18 and 6/9	6/9 and 6/6	Oral steroid, methotrexate	Cataract surgery, glaucoma filtration surgery

M: male; F: female; IV: intravenous; ATT: antitubercular treatment; HM: hand movement. Intravenous corticosteroid as a 500 mg injection of methylprednisolone, twice a day for 3 days. Oral corticosteroid as prednisolone tablet at a dose of 1 mg/kg. Azathioprine tablet at a dose of 1.5 mg/kg/day. Methotrexate tablet at a dose of 7.5 mg once a week along with 5 days of supplementary folic acid 5 mg a week after initial liver function testing.

The fluorescent angiography (FA) findings in most of the eyes were multiple spots of pinpoint hyperfluorescence in the early arteriovenous phase (Figure 4) with pooling of the dye within the serous RD in the late phase of the angiogram.

At the first presentation, four out of six cases (66.7%) received oral and topical corticosteroids, while two cases (33.3%) received intravenous corticosteroids. Immunomodulator therapy either with azathioprine or methotrexate was given later to control recurrence in cases 2 and 3, respectively (Table 2). Two of the cases, in addition to the immunomodulator therapy, also received antitubercular treatment (ATT) for 9 months due to a mixed picture of the disease.

The most common complication was cataract, comprising 50% (6 out of 12 eyes), for which cataract surgery was done. Glaucoma filtration surgery was done in two eyes (33.3%) for secondary glaucoma not controlled with topical medications. All the patients in the series attained a final visual acuity of ≥6/24 (Table 1).

4. Discussion

Vogt-Koyanagi-Harada disease is relatively uncommon among the Nepalese population, and extraocular manifestation of the disease is even rare [2]. The prognosis in terms of vision remain good when proper treatment is provided even if there is presence of structural changes in the retinal outer layers [3].

The mean age and the female predominance in our series correlates with those presented in other literature. Disc hyperemia and serous retinal detachment were the most common posterior segment presentation similar to comparative literature [1]. Only few cases had extraocular manifestation in this series even though they presented with a typical fundus finding, the possibility of which has been explored in the study by Beniz et al. [9].

Optical coherence tomography could prove to be an invaluable imaging modality for early detection of macula-related complications and detection of the subretinal fluids [10]. In addition, if enhanced depth imaging (EDI) is available, the amount of choroidal inflammation could also be assessed depending on the stage of the disease [11].

Similar to the finding of Paredes et al. [12], immunomodulator therapy along with tapered systemic and topical application of a corticosteroid resulted in a better visual outcome. In this series, two cases were receiving antitubercular therapy along with an immunomodulator due to the possibility of the antigenic mimicry and cross-reactivity between the two conditions [13].

5. Conclusion

VKH is a multisystem disorder, and diagnosis is mainly clinical. The mainstay of treatment is aggressive corticosteroid therapy in the acute phase and an additional immunosuppressive agent. There is a potential for significant visual loss, but timely identification and treatment can minimize ocular morbidity.

Consent

Consent for use of images was obtained.

References

[1] S. Lodhi, J. Reddy, and V. Peram, "Clinical spectrum and management options in Vogt-Koyanagi-Harada disease," *Clinical Ophthalmology*, vol. 11, pp. 1399–1406, 2017.

[2] R. Kharel, D. N. Shah, and M. Chaudhary, "Presumed Vogt-Koyanagi-Harada (VKH) disease in Nepalese population: a rare entity," *Journal of Clinical Ophthalmology and Research.*, vol. 4, no. 2, p. 97, 2016.

[3] B. Liu, T. Deng, L. Zhu, and J. Zhong, "Association of human leukocyte antigen (HLA)-DQ and HLA-DQA1/DQB1 alleles with Vogt-Koyanagi-Harada disease: a systematic review and meta-analysis," *Medicine*, vol. 97, no. 7, article e9914, 2018.

[4] A. Agrawal and J. Biswas, "Unilateral Vogt-Koyanagi-Harada disease: report of two cases," *Middle East African Journal of Ophthalmology*, vol. 18, no. 1, pp. 82–84, 2011.

[5] Y. Usui and H. Goto, "Presumed Vogt-Koyanagi-Harada disease with unilateral ocular involvement: report of three cases," *Graefe's Archive for Clinical and Experimental Ophthalmology*, vol. 247, no. 8, pp. 1127–1132, 2009.

[6] R. S. Moorthy, H. Inomata, and N. A. Rao, "Vogt-Koyanagi-Harada syndrome," *Survey of Ophthalmology*, vol. 39, no. 4, pp. 265–292, 1995.

[7] A. Neves, A. Cardoso, M. Almeida, J. Campos, A. Campos, and J. P. C. Sousa, "Unilateral Vogt-Koyanagi-Harada disease: a clinical case report," *Case Reports in Ophthalmology.*, vol. 6, no. 3, pp. 361–365, 2015.

[8] D. J. Forster, R. L. Green, and N. A. Rao, "Unilateral manifestation of the Vogt-Koyanagi-Harada syndrome in a 7-year-old child," *American Journal of Ophthalmology*, vol. 111, no. 3, pp. 380–382, 1991.

[9] J. Beniz, D. J. Forster, J. S. Lean, R. E. Smith, and N. A. Rao, "Variations in clinical features of the Vogt-Koyanagi-Harada syndrome," *Retina*, vol. 11, no. 3, pp. 275–280, 1991.

[10] M. Agarwal, A. Radosavljevic, G. Patnaik, E. Rishi, and F. Pichi, "Diagnostic value of optical coherence tomography in the early diagnosis of macular complications in chronic Vogt-Koyanagi-Harada disease," *Ocular Immunology and Inflammation*, pp. 1–8, 2020.

[11] V. M. Sakata, F. T. da Silva, C. E. Hirata, W. Y. Takahashi, R. A. Costa, and J. H. Yamamoto, "Choroidal bulging in patients with Vogt-Koyanagi-Harada disease in the non-acute uveitic stage," *Journal of Ophthalmic Inflammation and Infection.*, vol. 4, no. 1, p. 6, 2014.

[12] I. Paredes, M. Ahmed, and C. Foster, "Immunomodulatory therapy for Vogt-Koyanagi-Harada patients as first-line therapy," *Ocular Immunology and Inflammation*, vol. 14, no. 2, pp. 87–90, 2006.

[13] B. Dogan, M. K. Erol, and A. Cengiz, "Vogt-Koyanagi-Harada disease following BCG vaccination and tuberculosis," *Springerplus*, vol. 5, no. 1, pp. 1–11, 2016.

18

The Use of Inner Retinectomy to Relieve Inner Retinal Foreshortening Causing Retinal Detachment in the Setting of Branch Retinal Vein Occlusion

Katsuya Yagisawa, Takayuki Baba, Tomomi Kaiho, Hirotaka Yokouchi, and Shuichi Yamamoto

Department of Ophthalmology and Visual Science, Chiba University Graduate School of Medicine, Chiba, Japan

Correspondence should be addressed to Takayuki Baba; babatakayuki@nifty.com

Academic Editor: Stephen G. Schwartz

A 61-year-old Japanese woman presented with impairment of her left vision due to macular schisis secondary to branch retinal vein occlusion. Her left vision was 20/50, and schisis was observed inferotemporally. She underwent phacoemulsification and aspiration, implantation of the intraocular lens, and removal of the epiretinal membrane and internal limiting membrane. Her visual acuity stabilized ~20/50 for two and a half years after the initial surgery. However, she developed macula-involving retinal detachment, and her visual acuity declined to counting fingers. She underwent pars plana vitrectomy and removal of the residual vitreous cortex together with the inner retina within the area of vein occlusion. After the removal of silicone oil and the addition of an encircling buckle, the retina remained attached and visual acuity improved to 20/60 at one year after the final surgery. The combination of rhegmatogenous and tractional detachment in the area of schisis was suspected, and vitrectomy with inner retinectomy was effective.

1. Introduction

Branch retinal vein occlusion (BRVO) is known to occur in 0.5 to 1.2 per 100 persons [1]. The pathogenesis of BRVO is mainly compression of veins at A-V crossings, degenerative changes of vessel walls of the vein, and hypercoagulability. Hypertension is the most common risk factor, and hyperlipidemia and diabetes follow. Age is also associated with the occurrence of BRVO, and the prevalence is 1.57 per 1000 in ages 40-49, 4.58 per 1000 in 50-59, 11.11 per 1000 in 60-69, and 12.76 per 1000 in 70-79 [2].

Reported complications of BRVO include macular edema [3], retinal neovascularization [4], vitreous hemorrhage [5], retinal break [6], and retinal detachment [7]. Serous retinal detachment is observed in 63% of major BRVO cases [8] and is more common than rhegmatogenous retinal detachment (RRD), which was reported as 1.3% [6] to 3% [9, 10]. On the other hand, retinal schisis is a rare condition, and there is no systematic study reporting the prevalence and treatment for the pathology.

In this case report, we presented a case with macula-involving retinal schisis secondary to BRVO that was treated with pars plana vitrectomy (PPV). In the postoperative period, the case developed RRD that was finally reattached by PPV with inner retinectomy.

2. Case Report

A 61-year-old Japanese woman presented with declining vision in her left eye. She was diagnosed with BRVO in her left eye and underwent photocoagulation of the retinal periphery five years before this event. She had no history of systemic disease except for hypertension, controlled by medications. She developed retinal schisis extending to the macula and was referred to Chiba University Hospital for treatment. Her visual acuity was 20/20 in the right eye and

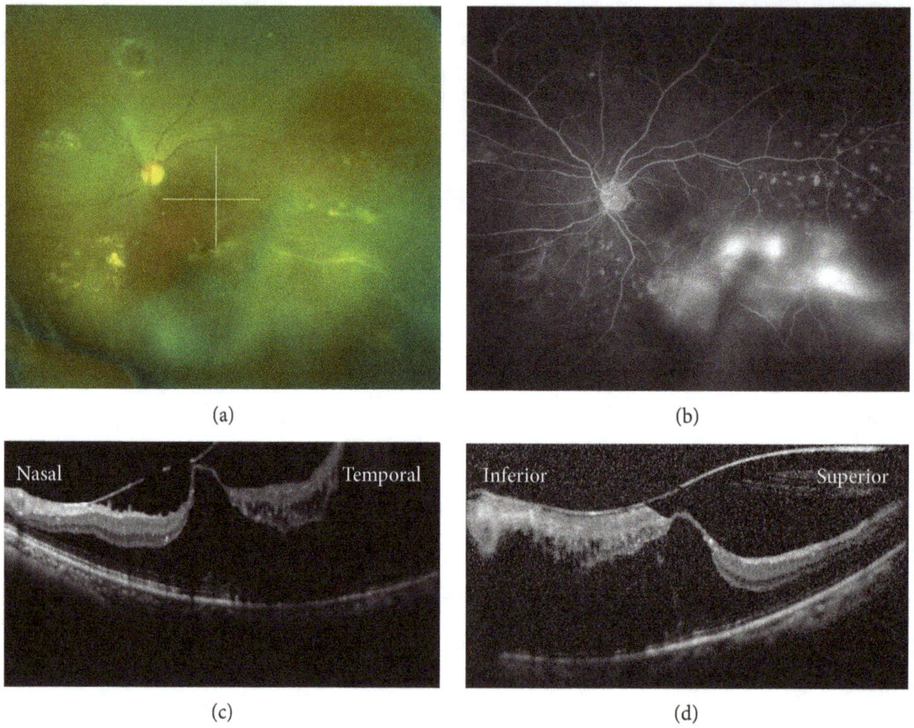

Figure 1: Preoperative images of a 61-year-old Japanese woman with macula-involving retinal schisis secondary to branch retinal vein occlusion (BRVO). (a) An ultrawidefield fundus photograph showing BRVO with white vessels at the inferior temporal retina. The visual acuity in the left eye was 20/50. The lines indicate the location of OCT scans presented in (c) and (d). (b) Fluorescein angiography showing retinal neovascularization in the area of BRVO. (c) A horizontal optical coherence tomography (OCT) image through the macula showing macular traction and extensive retinal schisis. (d) A vertical OCT image through the macula showing broad adhesion of the vitreous and retinal schisis.

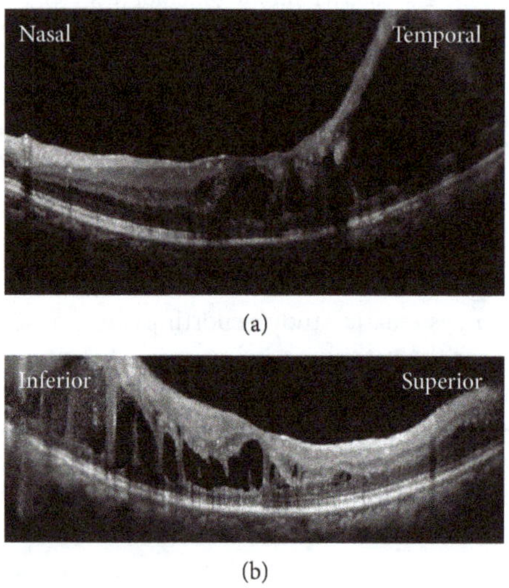

Figure 2: Postoperative images at two months after phacovitrectomy and membrane peeling for retinal schisis. (a) A horizontal optical coherence tomography (OCT) image showing the decreased height of retinal schisis. The schisis cavity is still wide in the temporal retina. (b) A vertical OCT image showing decreased but persistent retinal schisis.

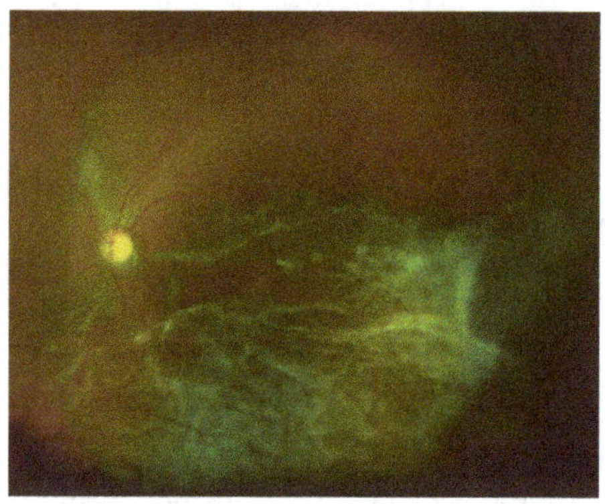

Figure 3: A preoperative image before the second vitrectomy. An ultrawidefield fundus photograph showing the retinal detachment involving the macula at two and a half years after the initial surgery. The visual acuity in the left eye was counting fingers.

20/50 in the left eye at the initial presentation. The intraocular pressure was 12 mmHg in the right eye and 11 mmHg in the left eye. The axial length was 21.53 and 21.75 mm in the right and left eyes, respectively. The retinal schisis was observed at the inferior temporal retina with white vessels. Optical coherence tomography (OCT) showed macular traction and schisis. The posterior vitreous detachment was incomplete. The fluorescein angiogram showed retinal neovascularization in the nonperfused retina (Figure 1). She underwent phacovitrectomy with implantation of intraocular lens. During the surgery, the epiretinal membrane and internal limiting membrane were removed from the macula using Brilliant Blue G. The posterior hyaloid was separated except for the inferior temporal area where the vitreous is firmly

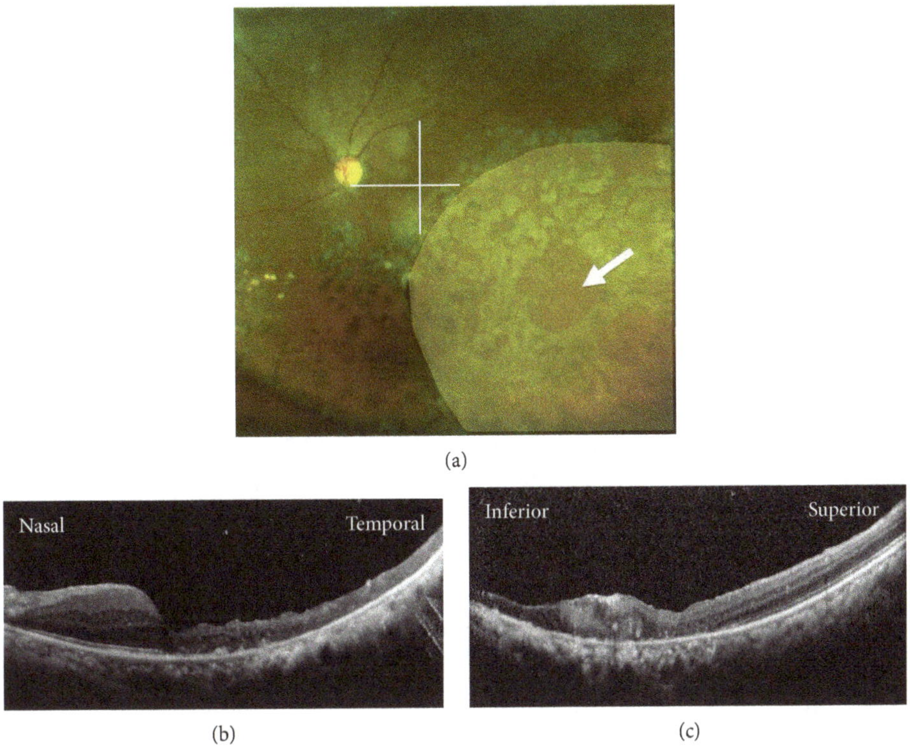

FIGURE 4: Postoperative images at one and a half years after the removal of silicone oil. (a) An ultrawidefield fundus photograph showing retinal reattachment with retinal scars after photocoagulation. An outer retinal break is observed (arrow). The pale area indicates the location of the inner retinectomy. The visual acuity in the left eye was 20/60. The lines indicate the location of OCT scans presented in (b) and (c). (b) A horizontal optical coherence tomography (OCT) image showing the attached macula and thinning of the temporal retina. (c) A vertical OCT image showing the attached macula and a scar formation at the inferior macula.

attached to the retina. After the surgery, the decrease in the schisis cavity was observed with stable visual acuity between 20/50 and 20/40 (Figure 2). Two and a half years after the initial surgery, she presented with macula-involving bullous retinal detachment (Figure 3). Her visual acuity decreased to counting fingers. The outer retinal break was suspected posterior to the equator in the retina with BRVO. She underwent PPV with inner retinectomy at the BRVO area to reduce vitreous traction because the hyaloid was impossible to be separated from retina. The retinectomy encompassed the inferotemporal peripheral retina and extended posteriorly into the macula, almost to the fovea (Figure 4); note that the inferotemporal arcade was truncated by the retinectomy. Subretinal fluid was drained through the outer retinal break, and the retina was attached with silicone oil tamponade. The retina remained attached after the removal of silicone oil and the addition of the 7 mm width encircling buckle to support the peripheral retina. Her visual acuity was 20/60, and intraocular pressure was 10 mmHg at one and a half years after the last surgery (Figure 4). The defect in her visual field slightly enlarged after the inner retinectomy (Figure 5).

3. Discussion

RRD is a rare complication of BRVO [6, 9, 10]. The detachment can occur due to retinal breaks secondary to vitreous traction in the vicinity of retinal neovascularization [11–13]. In our case, the chronic BRVO developed retinal schisis, and the schisis gradually extended into the macula. We treated this patient with phacovitrectomy and removed the epiretinal membrane and internal limiting membrane to reduce macular traction. The schisis improved; however, retinal detachment developed later. We speculated that the residual vitreous caused traction and outer retinal break in the area of schisis. We had already known that the visual field was lost within the schisis and performed inner retinectomy to eliminate the vitreous traction. Since scleral buckling could support the vitreous base but not posterior traction, we suggest that the inner retinectomy plays a more important role in the reattachment of the retina in this case. The usefulness of inner retinectomy has been reported in the eyes with congenital schisis [14] and schisis associated with retinopathy of prematurity [15]. In our BRVO case, the procedure was effective, resulting in the reattachment of the retina with favorable visual recovery and minimal loss of the visual field. We suggest that the inner retinotomy is tolerable when the visual function disappeared in the area of schisis with persistent vitreoretinal traction. The efficacy of PPV for the treatment of RRD in BRVO cases has been reported [16], with better visual outcome in cases that lack vitreous adhesion [17]. Eyes with tractional tear more frequently presented macula-off RRD which required reoperation more often. Our case also showed firm adhesion of the vitreous, and late development

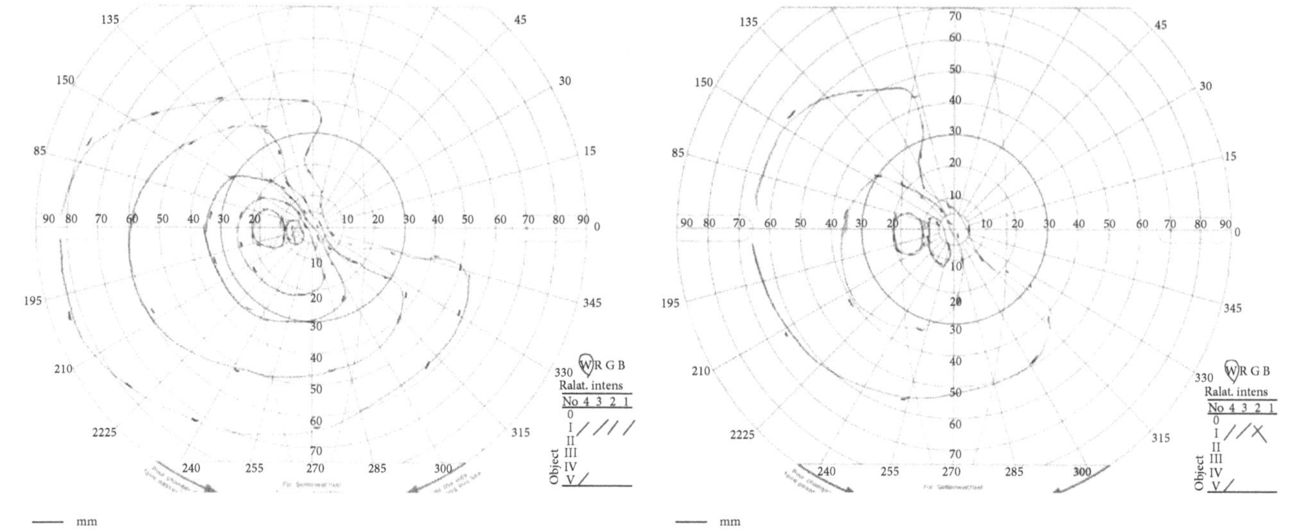

(a) (b)

Figure 5: The visual field of the left eye before and after surgeries. (a) A preoperative Goldmann perimetry test before the initial surgery showing the defect of the superior nasal visual field corresponding to the area with branch retinal vein occlusion. (b) A postoperative Goldmann perimetry test at three months after the silicone removal showing narrowing of the nasal visual field slightly, but the majority of the visual field was retained.

of RRD occurred. It seems essential to follow cases where vitreous traction was not completely released.

In conclusion, we experienced a BRVO case with macula-involving retinal schisis treated with PPV. After the initial surgery, RRD developed and was successfully treated with PPV with inner retinectomy extending into the temporal macula. Retinal schisis is a rare complication of BRVO and may contribute to the risk of RRD via vitreoretinal traction.

References

[1] A. Jaulim, B. Ahmed, T. Khanam, and I. P. Chatziralli, "Branch retinal vein occlusion: epidemiology, pathogenesis, risk factors, clinical features, diagnosis, and complications. An update of the literature," *Retina*, vol. 33, no. 5, pp. 901–910, 2013.

[2] S. Rogers, R. L. McIntosh, N. Cheung et al., "The prevalence of retinal vein occlusion: pooled data from population studies from the United States, Europe, Asia, and Australia," *Ophthalmology*, vol. 117, no. 2, pp. 313–319.e1, 2010.

[3] D. H. Orth and A. Patz, "Retinal branch vein occlusion," *Survey of Ophthalmology*, vol. 22, no. 6, pp. 357–376, 1978.

[4] J. S. Shilling and E. M. Kohner, "New vessel formation in retinal branch vein occlusion," *British Journal of Ophthalmology*, vol. 60, no. 12, pp. 810–815, 1976.

[5] C. L. Trempe, M. Takahashi, and H. W. Topilow, "Vitreous changes in retinal branch vein occlusion," *Ophthalmology*, vol. 88, no. 7, pp. 681–687, 1981.

[6] E. Kir, A. O. Saatci, Z. Ozbek, S. Kaynak, and M. H. Ergin, "Retinal breaks and rhegmatogenous retinal detachment in association with branch retinal vein occlusion," *Ophthalmic Surgery and Lasers*, vol. 30, no. 4, pp. 285–288, 1999.

[7] A. Amirikia, I. U. Scott, T. G. Murray, H. W. Flynn Jr., W. E. Smiddy, and W. J. Feuer, "Outcomes of vitreoretinal surgery for complications of branch retinal vein occlusion," *Ophthalmology*, vol. 108, no. 2, pp. 372–375, 2001.

[8] Y. Yamaguchi, T. Otani, and S. Kishi, "Serous macular detachment in branch retinal vein occlusion," *Retina*, vol. 26, no. 9, pp. 1029–1033, 2006.

[9] F. A. Gutman and H. Zegarra, "The natural course of temporal retinal branch vein occlusion," *Transactions-American Academy of Ophthalology and Otolaryngology*, vol. 78, no. 2, pp. OP178–OP192, 1978.

[10] F. A. Gutman and H. Zegarra, "Retinal detachment secondary to retinal branch vein occlusions," *Transactions. Section on Ophthalmology American Academy of Ophthalmology and Otolaryngology*, vol. 81, 3, Part 1, pp. 491–496, 1976.

[11] H. C. Joondeph and M. F. Goldberg, "Rhegmatogenous retinal detachment after tributary retinal vein occlusion," *American Journal of Ophthalmology*, vol. 80, no. 2, pp. 253–257, 1975.

[12] M. Singh, L. Dhir, C. Kon, and S. Rassam, "Tractional retinal break and rhegmatogenous retinal detachment consequent to branch retinal vein occlusion," *Eye*, vol. 20, no. 11, pp. 1326-1327, 2006.

[13] M. R. Martinez and A. Ophir, "Extrafoveal traction in retinal vein occlusion using spectral domain optical coherence tomography," *Graefes Archive for Clinical and Experimental Ophthalmology*, vol. 249, no. 6, pp. 811–820, 2011.

[14] P. J. Ferrone, M. T. Trese, and H. Lewis, "Vitreoretinal surgery for complications of congenital retinoschisis," *American Journal of Ophthalmology*, vol. 123, no. 6, pp. 742–747, 1997.

[15] B. Todorich, A. Thanos, Y. Yonekawa et al., "Surgical management of tractional retinoschisis associated with vitreous hemorrhage in retinopathy of prematurity," *Retinal Cases & Brief Reports*, vol. 13, no. 1, pp. 72–74, 1997.

[16] S. R. Russell, C. F. Blodi, and J. C. Folk, "Vitrectomy for complicated retinal detachments secondary to branch retinal vein occlusions," *American Journal of Ophthalmology*, vol. 108, no. 1, pp. 6–9, 1989.

[17] Y. Ikuno, Y. Tano, J. M. Lewis, T. Ikeda, and Y. Sato, "Retinal detachment after branch retinal vein occlusion: influence of the type of break on the outcome of vitreous surgery," *Ophthalmology*, vol. 104, no. 1, pp. 27–32, 1997.

19

Vitreous Hemorrhage as Presenting Sign of Retinal Arteriovenous Malformation

Geraldine P. B. M. Accou,[1] Fanny Nerinckx,[1] Bart P. Leroy,[2,3] and Julie De Zaeytijd[1]

[1]*Department of Ophthalmology, Ghent University Hospital, Ghent, Belgium*
[2]*Department of Ophthalmology & Center for Medical Genetics, Ghent University Hospital, Ghent, Belgium*
[3]*Children's Hospital of Philadelphia, Philadelphia, PA, USA*

Correspondence should be addressed to Geraldine P. B. M. Accou; geraldine.accou@uzgent.be

Academic Editor: Alexander A. Bialasiewicz

Objective. To describe a patient with vitreous hemorrhage and peripheral retinal ischemia, eventually diagnosed with an underlying retinal arteriovenous malformation. *Methods.* A 15-year-old girl presented with sudden-onset, painless visual loss in the right eye. She underwent a full ophthalmological work-up. *Results.* BCVA was less than 20/400 in the right eye and 20/20 in the left eye. Intraocular pressure and anterior segment examination were unremarkable. Fundoscopy was impossible due to an opaque vitreous hemorrhage in the right eye. The left eye was completely unremarkable. Examination during a 23-gauge pars plana vitrectomy showed dilated, tortuous arteriovenous vessels extending from the optic disc and silver wiring of the enlarged vessels. A clinical diagnosis of retinal arteriovenous malformation was made. During surgery, a peripheral retinal photocoagulation was executed to avoid rebleeding. Postoperatively, fluorescein angiography demonstrated additional macular microangiopathy and diffuse retinal nonperfusion in the periphery. The MRI brain revealed neither cerebral nor orbital vascular anomaly, confirming a group 2 retinal arteriovenous malformation. *Conclusion.* Retinal arteriovenous malformations are generally considered stable over time. However, complications due to retinal ischemia can occur. Hence, regular observation is warranted. In so doing, timely treatment can be offered to avoid complications.

1. Introduction

Retinal arteriovenous malformation is a rare, unilateral sporadic disorder. It is characterized by anomalous arteriovenous malformations of the retina, looking like tangle-like loops of small arteries entering into retinal veins. The malformations can be both local or extensive and can be distributed over the entire retina [1]. If local, they are predominantly found either close to the optic disc or in the temporal retinal periphery. If associated with cerebral arteriovenous malformations and facial nevi, the condition is known as the Wyburn-Mason syndrome [2, 3].

In 1973, Archer et al. published a classification of retinal arteriovenous malformations, which is still in use today. In short, group 1 is characterized by small lesions with an abnormal capillary plexus in between, group 2 by arteriovenous malformations without intervening capillary bed, and group 3 by extensive malformations where no distinction can be made between arteries and veins [3].

Retinal arteriovenous malformation can cause vision loss via various ocular complications [4, 5–7]. This case report presents a young patient in whom the AV malformation had been previously undiagnosed, who presented with a vitreous hemorrhage.

2. Case Description

A 15-year-old girl presented with a history of sudden-onset, painless visual loss in the right eye, since 3 months. Generally, she was in good health, and her family history was unremarkable. The best-corrected visual acuity was less than 20/400 in the right eye and 20/20 in the left eye. Intraocular pressure and slit-lamp examination were unremarkable in both eyes. Fundoscopy was impossible due to a dense

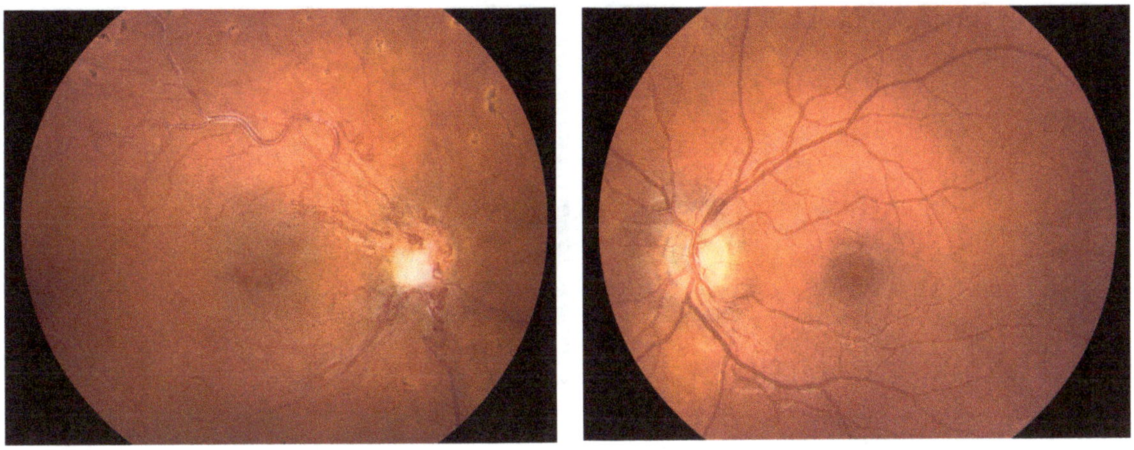

(a) (b)

Figure 1: (a) Fundus of the affected right eye of patient postsurgery, showing enlarged and tortuous vessels extending from the optic disc. A fibrous tuft is visible at the optic disc. (b) Normal fundus of the left eye.

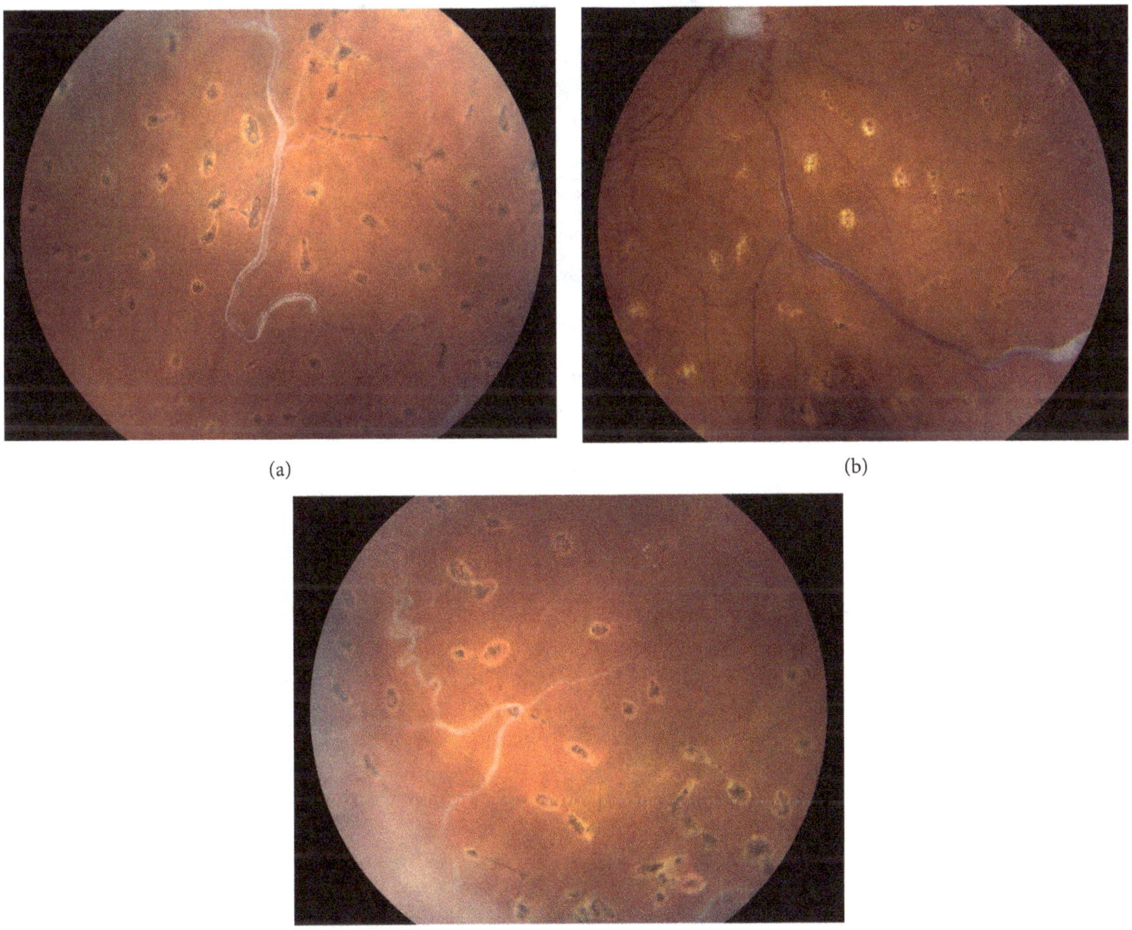

(a) (b) (c)

Figure 2: Silver wiring of the retinal veins in the superior (a), inferior (b), and temporal quadrant of the retina (c).

vitreous hemorrhage blocking the view of the fundus in the right eye. Ocular ultrasound confirmed the vitreous hemorrhage in the absence of a retinal detachment, a retinal tear, or an intraocular mass. A preoperative etiological work-up including fundoscopy and fluorescein angiography of the left eye to identify common retinal vascular or inflammatory pathologies was negative.

Without spontaneous clearing, the vitreous hemorrhage of the right eye was treated with a 23-gauge pars plana vitrectomy, which revealed dilated and tortuous retinal arteries as

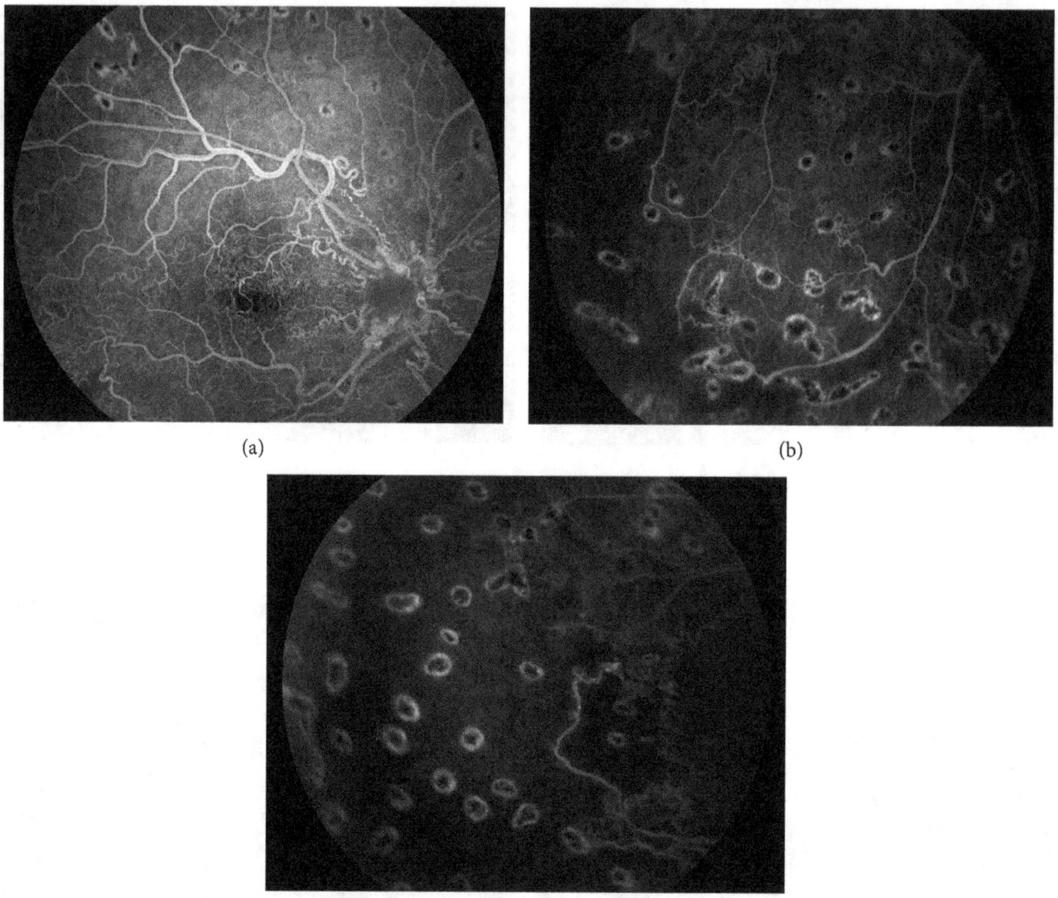

(a) (b) (c)

Figure 3: Fluorescein angiography of the affected right eye of the patient. (a) Abnormal arteriovenous communications with microangiopathy in the macula and an enlarged foveal avascular zone. (b, c) Diffuse capillary drop out in retinal periphery. No peripheral neovascularization is observed; however, pictures were taken 2 weeks after peroperative intravitreal anti-VEGF injection.

well as veins, extending from the optic disc with multiple communications and with some of them crossing the midline (Figure 1). There was an intraretinal hemorrhage in the temporal retinal periphery, but no exudations. Three neovascular tufts were visible in the inferior retinal periphery. Silver wiring of the retinal veins was pronounced in all four quadrants of the retina (Figure 2). Because of silver wiring, peripheral retinal ischemia was suspected. The combination of the retinal vascular malformation on the optic disc, with neovascular tufts in the inferior retinal periphery, led to a diagnosis of vitreous hemorrhage with neovascularization. An intravitreal injection of bevacizumab was given during surgery to avoid rebleeding. A peripheral pan-retinal photocoagulation was performed to aim for long-term stabilization.

Two weeks postsurgery, the BCVA in the right eye had improved to 20/60. Fluorescein angiography of the right eye demonstrated abnormal arteriovenous communications with an altered capillary network in the macula and diffuse ischemia in the retinal periphery (Figure 3). No peripheral retinal neovascularization was observed, possibly because of the intravitreal anti-VEGF injection administered during surgery.

Based on the above, a diagnosis of arteriovenous malformation group 2 (classification by Archer et al.) was made. Additional magnetic resonance imaging (MRI) of the brain revealed no abnormality.

3. Discussion

Arteriovenous malformations can remain stable over many years and are therefore usually thought of as benign and stationary lesions [8]. However, during follow-up, retinal complications cannot be considered rare, with a reported prevalence as high as 24.6%. Retinal hemorrhages are the most frequent (28.1%), followed by retinal vein occlusion (17.5%) and vitreous hemorrhage (10.5%). Evolution towards neovascular glaucoma on the other hand is rare (0.05%) [1, 9–11, 12].

Arteriovenous malformations are high-flow systems because of direct communication between retinal arteries and veins, with either an abnormal or completely absent interposing capillary plexus. Consequently, the hydrostatic pressure in the retinal veins is a lot higher than normal and exposes the veins to arterial blood pressure levels. Considering a majority of the complications imply ischemia related etiology, three hypothetical mechanisms have been put forward to explain the mechanism of the underlying retinal ischemia. The first mechanism states that this abnormally elevated hydrostatic venous pressure causes endothelial injury of the vessel wall, leading to thrombosis. The second hypothesis discusses a "steal phenomenon." Due to the increased venous flow in the absence of a capillary network, the retinal perfusion is decreased, leading to retinal and/or choroidal ischemia. The third mechanism states direct compression of the veins due to the arteriovenous malformation at arteriovenous crossing sites, the more common mechanism for retinal vein occlusion [1, 9, 11, 13, 14].

In the patient described in this report, the mechanism behind the vitreous hemorrhage is most likely a combination of the elevated hydrostatic pressure, given the amount of silver wiring vessels, and the steal phenomenon, leading to peripheral retinal ischemia. Indeed, the lack of numerous intraretinal hemorrhages and the absence of filling defects on fluorescein angiography argue against damage to the vessel wall with subsequent occlusion.

The ocular management of retinal arteriovenous malformations is observation of the lesions or, if required, treatment of the ocular complications. Gass already emphasized that relatively minor alterations of retinal vessels may occur in association with central nervous system vascular anomalies [15]. Thus, whenever confronted with a retinal arteriovenous malformation, the neurologic evaluation with MRI imaging of the brain is always indicated.

4. Conclusions

The etiology of a vitreous hemorrhage varies according to the characteristics of the patient population. In patients younger than 40 years, the most frequent cause is an ocular trauma. If there is no evidence of a trauma, a work-up, including laboratory testing and fluorescein angiography is indicated. If the etiology is unclear after work-up, and no visualization of the retina is possible, pars plana vitrectomy is indicated.

A retinal arteriovenous malformation is part of the differential diagnosis of a vitreous hemorrhage in an otherwise healthy person. Although retinal arteriovenous malformations are thought of to be stable over time, complications, especially due to retinal ischemia, might occur. Observation, in combination with fluorescein angiography, is warranted. As such, timely treatment can be offered to avoid complications.

References

[1] P. N. Dayani and A. A. Sadun, "A case report of Wyburn-Mason syndrome and review of the literature," *Neuroradiology*, vol. 49, no. 5, pp. 445–456, 2007.

[2] R. Wyburn-Mason, "Arteriovenous aneurysm of mid-brain and retina, facial naevi and mental changes," *Brain*, vol. 66, no. 3, pp. 163–203, 1943.

[3] D. B. Archer, A. Deutman, J. T. Ernest, and A. E. Krill, "Arteriovenous communications of the retina," *American Journal of Ophthalmology*, vol. 75, no. 2, pp. 224–241, 1973.

[4] D. Karagiannis, D. Panagiotidis, I. Tsoubris, and P. Theodossiadis, "Spontaneous development of macular ischemia in a case of racemose hemangioma," *Clinical Ophthalmology*, vol. 5, pp. 931-932, 2011.

[5] P. Rao, B. J. Thomas, Y. Yonekawa, J. Robinson, and A. Capone Jr., "Peripheral retinal ischemia, neovascularization, and choroidal infarction in Wyburn-Mason syndrome," *JAMA Ophthalmology*, vol. 133, no. 7, pp. 852–854, 2015.

[6] M. A. Materin, C. L. Shields, B. P. Marr, H. Demirci, and J. A. Shields, "Retinal racemose hemangioma," *Retina*, vol. 25, no. 7, pp. 936-937, 2005.

[7] K. I. Papageorgiou, S. M. S. Ghazi-Nouri, and P. S. Andreou, "Vitreous and subretinal haemorrhage: an unusual complication of retinal racemose haemangioma," *Clinical and Experimental Ophthalmology*, vol. 34, no. 2, pp. 176-177, 2006.

[8] J. J. Augsburger, R. E. Goldberg, J. A. Shields, R. D. Mulberger, and L. E. Magargal, "Changing appearance of retinal arteriovenous malformation," *Albrecht von Graefe's Archive for Clinical and Experimental Ophthalmology*, vol. 215, no. 1, pp. 65–70, 1980.

[9] X. J. Qin, C. Huang, and K. Lai, "Retinal vein occlusion in retinal racemose hemangioma: a case report and literature review of ocular complications in this rare retinal vascular disorder," *BMC Ophthalmology*, vol. 14, no. 1, 2014.

[10] P. A. Bloom, A. Laidlaw, and D. L. Easty, "Spontaneous development of retinal ischaemia and rubeosis in eyes with retinal racemose angioma," *British Journal of Ophthalmology*, vol. 77, no. 2, pp. 124-125, 1993.

[11] D. Schmidt, M. Pache, and M. Schumacher, "The congenital unilateral retinocephalic vascular malformation syndrome (Bonnet-Dechaume-Blanc syndrome or Wyburn-Mason syndrome): review of the literature," *Survey of Ophthalmology*, vol. 53, no. 3, pp. 227–249, 2008.

[12] A. M. Mansour, C. G. Wells, L. M. Jampol, and R. E. Kalina, "Ocular complications of arteriovenous communications of the retina," *Archives of Ophthalmology*, vol. 107, no. 2, pp. 232–236, 1989.

[13] C. Yang, Y. L. Liu, H. L. Dou, X. R. Lu, F. Qian, and L. Zhao, "Unilateral hemi-central retinal vein obstruction associated with retinal racemose angioma," *Japanese Journal of Ophthalmology*, vol. 53, no. 4, pp. 435-436, 2009.

[14] C. Salati, E. Ferrari, R. Basile, G. Virgili, and U. Menchini, "Retinal vein occlusion: late complication of a congenital arteriovenous anomaly," *Ophthalmologica*, vol. 216, no. 2, pp. 151-152, 2002.

[15] J. D. Gass, "Treatment of retinal vascular anomalies," *Transactions - American Academy of Ophthalmology and Otolaryngology*, vol. 83, pp. 432–442, 1977.

20

Endophthalmitis in Retinopathy of Prematurity after Intravitreal Aflibercept Injection

Elcin Suren,[1] Ersan Cetinkaya,[1] Mustafa Kalayci,[1] Sariye Elif Özyazıcı Özkan,[2] Mehmet Fatih Kucuk,[1] and Muhammet Kazim Erol[1]

[1]University of Health Sciences, Antalya Training and Research Hospital, Department of Ophthalmology, Antalya, Turkey
[2]University of Health Sciences, Antalya Training and Research Hospital, Department of Pediatrics, Antalya, Turkey

Correspondence should be addressed to Mustafa Kalayci; drkalayci07@hotmail.com

Academic Editor: Nicola Rosa

We report the case of a male infant who had an intravitreal anti-VEGF (aflibercept) injection for the treatment of retinopathy of prematurity at 35-week postmenstrual age. Four days following the injection, retinal imaging demonstrated a yellowish gray blurred mass that extended into the vitreous in the right eye, and the vitreous body was blurred. After two days, despite starting endophthalmitis treatment, there was still no improvement in the retinal lesion. Due to the worsening of the clinical signs, we decided to perform 25-gauge lens-sparing pars plana vitrectomy.

1. Introduction

Retinopathy of prematurity (ROP) is caused by an abnormality in the development of blood vessels in premature babies. This leads to potential vision loss. It is an important cause of childhood blindness in both developed and developing countries [1]. Peripheral retinal ablation with confluent pattern laser therapy is the traditional treatment for ROP; however, this therapy is destructive, invasive, and not entirely effective against blindness in premature babies [2]. Today, antivascular endothelial growth factor (VEGF) injections stand out as an alternative and up-to-date therapy with good results [3].

Infectious endophthalmitis is the most destructive and scary complication of intravitreal anti-VEGF injections [4]. To our knowledge, the literature contains only two case reports on infectious endophthalmitis after anti-VEGF injections in ROP [4, 5]. Our purpose in this case report is to report the first case of endophthalmitis that developed after aflibercept injection in ROP and to discuss the management of this complication.

2. Case Report

A male infant with a gestational age of 27 weeks and a birth weight of 1,200 g was admitted to the ROP unit of ATR Hospital. A routine retinal screening at 31-week postmenstrual age (PMA) indicated a demarcation line in the posterior retina. Two weeks later, the ridge became marked, and stage 1-2 ROP without plus disease was defined. At 35-week PMA, retinal disease progressed with the retinal image demonstrating stage 2-3 ROP in zone 2 with plus disease (tortuous arteries and dilated veins) in the posterior retina. At this visit, we decided to treat the patient. The parents of the patient were written and verbally informed about the side effects of the treatment options, and it was decided to apply an intravitreal anti-VEGF (aflibercept) injection for the treatment of ROP.

Written informed consent was obtained from the parents before the intravitreal injection. The injection was administered in an operating room. A topical anesthetic, 5 mg proparacaine HCl (Alcaine), was applied to both eyes, and a 5% povidone-iodine solution was applied for surgical asepsis. Then, aflibercept was injected 1.5 mm posterior to the limbus

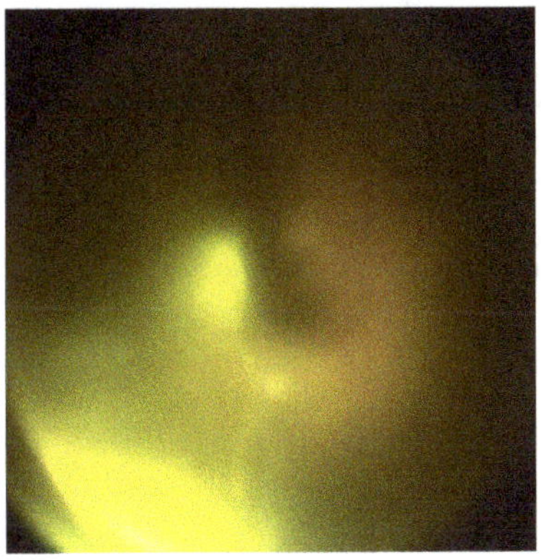

FIGURE 1: Yellowish-gray blurred mass that extended into the vitreous.

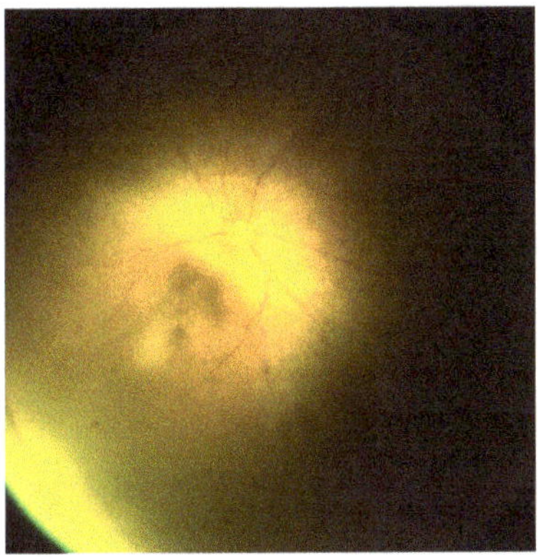

FIGURE 2: Favorable anatomic result was achieved four weeks after the pars plana vitrectomy.

in each eye. As followed in our routine procedure after surgery, a topical antibiotic (moxifloxacin [0.5%] ophthalmic solution) and steroid (dexamethasone ophthalmic solution) combination drop was recommended eight times daily. No systemic antibiotic was applied. Four days following the injection, plus disease and ROP stage were regressed in the left eye but retinal imaging demonstrated a yellowish-gray blurred mass that extended into the vitreous in the right eye, and the vitreous body was blurred (Figure 1). In the right eye, no conjunctival congestion or hypopyon was observed. We diagnosed endophthalmitis based on the characteristics of the retinal lesion and immediately administered empirical therapy through an intravitreal injection of vancomycin (0.5 mg) and ceftazidime (1 mg) to the right eye (half of the adult dosage) after a vitreous tap. Intravenous meropenem (40 mg/kg * 3), vancomycin (15 mg/kg * 3), and amikacin (15 mg single dose) were also started in the neonatal intensive care unit after requesting blood culture analysis. After two days, despite starting endophthalmitis treatment, there was still no improvement in the retinal lesion. The vitreous sample and blood culture were negative for microbiological analysis. Corneal edema started. Due to the worsening of the clinical signs, we decided to perform 25-gauge lens-sparing pars plana vitrectomy (PPV) in the right eye after obtaining informed consent from the parents. The vitreous membranes were removed. Three days after the surgery, retinal imaging demonstrated a decrease in the size of the retinal lesion, the retina was partially clearly seen, and neither ROP nor plus disease was noted. Topical drops and intravenous antibiotics were continued for 10 days. A favorable and satisfactory anatomic result was achieved four weeks after the surgery (Figure 2).

3. Discussion

Anti-VEGF treatment has numerous advantages for the treatment of ROP. However, intravitreal injections may cause noninfectious or infectious intraocular inflammatory reactions [6]. In major studies, no endophthalmitis associated with intravitreal injection has been reported in ROP. To our knowledge, there are two reported cases of endophthalmitis in ROP. Wang and Xiang [4] defined bacterial endophthalmitis in ROP after an intravitreal bevacizumab injection, and Chandra et al. [5] presented a case after an intravitreal ranibizumab injection. We reported the first case of postaflibercept injection endophthalmitis in ROP. Endophthalmitis in infants may involve many challenges, such as the lack of prominent clinical features (e.g., pain, chemosis, edema, and hypopyon), delayed presentation, and difficulty in differentiating between sterile and infectious inflammation. In adults, there are numerous studies showing sterile inflammation after an intravitreal aflibercept injection with favorable outcomes [7]. In contrast, even a suspect of endophthalmitis in ROP should be managed by hospitalization. In our case, only the right eye was inflamed, and despite the absence of other features in endophthalmitis, the case did not appear to have sterile inflammation; thus, it was evaluated as endophthalmitis induced by the intravitreal aflibercept injection. As endophthalmitis may seriously damage vision, it has been suggested that broad-spectrum intravitreal antibiotics, ceftazidime plus vancomycin, should be applied to treat this condition before the differentiation of infective organisms. In addition, intravenous therapy with a wide antimicrobial coverage should be started. Amikacin, meropenem, and tazobactam–piperacillin seem to be ideal empirical systemic antibiotics with higher intravitreal penetration in infants. Studies have shown that an early intravitreal injection of broad-spectrum antibiotics may be an effective and important treatment for premature infants with bacterial endophthalmitis [7, 8]. However, endophthalmitis in ROP necessitates early surgery if the patient does not respond to medical therapy. In our present case, the infection could not be controlled by medical therapy. In cases involving postoperative bacterial endophthalmitis, only 69% of the cultures show positive bacterial growth [9]. Therefore, despite the negative results obtained from the vitreous and blood culture, we accepted the case as infectious. We evaluated no clinical improvement and performed PPV. The role of PPV in the management of endophthalmitis in the pediatric population has been emphasized in previous studies [9]. PPV may be reserved because of higher risk of ocular complications and anesthesia-related mortality and morbidity of endophthalmitis in infants but early PPV and intravitreal vancomycin plus ceftazidime injections have been shown to improve functional and anatomic success in pediatric eyes with exogenous endophthalmitis [10].

The current case also indicates that early PPV may be effective for the management of endophthalmitis in ROP after an intravitreal injection. In conclusion, an intravitreal injection of broad-spectrum antibiotics is administered in medical therapy for endophthalmitis in ROP as the first-line treatment but infants who are unable to complain of a loss of visual acuity may need to be treated by early PPV and intravitreal vancomycin plus ceftazidime injections to improve positive outcomes.

Disclosure

The study was conducted at the Department of Ophthalmology, Antalya Training and Research Hospital, Antalya, Turkey.

Authors' Contributions

The manuscript has been read and approved by all the authors.

References

[1] International Committee for the Classification of Retinopathy of Prematurity, "The international classification of retinopathy of prematurity revisited," *Archives of Ophthalmology*, vol. 123, no. 7, pp. 991–999, 2005.

[2] K. A. Rezai, "Near confluent laser photocoagulation for the treatment of threshold retinopathy of prematurity," *Archives of Ophthalmology*, vol. 123, no. 5, pp. 621-626, 2005.

[3] E. J. Chung, J. H. Kim, H. S. Ahn, and H. J. Koh, "Combination of laser photocoagulation and intravitreal bevacizumab (Avastin®) for aggressive zone I retinopathy of prematurity," *Graefe's Arch Clin Exp Ophthalmol*, vol. 245, no. 11, pp. 1727–1730, 2007.

[4] J. Wang and D. Xiang, "Early clinical characteristics of bacterial endophthalmitis in retinopathy of prematurity after intravitreal bevacizumab injection: a case report," *Experimental and Therapeutic Medicine*, vol. 13, no. 6, pp. 3563–3566, 2017.

[5] P. Chandra, D. Kumawat, R. Tewari, and S. Azimeera, "Post-ranibizumab injection endophthalmitis in aggressive posterior retinopathy of prematurity," *Indian Journal of Ophthalmology*, vol. 67, no. 6, pp. 967–969, 2019.

[6] C. A. Mccannel, "Meta-analysis of endophthalmitis after intravitreal injection of anti-vascular endothelial growth factor agents," *Retina*, vol. 31, no. 4, pp. 654–661, 2011.

[7] P. Hahn, J. E. Kim, S. Stinnett et al., "Aflibercept-related sterile inflammation," *Ophthalmology*, vol. 120, no. 5, pp. 1100-1101.e5, 2013.

[8] S. Basu, A. Kumar, K. Kapoor, N. K. Bagri, and A. Chandra, "Neonatal endogenous endophthalmitis: a report of six cases," *Pediatrics*, vol. 131, no. 4, pp. e1292–e1297, 2013.

[9] "Results of the Endophthalmitis Vitrectomy Study. A randomized trial of immediate vitrectomy and of intravenous antibiotics for the treatment of postoperative bacterial endophthalmitis. Endophthalmitis Vitrectomy Study Group," *Archives of Ophthalmology*, vol. 113, no. 12, pp. 1479–1496, 1995.

[10] M. Çakir, O. Çekiç, G. Pekel, and Ö. F. Yilmaz, "Pars plana vitrectomy results of exogenous endophthalmitis in children," *European Journal of Ophthalmology*, vol. 20, no. 2, pp. 424–428, 2018.

21

Recurrent Herpes Zoster Ophthalmicus Preceded by Anabolic Steroids and High-Dose L-Arginine

Stephen A. LoBue,[1,2] Adam Goldman,[1] Richard A. Giovane,[3] Stacy M. Carlson,[4] Michael Bivona,[1] Sinan Albear,[1] and Thomas D. LoBue[2]

[1]*Department of Ophthalmology, SUNY Downstate, Brooklyn, NY 11203, USA*
[2]*LoBue Laser & Eye Medical Centers, Murrieta, CA 92562, USA*
[3]*LV Stabler Hospital, Greenville, AL 36037, USA*
[4]*Montefiore Medical Center, Bronx, NY 10467, USA*

Correspondence should be addressed to Stephen A. LoBue; slobue87@gmail.com

Academic Editor: Nicola Rosa

Purpose. To report a case of a 34-year-old male with recurrent herpes zoster ophthalmicus (HZO) preceded by a 6-week cycle of anabolic steroids and high-dose amino acid supplementation. *Case Presentation.* A 34-year-old man presented to our institution for left eye pain for one week associated with a vesicular rash in the V1 dermatome, respecting the midline. The patient had no significant past medical or past ocular history, including systemic immunosuppressive agents or HIV. However, prior to the onset of his symptoms the patient had completed a 6-week course of anabolic steroids including trenbolone, deca-durabolin, and testosterone as well as high-dose arginine supplementation averaging more than 40 grams a day. The best-corrected vision was 20/25 OS with slit-lamp examination remarkable for punctate staining and pseudodendrites at 6 o'clock, outside the visual axis. The patient was treated with oral acyclovir 800 mg five times a day for seven days along with prednisolone QID and moxifloxacin QID which was tapered over a month. Four months after resolution, the patient developed a recurrent HZO keratitis preceded by another cycle of anabolic steroids and amino acid supplementation. *Conclusion.* In vitro L-arginine supplementation has been associated with the proliferation and virulence of a variety of herpes viruses. Anabolic steroids have also been demonstrated by various studies to negatively affect cell-mediated immunity necessary to prevent viral infection. Thus, it is possible that anabolic steroids in conjunction with increased L-arginine intake may have precipitated a recurrent HZO in a previously healthy, immunocompetent individual.

1. Introduction

Anabolic-androgenic steroids (AAS), or performance-enhancing drugs, have been used by elite professional athletes and general fitness enthusiasts in order to increase strength and muscle growth. However, the prevalence of anabolic abuse within the USA is not known. Several factors may contribute to the underestimation of anabolic steroid users including insufficient drug tests, on and off cycling of AAS, and taboo or illegal connotation associated with AAS.

AAS comprises a group of synthetic and natural hormones which are structurally and functionally similar to testosterone. Despite the benefits associated with AAS, there are numerous well-known side effects including psychosis, organ damage (e.g., heart, liver, and kidney), hair loss, severe acne, increased risk of tendinitis or tendon rupture, and liver tumors [1]. Also, certain types of AAS have been documented to have immunosuppressive features, impairing B and T cell functions necessary for viral infections [2, 3].

Herpes zoster or shingles is the product of the reactivation of latent varicella zoster virus (VZV). Reactivation of the virus is common in the elderly and immunocompromised, with the rate of incidence increasing in each decade of life and peaking around 80 years old. Approximately 30% of all individuals will develop at least one shingles outbreak in their lifetime [4]. VZV can also affect the eye during the involvement of the ophthalmic division of the fifth cranial nerve (V1), known as herpes zoster ophthalmicus (HZO).

Nevertheless, we noticed an unusual presentation of recurrent HZO in a 34-year-old male, preceded by a 6-week cycle of anabolic steroids and high-dose amino acid supplementation prior to each episode.

2. Case Presentation

A 34-year-old man with no past medical history presented to our clinic complaining of left eye pain and pressure for one week. He was referred by his primary care doctor for suspected HZO, who had started the patient on acyclovir 800 mg 5 times a day prior to his visit to our clinic.

The patient denied any relevant past medical history including diabetes and HIV. He denied smoking, alcohol, or illicit drug use. The patient also denied taking any immunosuppressant agents including prednisone. However, the patient was an active weightlifter who reported having completed a 6-week course of AAS two weeks prior to the onset of his symptoms. His regimen consisted of trenbolone 200 mg, deca-durabolin 200 mg, and testosterone 500 mg a week (Table 1) along with a diet high in protein and supplemental amino acids including arginine. A diet recall averaged above 40 grams of L-arginine a day (Table 2).

On external exam, vesicles were noted over the left eyebrow and upper lid. Anterior segment exam was notable for decreased corneal sensation OS. Slit-lamp examination was remarkable for punctate staining and pseudodendrites at 6 o'clock, outside the visual axis OS. No anterior segment inflammation was noted with intraocular pressure within normal limits. The fundus exam was unremarkable for both eyes.

The patient was continued on oral acyclovir as well as moxifloxacin 0.5% QID and prednisone 1% QID OS which was tapered over a month. The patient was strongly encouraged to stop his AAS regiment as well as high-dose arginine diet/supplementation. HZO keratitis resolved over the course of a month.

Four months later, the patient presented to the clinic with new eye pain OS after completing another cycle of the above AAS and high-arginine diet. Uncorrected visual acuity was 20/40. Slit-lamp examination revealed deep stromal vessels with a 2 × 2 mm infiltrate just inferior to the visual axis at 5 o'clock. Intraocular pressure and fundus exam were unremarkable. The patient was started on acyclovir 800 mg 5 times a day for the next seven days with prednisolone 1% QID. The patient was counseled on stopping AAS as well as the need for a lifelong prophylaxis dose of acyclovir. However, after interval improvement, the patient was lost to follow-up.

3. Discussion

HZO can occur with or without ocular involvement in 10-20% of patients with a vesicular rash in the V1 dermatome [5]. Ocular findings most commonly include conjunctivitis, episcleritis/scleritis, keratitis, uveitis, and less commonly

Table 1: The route, dosage, frequency, and schedule of anabolic-androgenic steroid (AAS) supplementation by the patient prior to each episode of HZO.

Anabolic androgenic steroid	Route	Amount	Frequency	Cycle
Trenbolone	Intramuscular	200 mg	1x week	4 weeks on 2 weeks off
Deca-durabolin	Intramuscular	200 mg	1x week	
Testosterone	Intramuscular	500 mg	1x week	

retinal necrosis which is often seen in immunocompromised patients [6].

VZV is considered a disease of late adulthood, with the rate of incidence increasing in each decade of life, especially when combined with immunocompromised individuals [7]. Although the majority of individuals affected by herpes zoster are over the age of 60 [8], recent trends show a decreasing mean age of onset which is likely due to widespread childhood varicella vaccination [9]. However, other risk factors have been documented for earlier age of onset including immunosuppression from either pharmacological or pathological etiologies (e.g., leukemia/lymphoma, HIV, transplant recipients, and corticosteroids or chemotherapy agents), autoimmune disorders, female gender, smoking, and diabetes [9].

In particular, smoking was the strongest risk factor for earlier age of onset, presenting on average 11.5 years earlier than nonsmokers [9]. Although approximately 30% of all individuals will develop at least one shingles outbreak in their lifetime, recurrent zoster infections are uncommon, ranging from 1.3% to 6.2% [10].

Our patient was a young, healthy 34-year-old individual who developed a recurrent HZO keratitis. He was not an active smoker, diabetic, or immunocompromised via the numerous etiologies listed above. Thus, it is possible that other factors may have contributed to his clinical presentation.

As an active weightlifter, our patient supplemented his diet with high-dose amino acids as well as anabolic steroids. We previously documented a case of recurrent HZO in a young, immunocompetent individual, preceded by high-dose L-arginine at 46.5 g/day [11]. L-arginine is a semiessential amino acid which has been found to have beneficial effects in wound healing, immune function, and metabolism at 4.2 to 20 g/day [12]. Nevertheless, the adverse effects of long-term supplementation above these recommended values have not been well studied [12].

L-Arginine also serves as an essential role in viral replication. Herpes simplex viruses (HSV-1 and HSV-2), varicella-zoster virus (VZV), cytomegalovirus (CMV), and adenovirus require arginine to replicate [13–16]. In vitro studies have demonstrated a decrease in HSV 1-2 replication, cell-to-cell transmission, and virus-mediated cytopathic effects in mediums deficient in L-arginine [13, 17]. Arginase, an enzyme that degrades L-arginine to L-ornithine and urea, was also found to be increased tenfold in a murine model

TABLE 2: A diet recall highlighting food and supplements containing high levels of L-arginine. The daily arginine intake ranged from 29.8–50.7 grams, averaging 40.2 grams/day. Arginine amount derived from the USDA National Nutrient Database (http://www.ars.usda.gov/nutrientdata).

Typical diet	Average amount	Arginine (grams)
Dry roasted nuts (peanuts, almonds, or walnuts)	2 cups	7.65-10.13
Meat (chicken, fish, pork, or beef)	4 cups	9.6-24.0
Whole cooked eggs	3 large	1.22
Cottage cheese	1 cup	2.56
Rice	2 cups	0.76
Supplements (protein powder, preworkout drinks, and amino acids)	Na*	8.0-12.0
Patient range		29.8-50.7
Normal range		6.0-20.0

of HSV-1-induced stromal keratitis infection [17], potentially linking arginine concentrations with symptom resolution. Other researchers also found an accumulation of arginine in the corneal epithelium during herpetic infections, a finding which was attributed to increased viral virulence and replication [17]. Additionally, the use of topical arginase led to a resolution of the herpetic episode, supporting arginine's role in infection and disease progression [18].

Despite these instances where arginine was associated with viral proliferation, other studies have shown that arginine and its derivatives can be viricidal. Naito et al. showed that arginine was effective against inhibiting HSV-1 replication in moderate concentrations while Yamasaki et al. reported that the arginine derivative Nα-Cocoyl-L-arginine ethyl ester was effective at inhibiting HSV extracellular virus particles and replication [19, 20]. The contrasting results of these studies may be due to the variances of arginine being utilized. Isomers of arginine versus arginine complexes are likely to affect the structure and thus function of the amino acid. In most studies, supplementation of arginine did not exceed 30 g/day. Thus, there may be a critical threshold in which arginine dosage can lead to adverse effects which has not been clearly documented in the literature.

The other variable we believe may have influenced the recurrent episodes of HZO in our patient is his use of AAS. Anabolic steroids are not a commonly associated risk factor in HZV outbreaks. Nevertheless, these hormones have been documented to cause immunosuppressive effects. Grossman and Roselle found that one of the biological actions of androgen steroid hormones is the modulation of the immune system through the regulation of T lymphocyte function [2]. In particular, AAS with intact steroid nucleus exhibited a persistent immunosuppressive effect while those with nuclear alterations elicited a delayed immunostimulatory effect [2]. This distinction is important in this case, as our patient reported only taking AAS that had intact steroid nuclei.

The cells most adversely influenced by AAS with an intact steroid nucleus are lymphocytes (T cells) whose differentiation and proliferation are curtailed by reduced natural killer cytotoxic activity and the diminished production of certain cytokines such as IL-2, interferon-gamma (IFN-γ), and corticotropin [21]. These findings are supported in a separate study examining the impact of oxymetholone, another AAS with an intact steroid nucleus. Researchers found a 15% decrease in cytotoxic T cell activity measured in mice taking 300 mg/kg of oxymetholone for fourteen days, indicating that cell-mediated immunity was impaired following exposure [22]. Another study analyzed the role of testosterone in response to the influenza vaccine in animals. Furman et al. found that testosterone was immunosuppressive in vivo, downregulating transcription factors (such as FOS and JUN) implicated in immune activation [3]. One group of experiments demonstrated that orchiectomies of mice led to increased protection against viral, fungal, bacterial, and parasitic infestations [23]. Orchiectomized animals also rejected allografts more rapidly and had accelerated graft-versus-host reactions [23].

Lastly, the role of VZV reactivation within immunosuppressed patients has been analyzed. Patients with depressed cell-mediated immune function from hematopoietic stem cell transplantation were assessed for VZV reactivation while receiving intravenous γ-globulin antibodies. It was observed that the incidence of shingles markedly increased in the study patients, highlighting the importance of cell-mediated immune function in preventing viral reactivation [24].

Therefore, we hypothesize that AAS used by the patient may have compromised his cell-mediated immunity necessary to prevent VZV reactivation. Also, high-dose L-arginine supplementation may have also facilitated increased viral replication and virulence within a potentially immunocompromised individual. Nevertheless, we have only documented two similar cases and require further studies to deem if a real association exists.

4. Conclusion

In summary, we present a 34-year-old, healthy individual who developed recurrent HZO preceded by anabolic steroid abuse and high-dose L-arginine supplementation. In vitro experiments have demonstrated conflicting results between stimulatory versus inhibitory effects on herpes virus replication and virulence with L-arginine. Although data on arginine supplementation is limited, no long-term studies have documented the effects of high-dose arginine supplementation, greater than 20 grams a day, on immune function.

Additionally, the immunosuppressive effects of AAS with intact steroid nucleus on the cell-mediated immune response have been documented in the literature. Increased rates of zoster reactivation have been witnessed in individuals who lack cell-mediated immune systems. Nevertheless, larger, prospective studies are needed to deem if a true association exists between recurrent HZO, L-arginine, and AAS.

Consent

The patient consented to publication of the case in writing. This report does not contain any personal information that could lead to the identification of the patient.

Disclosure

All authors attest that they meet the current ICMJE criteria for Authorship.

References

[1] H.-L. KRÜSKEMPER, "Side effects of anabolic steroids," in *Anabolic Steroids*, pp. 167–183, Academic Press, Cambridge, MA, USA, 1968.

[2] C. L. Mendenhall, C. J. Grossman, G. A. Roselle et al., "Anabolic steroid effects on immune function: differences between analogues," *The Journal of Steroid Biochemistry and Molecular Biology*, vol. 37, no. 1, pp. 71–76, 1990.

[3] D. Furman, B. P. Hejblum, N. Simon et al., "Systems analysis of sex differences reveals an immunosuppressive role for testosterone in the response to influenza vaccination," *Proceedings of the National Academy of Sciences*, vol. 111, no. 2, pp. 869–874, 2014.

[4] Shingles, *Centers for Disease Control and Prevention, Centers for Disease Control and Prevention*, 2019, http://www.cdc.gov/shingles/surveillance.html.

[5] T. J. Liesegang, "Herpes zoster ophthalmicus natural history, risk factors, clinical presentation, and morbidity," *Ophthalmology*, vol. 115, no. 2, pp. S3–12, 2008.

[6] B. P. Yawn, P. C. Wollan, J. L. St Sauver, and L. C. Butterfield, "Herpes zoster eye complications: rates and trends," *Mayo Clinic Proceedings*, vol. 88, no. 6, pp. 562–570, 2013.

[7] R. P. Insinga, R. F. Itzler, J. M. Pellissier, P. Saddier, and A. A. Nikas, "The incidence of herpes zoster in a United States administrative database," *Journal of General Internal Medicine*, vol. 20, no. 8, pp. 748–753, 2005.

[8] R. Harpaz, I. R. Ortega-Sanchez, J. F. Seward, and Advisory Committee on Immunization Practices (ACIP) Centers for Disease Control and Prevention (CDC), "Prevention of herpes zoster: recommendations of the Advisory Committee on Immunization Practices (ACIP)," *MMWR Recomm Rep*, vol. 57, no. RR-5, pp. 1–30, 2008.

[9] A. Y. Chan, C. D. Conrady, K. Ding, J. D. Dvorak, and D. U. Stone, "Factors associated with age of onset of herpes zoster ophthalmicus," *Cornea*, vol. 34, no. 5, pp. 535–540, 2015.

[10] B. P. Yawn, P. C. Wollan, M. J. Kurland, J. L. St Sauver, and P. Saddier, "Herpes zoster recurrences more frequent than previously reported," *Mayo Clinic Proceedings*, vol. 86, no. 2, pp. 88–93, 2011.

[11] S. A. LoBue, P. Tailor, S. M. Carlson et al., "Recurrent herpes zoster ophthalmicus in a young, healthy individual taking high doses of l-arginine," *American Journal of Ophthalmology Case Reports*, vol. 16, p. 100547, 2019.

[12] A. Shao and J. N. Hathcock, "Risk assessment for the amino acids taurine, L-glutamine and L-arginine," *Regulatory Toxicology and Pharmacology*, vol. 50, no. 3, pp. 376–399, 2008.

[13] R. W. Tankersley, "Amino acid requirements of herpes simplex virus in human cells," *Journal of Bacteriology*, vol. 87, no. 3, pp. 609–613, 1964.

[14] E. Gönczöl, I. Boldogh, and L. Váczi, "Effect of arginine deficiency on the reproduction of human cytomegalovirus," *Acta Microbiologica Academiae Scientiarum Hungaricae*, vol. 22, no. 3, pp. 263–270, 1975.

[15] R. Wigand and G. Kümel, "Amino acid requirement of adenovirus multiplication," *The Journal of General Virology*, vol. 39, no. 2, pp. 281–292, 1978.

[16] M. D. Sanchez, A. C. Ochoa, and T. P. Foster, "Development and evaluation of a host-targeted antiviral that abrogates herpes simplex virus replication through modulation of arginine-associated metabolic pathways," *Antiviral Research*, vol. 132, pp. 13–25, 2016.

[17] S. K. Mistry, M. Zheng, B. T. Rouse, and S. M. Morris, "Induction of arginases I and II in cornea during herpes simplex virus infection," *Virus Research*, vol. 73, no. 2, pp. 177–182, 2001.

[18] I. L. Kahán, K. Hajas, and A. Halász, "The significance of the arginine and arginase of tears in experimentally-induced herpes simplex corneae," *Albrecht von Graefes Archiv für Klinische und Experimentelle Ophthalmologie*, vol. 209, no. 3, pp. 219–224, 1979.

[19] T. Naito, H. Irie, K. Tsujimoto, K. Ikeda, T. Arakawa, and A. H. Koyama, "Antiviral effect of arginine against herpes simplex virus type 1," *International Journal of Molecular Medicine*, vol. 23, no. 4, pp. 495–499, 2009.

[20] H. Yamasaki, K. Tsujimoto, K. Ikeda, Y. Suzuki, T. Arakawa, and A. H. Koyama, "Antiviral and virucidal activities of nα-cocoyl-L-arginine ethyl ester," *Adv Virol*, vol. 2011, pp. 1–6, 2011.

[21] T. K. Hughes, E. Fulep, T. Juelich, E. M. Smith, and G. J. Stanton, "Modulation of immune responses by anaboloic androgenic steroids," *International Journal of Immunopharmacology*, vol. 17, pp. 857–863, 1995.

[22] N. A. Karrow, J. A. McCay, R. Brown et al., "Oxymetholone modulates cell-mediated immunity in male B6C3F1 mice," *Drug and Chemical Toxicology*, vol. 23, no. 4, pp. 621–644, 2000.

[23] S. A. Ahmed and N. Talal, "Effects of sex hormones on immune responses and autoimmune diseases: an update," *American Journal of Pathology*, pp. 333–337, 1999.

[24] M. Oxman, "Herpes zoster pathogenesis and cell-mediated immunity and immunosenescence," *Journal of the American Osteopathic Association*, vol. 109, no. 6, pp. S13–S17, 2009.

22

Sodium-Glucose Cotransporter 2 Inhibitors Improve Chronic Diabetic Macular Edema

Yoko Takatsuna,[1,2] Ryoichi Ishibashi,[3,4] Tomoaki Tatsumi,[2] Masaya Koshizaka,[5] Takayuki Baba,[2] Shuichi Yamamoto,[2] and Koutaro Yokote[4,5]

[1]*Department of Ophthalmology, Chiba Rosai Hospital, Ichihara, Chiba, Japan*
[2]*Department of Ophthalmology and Visual Science, Chiba University Graduate School of Medicine, Chiba, Japan*
[3]*Department of Medicine, Division of Diabetes, Endocrinology and Metabolism, Kimitsu Chuo Hospital, Kisarazu, Chiba, Japan*
[4]*Department of Endocrinology, Hematology and Gerontology, Graduate School of Medicine, Chiba University, Chiba, Japan*
[5]*Division of Diabetes, Metabolism and Endocrinology, Chiba University Hospital, Chiba, Japan*

Correspondence should be addressed to Yoko Takatsuna; yoko_takatsuna@chibah.johas.go.jp

Academic Editor: Stephen G. Schwartz

Purpose. Diabetic macular edema (DME) is a vision-threatening condition that develops in diabetic patients. The first-line therapy for DME is intravitreal injections of antivascular endothelial growth factor (anti-VEGF) agents; however, the high frequency of repeat injections, invasiveness of the procedure, and high cost are drawbacks for this treatment. The purpose of this report is to present our findings in 3 patients with chronic DME whose edema was resolved soon after oral doses of sodium-glucose cotransporter-2 (SGLT2) inhibitors were used. *Case Presentation*. Case 1 was a 66-year-old woman diagnosed with moderate nonproliferative diabetic retinopathy (DR) with DME that had developed a decade earlier. The DME persisted for 4 years in the left eye. The addition of oral empagliflozin, a SGLT2 inhibitor, led to a marked improvement of the DME after one month, and this improvement continued over two years. Case 2 was a 68-year-old woman who was diagnosed with preproliferative DR with bilateral DME. The addition of oral dapagliflozin led to the improvement of the DME after two months, and this improvement continued over one year. Case 3 was a 61-year-old woman who was diagnosed with moderate nonproliferative DR with DME. Oral luseogliflozin was given which led to better glycemic control, and her left central retinal thickness (CRT) was markedly reduced after only two weeks. This reduction was maintained in her left eye for six months without any additional ophthalmic procedures. *Conclusions*. Although this study involved only three cases, our findings indicate that SGLT2 inhibitors might have possible efficacy for chronic DME.

1. Introduction

Diabetic retinopathy (DR) is a frequent cause of blindness in working-age individuals. Diabetic macular edema (DME) is one of the vision-reducing conditions that is associated with DR, and the number of patients with DME increases with the advancement of the retinopathy.

At present, the standard treatment for DME is intravitreal injections of anti-vascular endothelial growth factor (VEGF) agents. A number of clinical studies have shown the superiority of anti-VEGF therapy over laser photocoagulation or steroid injections to treat DME [1, 2]. However, there are some problems with the anti-VEGF therapy; the need for frequent repeat injections and the high cost of anti-VEGF agents are obstacles for their more frequent use. In addition, DME can persist even after the anti-VEGF treatment in approximately 31.6 to 65.6% of the patients [3].

Sodium-glucose cotransporter 2 (SGLT2) inhibitors are a new treatment option for patients with type 2 diabetes mellitus that improves the glycemic control by inhibiting the reabsorption of glucose in the proximal renal tubules leading to an increase in renal glucose extraction [4]. Approximately 90% of the glucose in glomerular filtrates is reabsorbed by the proximal renal tubule and returned to the blood. SGLT2 is present in the proximal renal tubule, and it cotransports glucose and sodium from the glomerular filtrate back into

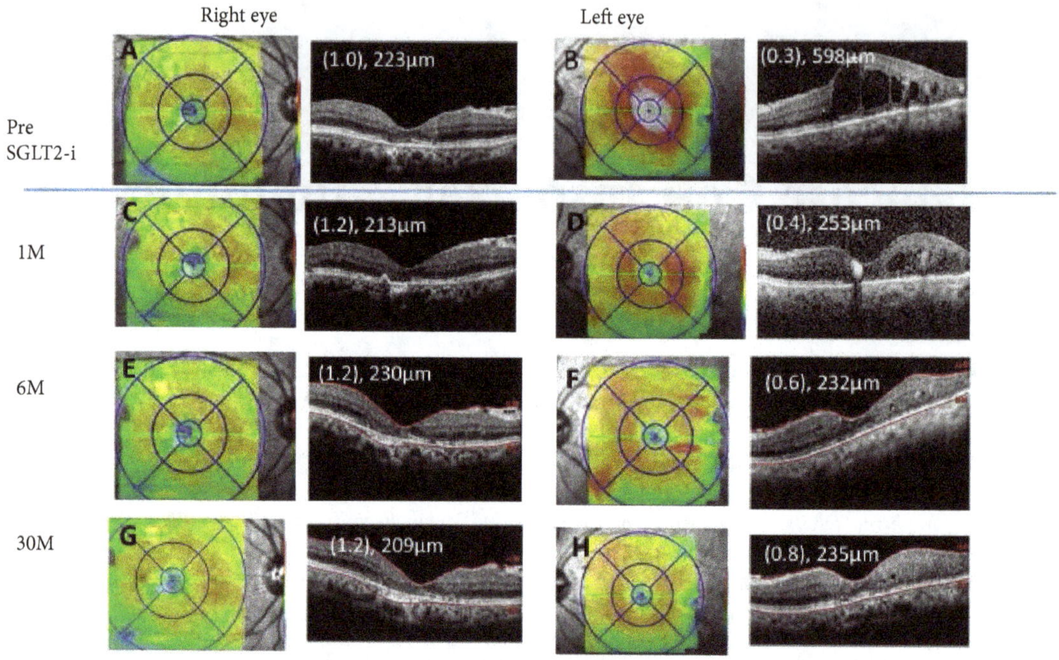

FIGURE 1: Case 1. Optical coherence tomographic images and fundus photographs showing the central retinal thickness (CRT) pre (A, B), at 1 month (M) (C, D), 6 M (E, F), and 30 M (G, H) after commencing the oral sodium-glucose cotransporter 2 inhibitor (SGLT2i).

the blood. SGLT2 inhibitors interfere with the glucose reabsorption, and the glucose is excreted in the urine. Recent large-scale clinical trials have demonstrated that SGLT2 inhibitors prevent or reduce mortality, heart failures [5], and the progression of renal impairment [6] in diabetic patients. In addition, studies have shown the presence of SGLT2 in retinal pericytes and mesangial cells [7]. Hyperglycemia results in functional and morphological changes in these cells, but these effects are attenuated by SGLT inhibitors. Although SGLT inhibitors have been shown to be helpful in maintaining the general condition in diabetic patients, their effect on the DME in patients with DR has not been determined.

We report our findings in three patients with type 2 diabetes with chronic DME who were refractory to anti-VEGF therapies and other therapies. However, the three cases had a marked improvement of the DME soon after an oral SGLT2 inhibitor was begun. All patients had chronic DME lasting for more than 5 years and had undergone laser and/or anti-VEGF and/or steroid injections.

2. Case Presentation

2.1. Case 1. A 66-year-old woman was diagnosed with moderate nonproliferative DR with DME bilaterally a decade earlier. She underwent focal laser photocoagulation in both eyes, and the decimal best-corrected visual acuity (BCVA) in her right eye improved to 1.0, but it did not improve in her left eye. She did not agree to further therapy such as anti-VEGF for the left eye, because the BCVA in her right eye was good and the high cost of anti-VEGF agents. The macular edema in the left eye persisted for 4 years with a decimal BCVA of 0.3 and a central retinal thickness (CRT) of 598 μm (Figure 1(B)). Six months later, the macular edema was completely resolved (Figure 1(D)). One month before this ophthalmic visit, her glycemic control deteriorated to a glycated hemoglobin A1c of 7.4%, and her general physician prescribed 25 mg of oral empagliflozin, an SGLT2 inhibitor. The CRT in her left eye decreased to 253 μm (Figure 1(D)) at one month after beginning the SGLT2 inhibitor treatment. Six months later (Figure 1(F)), her body weight was reduced, and the glycemic control was improved with the glycated hemoglobin A1c of 6.5% (Table 1). The CRT reduction was maintained for over two years without other ophthalmic therapy. The clinical course of the macular edema before and after the administration of the SGLT2 inhibitor is shown in Figure 1. The final decimal BCVA improved to 0.8, and the CRT measured by optical coherence tomography (OCT) was 235 μm (Figure 1(H)) at 30 months after commencing the SGLT2 inhibitor.

2.2. Case 2. A 68-year-old woman was diagnosed with preproliferative DR 6 years earlier, and panretinal photocoagulation had been performed. However, the DME gradually developed beginning 5 years earlier. She was treated twice with intravitreal injections of ranibizumab and a sub-Tenon injection of triamcinolone acetonide in her left eye. In her right eye, she received 7 intravitreal injections of aflibercept and focal-grid laser photocoagulation. However, the DME persisted, and her decimal BCVA was 0.6 in the right eye and 0.3 in the left eye. The CRT was 519 μm in the right eye and 467 μm in the left eye (Figure 2(A) and (B)). Oral dapagliflozin was administered to improve the glycemic control. At the beginning of the dapagliflozin, her glycated hemoglobin A1c was 7.0%; however, her glycemic control was exacerbated by overconsumption; although, the refractory DME was improved. Two months later, the CRT was thinner in her left eye (Figure 2(D)), and six months later,

Table 1: Summary of three cases of DME pre and 6 months (M) after the SGLT2-i administration.

	Case 1		Case 2		Case 3	
	Pre	6 M after SGLT2-i	Pre	6 M after SGLT2-i	Pre	6 M after SGLT2-i
Age (yrs)/sex	66/F		68/F		61/F	
Body height (cm)	158		156		153	
Body weight (kg)	49.1	45.2	43	41.1	46.1	45
Blood pressure (mmHg)	150/82	136/62	128/70	126/74	124/77	121/70
SGLT2 inhibitor	—	Empagliflozin 25 mg	—	Dapagliflozin 5 mg	—	Luseogliflozin 2.5 mg
Diabetes treatment	Vildagliptin 100 mg Glimepiride 1.5 mg	Vildagliptin 100 mg	Alogliptin 25 mg Acarbose 300 mg Metformin 500 mg	Acarbose 300 mg Metformin 500 mg	—	—
Ophthalmic treatment; OD	Focal laser	—	Focal/grid laser IVA ×7	—	Focal laser, IVA ×1	—
; OS	Focal laser	—	IVR ×2, STTA ×2	—	Focal laser ×3, IVA ×5, STTA ×2	—
Central retinal thickness (μm) OD/OS	223/598	230/232	519/467	491/326	613/412	451/273
Visual acuity OD/OS	(1.0)/(0.3)	(1.2)/(0.6)	(0.3)/(0.3)	(0.6)/(0.3)	(1.0)/(1.0)	(1.0)/(1.0)
HgA1c (%)	7.4	6.5	7.0	7.9	6.5	6.1
Blood glucose (mg/dL)	116	118	118	129	113	100
Total protein (g/dL)	ND	6.5	6.4	6.9	7.6	ND
Albumin (g/dL)	ND	ND	ND	4.1	4.2	ND
Aspartate aminotransferase (U/L)	ND	18	12	12	21	22
Alanine aminotransferase (U/L)	ND	13	11	11	18	18
Creatinine (mg/dL)	0.47	0.42	0.61	0.65	0.59	0.62
U-protein (qualitative analysis)	—	—	—	±	—	—
U-albumin (mg/g⊠Cre)	8.7	6.9	ND	ND	24.8	ND

DME: diabetic macular edema; SGLT2-i: SGLT2 inhibitor; OD: oculus dexter; OS: oculus sinister; IVA: intravitreal injection of aflibercept; IVR: intravitreal injection of ranibizumab; STTA: sub-Tenon injection of triamcinolone acetonide.

the CRT was reduced to 491 μm in the right eye (Figure 2(G)) and 326 μm in the left eye (Figure 2(H)). Her BCVA was 0.6 in the right eye and 0.3 in the left. At six months, her body weight was reduced; although, the glycated hemoglobin A1c was elevated to 7.9% (Table 1). The clinical course of the macular edema is shown in Figure 2. A sub-Tenon injection of triamcinolone acetonide was administered to her right eye at eight months. Her final BCVA was 0.8 in the right eye and 0.4 in the left eye, and the CRT was 378 μm in the right (Figure 2(I)), 305 μm in the left (Figure 2(J)) at twelve months.

2.3. Case 3. A 61-year-old woman was diagnosed with moderate nonproliferative DR without DME 7 years earlier. She had undergone bilateral cataract surgery 5 years earlier, and her BCVA had recovered to 1.0, but there was a gradual development of macular edema. She received 2 sub-Tenon injections of triamcinolone acetonide, 5 intravitreal injections of aflibercept, and focal laser treatment in her left eye. She received 1 intravitreal injection of aflibercept and a focal laser treatment in her right eye. Despite these treatments, the CRT was still 613 μm in the right eye (Figure 3(A)) and 412 μm in the left eye (Figure 3(B)); although, the decimal BCVA was 1.0 in both eyes. Her BCVAs were maintained, and she did not agree to continue anti-VEGF therapy. Oral luseogliflozin 2.5 mg was administered, and the CRT of both eyes (Figure 3(C) and (D)) began to decrease by two weeks after commencing the luseogliflozin. This reduction continued for six months. Six months later, her CRT was reduced to 451 μm in the right eye (Figure 3(I)) and 273 μm in the left eye (Figure 3(J)). The BCVA was maintained at 1.0 in both eyes. Her body weight was reduced at six months, and the glycated hemoglobin A1c was reduced from 6.5% to 6.1% at six months (Table 1).

3. Discussion

The findings in these three cases suggested that SGLT2 inhibitors can improve the chronic DME which was resistant to standard ophthalmic therapies. Anti-VEGF drugs are the

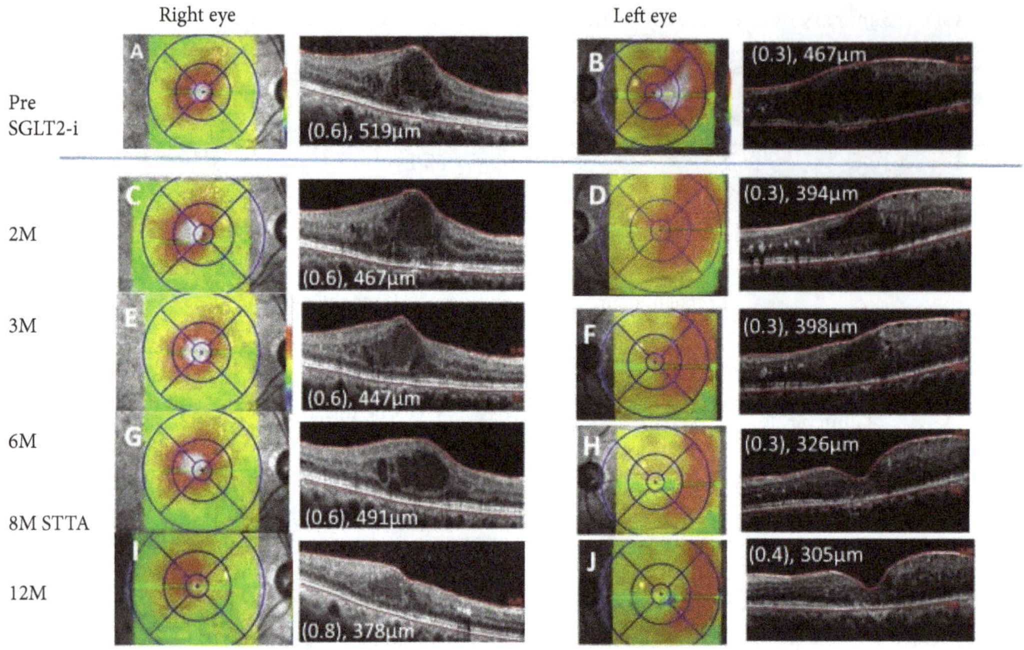

Figure 2: Case 2. Optical coherence tomographic images and fundus photographs showing the central retinal thickness (CRT) pre (A, B) and at 2 months (M) (C, D), 3 M (E, F), 6 M (G, H), and 12 M (I, J) after commencing the oral sodium-glucose cotransporter 2 inhibitor (SGLT2i). A sub-Tenon injection of triamcinolone acetonide (STTA) was administered in her right eye at eight months.

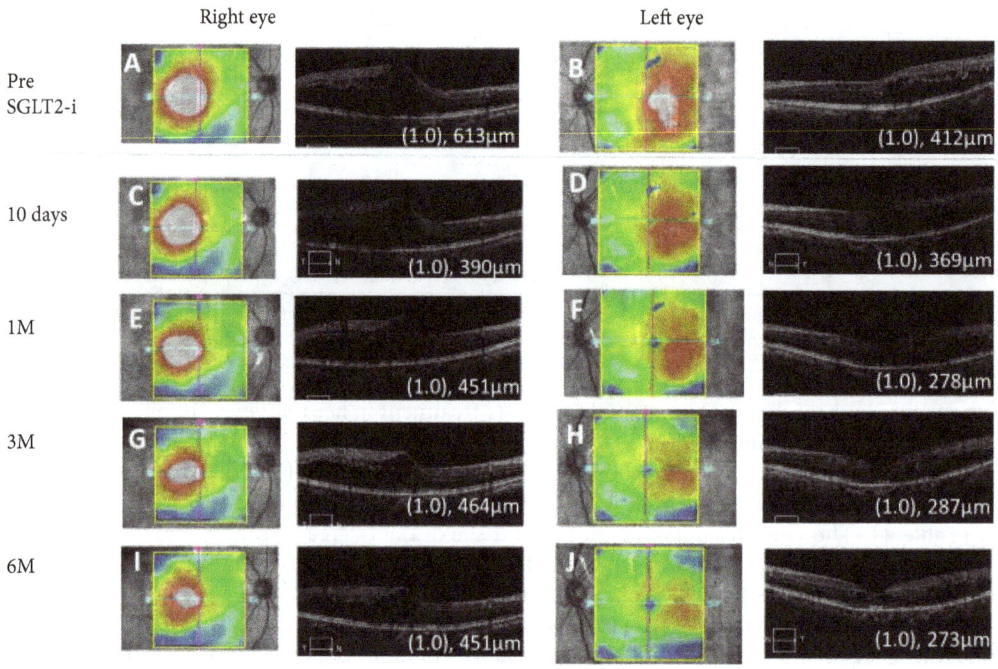

Figure 3: Case 3. Optical coherence tomographic images and fundus photographs showing the central macular thickness (CRT) pre (A, B) and at 10 days (C, D), 1 month (M) (E, F), 3 M (G, H), and 6 M (I, J) after commencing the oral sodium-glucose cotransporter 2 inhibitor (SGLT2i).

first-line therapy for center-involved DMEs [1, 2]; however, they are costly, and clinical patients receive approximately three injections per year in Japan [8]. Our three patients did not agree to the frequent anti-VEGF injections due to their high costs, and reducing the number of anti-VEGF injections can lead to an overall decrease in the efficacy as seen in randomized trials [1, 2]. DME pathology persisted in all three cases following the multimodal therapy including steroid injections and focal/grid laser photocoagulation in our cases. However, stabilization and recovery were observed soon after the oral administration of a SGLT2 inhibitor. Notably, the improvements were detected as soon as two weeks after the initiation of the SGLT2 inhibitor in Case 3, and the improvements were maintained for at least 2 years in Case 1.

There is no evidence that internal medications have positive effects on DME, but two studies have reported the effectiveness of SGLT2 inhibitors for the treatment of DME [9, 10]. One study reported on the efficacy of SGLT2 inhibitors on the vitrectomized eyes of five patients [9]. However, vitrectomy is not the standard or even the preferential treatment for DME, and anti-VEGF therapy or other standard treatments were omitted in that study. An additional study presented a case of a DME patient who was given ipragliflozin. The patient was not treated with any anti-VEGF before the SGLT2-inhibitor administration, and OCT showed no significant changes after 24 weeks of SGLT2-inhibitor administration [10].

The precise mechanism by which SGLT2 inhibitors resolve the DME was not determined. Weight loss was observed in all cases, and the rapid effects of the SGLT2 inhibitors may be related to its diuretic effects. In Case 2, however, the blood glycemic level did not improve, suggesting that a short period of glycemic control improvement by SGLT2 inhibitors may not have a direct effect on the DME.

Empagliflozin reduces the risk of major adverse cardiovascular events [5] and reduces the progression of kidney diseases [6]. SGLT2 inhibitors may improve DME via systemic fluid adjustments.

One in vitro study reported that phlorizin, an SGLT inhibitor, attenuated the high glucose-induced morphological and functional changes in cultured bovine retinal pericytes [11].The expression of SGLT1 and SGLT2 in the eye including the retina has been reported in several papers [7, 12]. SGLT2 inhibitors remove excess glucose from the retinal microcirculation and hence reduce glucotoxicity, oxidative stress, low-grade inflammation, and restore insulin signaling. By preventing continued glucose-induced vascular dysfunction, the progression of microangiopathy and especially DR is improved [13, 14]. The long-lasting effect of SGLT2 inhibitors might be related to the reduction of the glucose-induced vascular endothelial dysfunction.

It has been well established that anti-VEGF therapy is the mainstay treatment for DME, and oral SGLT2 inhibitors combined with anti-VEGF injections may be additive and a good option for refractory DME.

There are some limitations in this study. Only three cases with widely different histories were studied, and all cases were undertreated with anti-VEGF agents compared to the standardized regimens. Additionally, three different SGLT2 inhibitors were prescribed to the three patients; all were effective in reducing the degree of DME, but their mechanism of action has not been clearly determined.

Therefore, we are planning a multicenter, randomized, open-label trial to investigate the safety and efficacy of combination therapy of anti-VEGF drug injections and SGLT2 inhibitors in patients with type 2 diabetes and DME [15].

In conclusion, our results showed an improvement of chronic DME after the initiation of oral SGLT2 inhibitors. SGLT2 inhibitors might be a novel, noninvasive, and low-cost treatment for DME.

Acknowledgments

The authors thank Professor Emeritus Duco Hamasaki of the Bascom Palmer Eye Institute for discussions and for editing the manuscript.

References

[1] The Diabetic Retinopathy Clinical Research Network, "Aflibercept, bevacizumab, or ranibizumab for diabetic Macular edema," *New England Journal of Medicine*, vol. 372, no. 13, pp. 1193–1203, 2015.

[2] P. Mitchell, F. Bandello, U. Schmidt-Erfurth et al., "The RESTORE study: ranibizumab monotherapy or combined with laser versus laser monotherapy for diabetic macular edema," *Ophthalmology*, vol. 118, no. 4, pp. 615–625, 2011.

[3] N. M. Bressler, W. T. Beaulieu, A. R. Glassman et al., "Persistent macular thickening following intravitreous aflibercept, bevacizumab, or ranibizumab for central-involved diabetic macular edema with vision impairment: a secondary analysis of a randomized clinical trial," *JAMA Ophthalmology*, vol. 136, no. 3, pp. 257–269, 2018.

[4] G. E. Dailey, "Empagliflozin: a new treatment option for patients with type 2 diabetes mellitus," *Drugs of Today*, vol. 51, no. 9, pp. 519–535, 2015.

[5] B. Zinman, C. Wanner, J. M. Lachin et al., "Empagliflozin, cardiovascular outcomes, and mortality in type 2 diabetes," *New England Journal of Medicine*, vol. 373, no. 22, pp. 2117–2128, 2015.

[6] C. Wanner, S. E. Inzucchi, J. M. Lachin et al., "Empagliflozin and progression of kidney disease in type 2 diabetes," *New England Journal of Medicine*, vol. 375, no. 4, pp. 323–334, 2016.

[7] M. Wakisaka and T. Nagao, "Sodium glucose cotransporter 2 in mesangial cells and retinal pericytes and its implications for diabetic nephropathy and retinopathy," *Glycobiology*, vol. 27, no. 8, pp. 691–695, 2017.

[8] M. Sugimoto, H. Tsukitome, F. Okamoto et al., "Clinical preferences and trends of anti-vascular endothelial growth factor treatments for diabetic macular edema in Japan," *Journal of Diabetes Investigation*, vol. 10, no. 2, pp. 475–483, 2019.

[9] H. Mieno, K. Yoneda, M. Yamazaki, R. Sakai, C. Sotozono, and M. Fukui, "The efficacy of sodium-glucose cotransporter 2 (SGLT2) inhibitors for the treatment of chronic diabetic macular oedema in vitrectomised eyes: a retrospective study," *BMJ Open Opthalmology*, vol. 3, no. 1, article e000130, 2018.

[10] H. Yoshizumi, T. Ejima, T. Nagao, and M. Wakisaka, "Recovery from diabetic macular edema in a diabetic patient after minimal dose of a sodium glucose co-trasporter 2 inhibitor," *American Journal of Case Reports*, vol. 19, pp. 462–466, 2018.

[11] M. Wakisaka, M. Yoshinari, T. Asano et al., "Normalization of glucose entry under the high glucose condition by phlorizin attenuates the high glucose-induced morphological and functional changes of cultured bovine retinal pericytes," *Biochimica et Biophysica Acta*, vol. 1453, no. 1, pp. 83–91, 1999.

[12] L. Y. Herat, V. B. Matthews, P. E. Rakoczy, R. Carnagarin, and M. Schlaich, "Focusing on sodium glucose cotransporter-2 and the sympathetic nervous system: potential impact in diabetic retinopathy," *International Journal of Endocrinology*, vol. 2018, Article ID 9254126, 8 pages, 2018.

[13] M. Oelze, S. Kröller-Schön, P. Welschof et al., "The sodium-glucose co-transporter 2 inhibitor Empagliflozin improves diabetes-induced vascular dysfunction in the streptozotocin diabetes rat model by interfering with oxidative stress and glucotoxicity," *PLoS One*, vol. 9, no. 11, article e112394, 2014.

[14] M. May, T. Framke, B. Junker, C. Framme, A. Pielen, and C. Schindler, "How and why SGLT2 inhibitors should be explored as potential treatment option in diabetic retinopathy: clinical concept and methodology," *Therapeutic Advances in Endocrinology and Metabolism*, vol. 10, 2019.

[15] R. Ishibashi, Y. Takatsuna, M. Koshizaka et al., "Safety and efficacy of ranibizumab and luseogliflozin combination therapy in patients with diabetic macular edema: protocol for a multicenter, open-label randomized controlled trial," *Diabetes Therapy*, vol. 11, no. 8, pp. 1891–1905, 2020.

23

Exophiala Keratitis following Descemet Stripping Automated Endothelial Keratoplasty

Ana Marta, Paula Costa, Virgínia Lopes, Miguel Mesquita Neves, Miguel Gomes, and Luís Oliveira

Department of Ophthalmology, Centro Hospitalar e Universitário do Porto, Oporto, Portugal

Correspondence should be addressed to Ana Marta; analuisamarta2@gmail.com

Academic Editor: Sandra M. Johnson

Purpose. To report a case with *Exophiala spp.* keratitis in a Portuguese patient. *Methods.* A case report with deep corneal brown-pigmented infiltrates that developed 2 months after a Descemet Stripping Automated Endothelial Keratoplasty (DSAEK) for pseudophakic bullous keratopathy. *Results.* Diagnosis was established by positive direct examination and cultures from the surgically obtained corneal button. Slit-lamp images and anterior segment optical coherence tomography (AS-OCT) scans were obtained. *Conclusion.* This is the first described case of fungal keratitis caused by Exophiala spp. in Portugal and, to our knowledge, the first case following DSAEK in the literature.

1. Introduction

The black yeast genus *Exophiala* belongs to the order Chaetothyriales and represents over 40 different yeast species that occur as saprobes on plants [1]. *Exophiala xenobiotica* is a segregant of the *Exophiala jeanselmei* complex, frequently found in habitats rich in monoaromatic hydrocarbons and alkanes [2]. Eye infections due to *Exophiala* species are extremely rare but have been reported [3].

Fungal keratitis is responsible for approximately 40% of all corneal ulcers in certain tropical climate countries but has a much lower incidence in temperate climates [1]. Fungal infection is an exceedingly rare complication following Descemet Stripping Automated Endothelial Keratoplasty (DSAEK), and it is always severe [4]. These infections tend to present in the late postoperative period as one or multiple infiltrates at the graft-host interface of the deep stroma. They are difficult to manage because the interface provides a unique sheltered environment [5].

We report a case that developed *Exophiala* spp. interface keratitis after DSAEK. This is the first described case of fungal keratitis caused by Exophiala spp. in Portugal and, to our knowledge, the first case following DSAEK in the literature.

2. Case Report

A 68-year-old male, diagnosed with pseudophakic bullous keratopathy (PBK), underwent DSAEK in the right eye (RE). A postoperative follow-up was uneventful under a topical and systemic steroid regimen. The patient reported a history of eye infection caused by pine processionary (Thaumetopoea pityocampa), diagnosed and treated at a different hospital, 9 months before DSAEK. At the time of DSAEK, signs of eye infection were no longer reported. Two months after DSAEK, he was referred to our hospital due to keratitis on the RE (Figure 1). On examination, the best corrected visual acuity (BCVA) of the right eye (RE) was 20/200 and 20/20 in the LE. The pupils were isocoric and isoreactive, without afferent pupillary defect. He had no pain with ocular movements. The biomicroscopic examination of the RE revealed brown multilobular lesions within deep corneal

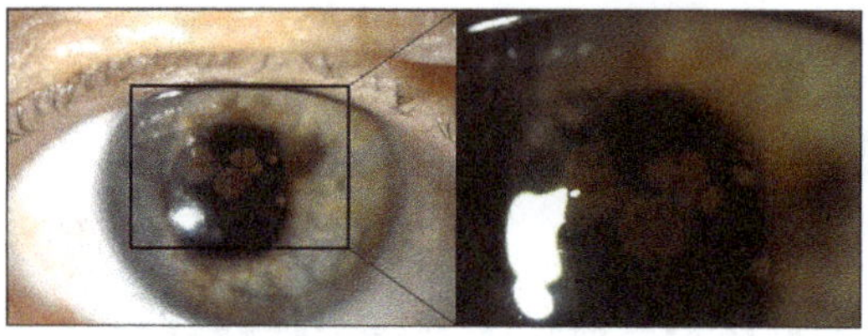

Figure 1: Slit-lamp image of the right eye at presentation. Dark multilobular lesions within deep stroma and a Descemet Stripping Automated Endothelial Keratoplasty graft as a subtle ring.

stroma, with no conjunctival hyperaemia, secretions, or epithelial defect. The anterior chamber was deep and clear. Intraocular pressure and fundus examination were normal. The examination of his LE revealed no abnormality. An anterior segment optical coherence tomography (AS-OCT) (Spectralis®; Heidelberg Engineering, Heidelberg, Germany) was used to document the stromal infiltrate, showing the central infiltrate affecting all layers and the peripheral infiltrate concentrating in deep stroma (Figure 2). Given the spread and extent of the infection, an urgent surgical approach was chosen; therefore, no topical or systemic antifungal was performed before surgery. The patient underwent therapeutic penetrating keratoplasty (PK) using 8.0 mm diameter graft over a 7.75 mm patient's cornea trephination and 16 interrupted nylon 10/00 sutures, with no incident. After PK, the medical treatment used included standard approach, but with lower doses of systemic and topical corticosteroids due to suspected fungal etiology. The storage medium of the graft and patient's corneal button were sent to microbiologic examination. Diagnosis was established by a positive direct examination and culture (Figure 3) of the same fungus from the surgically obtained corneal button. There were no signs of recurrence of the infection during an extremely frequent initial follow-up; it was therefore decided not to medicate with antifungals, avoiding their associated toxicity. At 6 months of follow-up, no clinical signs of fungal infection developed and visual acuity was 20/200 without correction, but not all sutures had been removed.

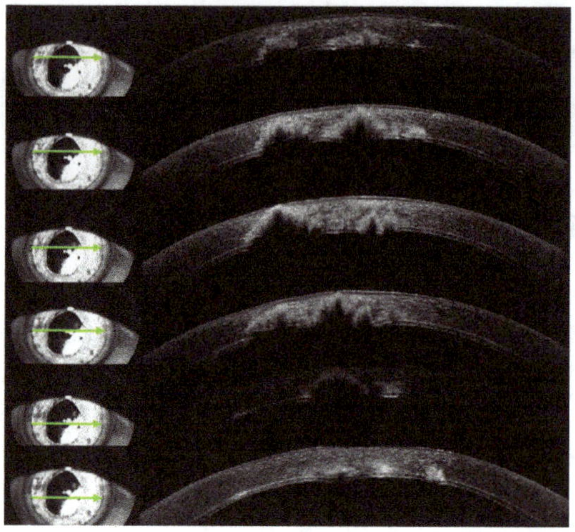

Figure 2: Anterior segment optical coherence tomography images of the patient at presentation. Graft-host interface and the stromal infiltrate with a shadow in the corneal stroma underlying the fungal lesion.

3. Discussion

Few cases of keratitis caused by *Exophiala spp.* have been reported: *E. dermatitidis* keratitis after keratoplasty [6] and after laser in situ keratomileusis [7], *E. jeanselmei* keratitis after minor trauma [8, 9], and soft contact lens use [10] and *E. phaeomuriformis* keratitis after severe ocular surface problems [1]. *Exophiala xenobiotica* is a rare strain of *Exophiala*, and no case of keratitis caused by this agent has been previously reported. Common risk factors predisposing of mycotic keratitis are refractive contact lens wear, ocular surface disease, ocular trauma, and chronic topical corticosteroid therapy. Corneal pigmented lesions could also be caused by corneal melanoma or corneal melanin deposition caused by topical epinephrine therapy. The medical history can be important to form differential diagnoses.

In our case, the origin of the fungal infection remained unknown. Potential sources of this particular fungal organism in this patient are susceptibility to infectious keratitis due to steroid therapy after DASEK in a previously asymptomatic carrier: infected donor cornea or contamination of the graft from airborne particles, irrigation solutions, or instruments. The characteristics of AS-OCT suggest the lesions started in the posterior corneal layers, making infected donor cornea or contamination during graft manipulation the most likely causes. Despite the patient's history of Thaumetopoea pityocampa infection, this is an unlikely source, due to no association with *Exophiala xenobiotica* being reported and the absence of infection reported at the time of DSAEK. Microbiological analysis of the donor corneal rim could allow the diagnosis of donor cornea infection; however, this was not performed. In fact, routine culture of donor corneal rims remains controversial. Fungi, when isolated from donor corneal rims, have more risk to lead a clinical infection than bacteria [11]. Thus, the culture of the donor corneal rim (special fungal culture) in cases of lamellar or endothelial keratoplasty could allow for an early detection and treatment [12, 13].

Due to the generally poor response to medical treatment or of graft lenticule removal, we opted to perform a therapeutic penetrating keratoplasty.

This case highlights the possibility of corneal infection by less common organisms in temperate regions such as *Exophiala spp.* and in less likely situations. We should suspect a fungal infection if an infiltrate appears in the graft-host interface several weeks after DSAEK. Donor rim cultures are useful for more complete diagnosis as long as culture times should be long enough for fastidious organism to grow.

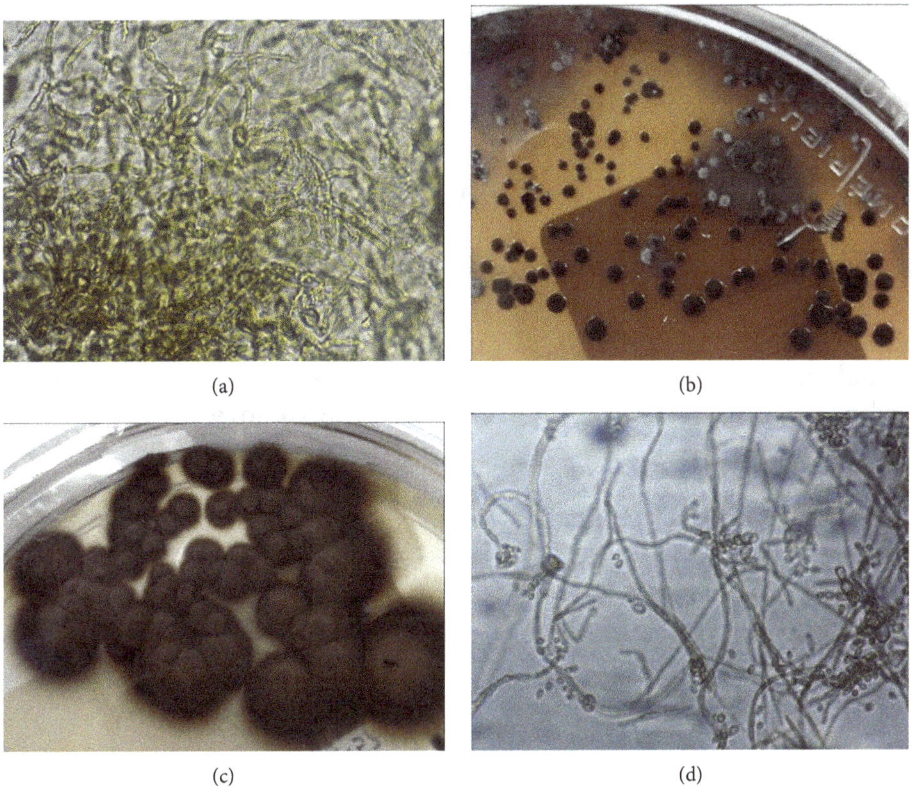

Figure 3: Microbiological examination. (a) Direct microscopy of ocular exudate: pigmented septate hyphae with some yeast cells. (b) Primary culture in blood agar medium and incubated at 37°C: black yeast colonies. (c) Primary culture in Sabouraud agar medium and incubated at 25°C: pigmented filamentous colonies. (d) Microscopic examination of the colonies.

References

[1] A. Vicente, F. Pedrosa Domellöf, and B. Byström, "*Exophiala phaeomuriformis* keratitis in a subarctic climate region: a case report," *Acta Ophthalmologica*, vol. 96, no. 4, pp. 425–428, 2018.

[2] G. S. de Hoog, J. S. Zeng, M. J. Harrak, and D. A. Sutton, "*Exophiala xenobiotica* sp. nov., an opportunistic black yeast inhabiting environments rich in hydrocarbons," *Antonie Van Leeuwenhoek*, vol. 90, no. 3, pp. 257–268, 2006.

[3] M. Homa, P. Manikandan, V. Saravanan et al., "*Exophiala dermatitidis* endophthalmitis: case report and literature review," *Mycopathologia*, vol. 183, no. 3, pp. 603–609, 2018.

[4] Q. Zhang, J. B. Randleman, R. D. Stulting et al., "Clinicopathologic findings in failed descemet stripping automated endothelial keratoplasty," *Archives of Ophthalmology*, vol. 128, no. 8, pp. 973–980, 2010.

[5] S. Palioura, K. Sivaraman, M. Joag et al., "Candida endophthalmitis after descemet stripping automated endothelial keratoplasty with grafts from both eyes of a donor with possible systemic candidiasis," *Cornea*, vol. 37, no. 4, pp. 515–518, 2018.

[6] F. Benaoudia, M. Assouline, Y. Pouliquen, A. Bouvet, and E. Guého, "*Exophiala (Wangiella) dermatitidis* keratitis after keratoplasty," *Medical Mycology*, vol. 37, no. 1, pp. 53–56, 1999.

[7] S. R. Patel, K. M. Hammersmith, C. J. Rapuano, and E. J. Cohen, "Exophiala dermatitidis keratitis after laser in situ keratomileusis," *Journal of Cataract and Refractive Surgery*, vol. 32, no. 4, pp. 681–684, 2006.

[8] O. J. Saeedi, S. A. Iyer, A. Z. Mohiuddin, and R. N. Hogan, "Exophiala jeanselmei keratitis," *Eye & Contact Lens*, vol. 39, no. 6, pp. 410–412, 2013.

[9] G. J. Ben-Simon, A. Grinbaum, and I. S. Barequet, "More than tears in your eyes (Exophiala jeanselmei keratitis)," *Cornea*, vol. 21, no. 2, pp. 230-231, 2002.

[10] J. Hay, S. Patel, and D. V. Seal, "Exophiala Jeanselmei: a potential ocular pathogen," *Journal of the British Contact Lens Association.*, vol. 18, no. 3, pp. 99–101, 1995.

[11] E. McElnea, B. Power, and C. Murphy, "Interface fungal keratitis after descemet stripping automated endothelial keratoplasty: a review of the literature with a focus on outcomes," *Cornea*, vol. 37, no. 9, pp. 1204–1211, 2018.

[12] V. A. Augustin, J. M. Weller, F. E. Kruse, and T. Tourtas, "Fungal interface keratitis after descemet membrane endothelial keratoplasty," *Cornea*, vol. 37, no. 11, pp. 1366–1369, 2018.

[13] Y. Nahum, C. Russo, S. Madi, and M. Busin, "Interface infection after descemet stripping automated endothelial keratoplasty: outcomes of therapeutic keratoplasty," *Cornea*, vol. 33, no. 9, pp. 893–898, 2014.

24

Image-Guided Intensity-Modulated Radiation Therapy for IgG4-Related Ophthalmic Disease

Rachel A. Sabol,[1] Virginia Bubenzer,[2] Krzysztof Moroz,[3] Shams Halat,[3] Audrey Dang,[2] Keith Ferdinand,[4] Angela Traylor,[5] Carol Boyd,[2] and Kendra Harris[2]

[1]*Tulane University School of Medicine, New Orleans, LA, USA*
[2]*Department of Radiation Oncology, Tulane University School of Medicine, New Orleans, LA, USA*
[3]*Department of Pathology, Tulane University School of Medicine, New Orleans, LA, USA*
[4]*Department of Cardiology, Tulane University School of Medicine, New Orleans, LA, USA*
[5]*Department of Psychiatry and Neurology, Tulane University School of Medicine, New Orleans, LA, USA*

Correspondence should be addressed to Kendra Harris; kharris11@tulane.edu

Academic Editor: Stephen G. Schwartz

Background. IgG4-related ophthalmic disease is a rare, newly recognized entity with high failure rates on first-line therapy of systemic corticosteroids and no other proven management options. *Case Presentation.* Here, we present the clinical course of a patient with IgG4 ophthalmic disease who achieved a favorable response from radiotherapy. Our patient initially presented with a history of recurrent painful flares of orbital inflammation, a pathologic diagnosis follicular lymphoid hyperplasia from a right lacrimal gland biopsy, and MRI imaging noting expansion of the lateral rectus muscle of the right eye. Initial treatment with dacryoadenectomy and multiple courses of corticosteroids failed to keep his symptoms at bay. Further evaluation revealed florid IgG4 staining. In this context, he was evaluated for image-guided intensity-modulated radiotherapy (IG-IMRT) to the orbit to 20 Gy in 10 fractions. His ophthalmic symptoms resolved. *Conclusions.* This treatment experience suggests radiotherapy may be a favorable option for symptom relief in patients with IgG4-related ophthalmic disease not controlled by corticosteroids.

1. Introduction

IgG4-related ophthalmic disease (IgG4-ROD) is a relatively recently recognized ocular inflammatory entity characterized by the infiltration of IgG4-positive plasma cells into tissues, typically ocular muscles. The etiology and pathogenesis of this process is currently unknown [1, 2]. IgG4-ROD can present as an inflammation limited to the orbit or can present as a systemic sclerosing inflammatory condition that can affect many different organs including the orbit, pancreas, liver, kidney, lung, and thyroid [3–5]. IgG4-ROD may be responsible for a significant proportion of what had previously been labeled idiopathic orbital inflammation/reactive lymphoid hyperplasia and should be in the differential for patients found to have ocular adnexal inflammation [2, 6–8].

Current treatments for IgG4-ROD limited to the orbit are guided by systemic agents used to address extraorbital multifocal disease. First-line therapy is often systemic corticosteroids, but retrospective data suggests progression/relapse rates as high as 72% [9]. Other systemic treatments for which there are published case series data include rituximab and other immunosuppressants such as azathioprine, methotrexate, mycophenolate, and cyclosporine [10]. Radiation has been described in the context of primary therapy and recurrent disease; however, variable responses have been described [7, 11–13].

Here, we describe the clinical course of a patient found to have IgG4-ROD, treated with image-guided intensity-modulated radiation therapy (IG-IMRT) who had an excellent and rapid clinical response at 3-month follow-up.

2. Case Presentation

The 39-year old patient initially presented in 2017 for recurrent episodes of dry, painful, swelling of the right eye (Figure 1(a)). Computerized tomography (CT) images at that

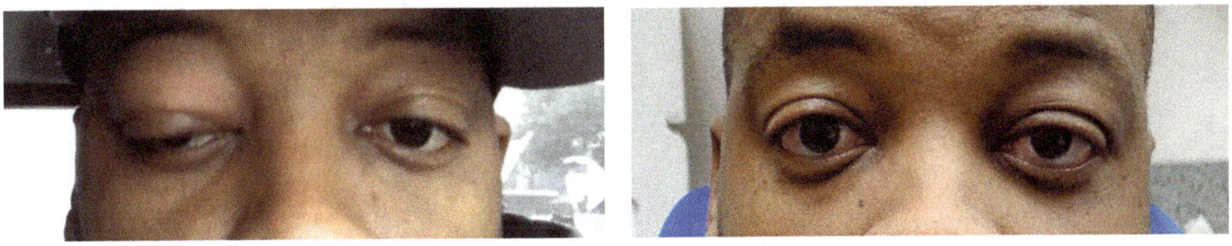

(a) (b)

FIGURE 1: (a) Patient with orbit inflammation after sugery and multiple rounds of steroids prior to radiation. (b) Follow-up: 3 months after radiation with resolution of inflammation and symptomatic improvement.

time demonstrated enlargement of the right lacrimal gland and increased size of the right lateral rectus muscle. The patient underwent right orbitotomy with tissue exploration with a biopsy of the posterior right lateral rectus muscle, right dacryoadenectomy, and right temporal tarsorrhaphy. Gross examination noted an abnormally hard lacrimal gland and pathology revealed intraglandular follicular lymphoid hyperplasia with no phenotypically abnormal lymphocytes on flow cytometric analysis. Pathology of the lateral recuts also demonstrated intramuscular follicular lymphoid hyperplasia. Of note, this patient's past medical history is significant for eosinophilic esophagitis without other known history of autoimmune diseases, and he is followed by cardiology for malignant hypertension treated with multiple antihypertensive agents. He denies ever having experienced unexplained weight loss, night sweats, or unexplained fevers.

The patient received dozens of courses of oral steroids over the course of the two years prior to presenting to radiation oncology. The steroid courses were of varying doses and duration and were not well tolerated due to medical comorbidities, mainly malignant hypertension. In 2019, he began to experience increased severity of symptoms during flares, rating pain 10/10 with no response to systemic steroids. Symptoms included new onset diplopia, severe ocular pain, and worsening upper and lower palpebral edema described by the patient as intermittently "so bad I can't open my eye at all." His physical exam was significant for mild right proptosis, right-ptosis, evoked diplopia with inability to fully medialize the right globe, and incomplete conjugate gaze at the far medial and lateral fields without appreciable impairment of visual acuity. The patient was referred to radiation oncology, where his constellation of findings prompted consideration of the possibility of IgG4-ROD and a request for IgG4 staining of tissue from his 2017 orbitotomy was sent and shown to be 100 per high-powered field (Figure 2). A number of blood tests were also ordered: EBV-, HIV-, and CMV-; quantitative systemic immunoglobulins (G, M, A) were all within the normal range.

Treatment options were reviewed. In the context of his comorbidities and polypharmacy, radiotherapy was selected as the preferred treatment approach by the patient over other second-line immunomodulators that have been described for use in IgG4-ROD to avoid the addition of another systemic therapy. We discussed that IgG4-ROD is one of a number of benign inflammatory conditions of the orbit including graves ophthalmopathy, orbital pseudotumor, and precursor lymphoproliferative process (up to and including lymphomas, in particular, mucosa-associated lymphoid tissue (MALT) lymphomas). We discussed that low-dose radiotherapy can be given to address the symptoms in the context of these other orbital processes and discussed the risks and benefits of a course of IG-IMRT with the goal of symptom control. After informed consent was obtained, the patient underwent IG-IMRT of 20 gray (Gy) in 10 fractions to the right orbit with attention to sparing the brain and lens.

Although he experienced an inflammatory flare during the first week of radiotherapy, he subsequently had an impressive clinical response (Figure 1). In the three months since treatment, no further orbital inflammatory flares have occurred and repeat imaging with orbital MRI confirms radiographic response. While 3-month follow-up is short to assess recurrence, it is notable in the context of symptom resolution and quality of life improvement reported by the patient.

3. Methods

3.1. Radiation Course. The patient was immobilized with a short aquaplast mask and underwent a CT simulation without IV contrast and an orbital MRI with gadolinium. The treatment field was defined as the bony orbit. An intensity-modulated radiotherapy plan with volumetric modulated arc radiotherapy (V-MAT) using 6 MV photos was created with two arcs delivered with the couch at 0 degrees and one arc delivered with the couch at 280 degrees. The quality of the plan was assessed for conformality and homogeneity. Daily image-guidance with cone beam CT was undertaken with a match to the bone. The dose was 20 Gy in 10 fractions.

4. Discussion

IgG4-ROD typically presents with fibro-inflammation of the orbit and symptoms of unilateral or bilateral proptosis, eyelid swelling, ocular pain, and impaired ocular movement [9, 10]. Other parts of the orbit, such as the extraocular muscles, orbital adipose and soft tissue, infraorbital nerve and canal, and nasolacrimal duct system, can be involved with key distinguishing features including a disproportionate involvement of the lateral rectus muscle and a typical tendon-spring morphology as well as lid retraction/lid lag [7, 10, 14]. The majority of published cases have described patients of Asian descent, and there is some controversy in the literature over

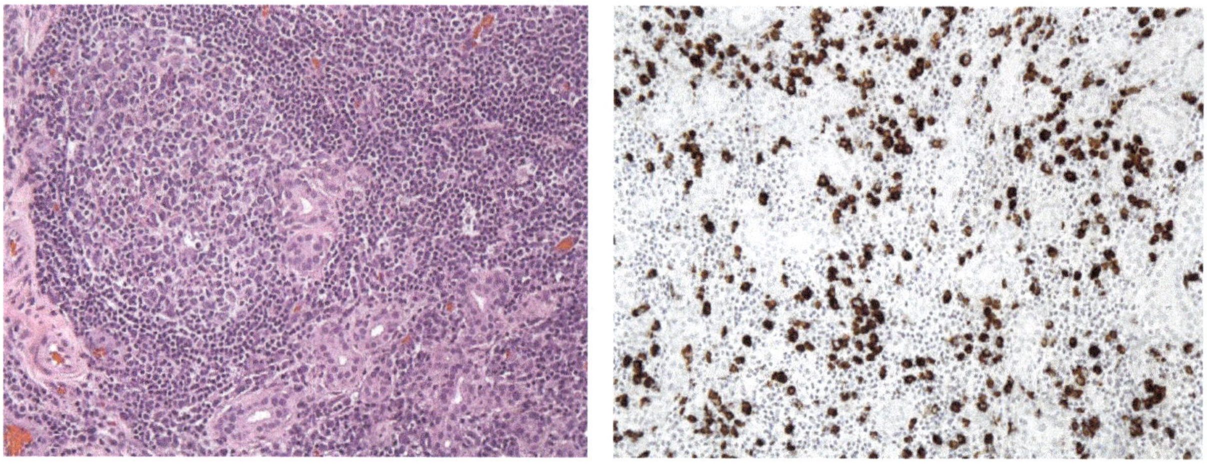

(a) (b)

Figure 2: (a) Lacrimal gland obliterated by dense lymphoplasmacytic infiltrate containing reactive lymphoid aggregate (H&E, 200x). (b) IgG4 immunohistochemical stain showing abundant IgG4+ plasma cells (IgG4, 200x).

the occurrence of IgG4-ROD in Western patients and if conclusions drawn from patients in Asia can be extrapolated more generally [8]. The clinic course of our patient contributes to the growing body of literature of IgG4-ROD in Western patients and offers evidence of a therapeutic response to low-dose radiotherapy.

Therapeutic options are important for this cohort of patients as recurrent symptoms are common and long-term steroids do not always produce the desired clinical relief. Additionally, inadequate steroid dose can lead to insufficient immunosuppression, and as was seen in this case, steroids could not be tolerated due to a history of malignant hyperthermia treated with multiple antihypertensives. Even when steroids do provide relief, long-term corticosteroid use is associated with many negative side effects including osteoporosis, hyperlipidemia, hyperglycemia, and adrenal insufficiency [15]. When steroids cannot be tolerated, and/or there is diminishing relief provided by steroids, alternative treatment options must be considered. In IgG4-ROD, immunomodulators including Rituximab are often considered as the second-line therapy. Additionally, radiation has been described in case reports as primary treatment, adjuvant therapy, or in combination with steroids and/or Rituximab, with variable responses and reported outcomes [7, 11–13, 16].

Given the variety of clinical scenarios in which radiotherapy has been used, as well as variable reported efficacy, this case report provides an important and unique perspective [11, 12]. This case adds an important additional perspective to the literature regarding IgG4-ROD describing symptom improvement and short-term response following 20 Gy radiotherapy. There are published experiences of treating IgG4-ROD with radiation; however, these reports demonstrate a variety of responses to radiation. Thus, there is a critical need to share our case report and experience to expound on other cases so clinicians can evaluate the body of experiences as a whole for clinical decision-making [11]. Here, we present an additional experience that expands upon and strengthens the growing body of literature by describing a patient with symptom improvement and short-term response to radiotherapy.

While there have been case reports of the use of radiotherapy in IgG4-ROD, the toxicities are often not described in the context of clinical decision-making in these cases. One of the most common side effects of radiotherapy to the orbit is dry eye syndrome. In this case, the patient had previously had a dacryoadenectomy in the affected eye that was to be treated with radiotherapy, which helped guide decision-making as the patient already had iatrogenically induced dry eye syndrome due to previous surgery. Radiation is often reserved as a second line therapy due to the increased risk of secondary malignancy following radiation.

Additionally, this case demonstrates a diagnosis of IgG4-ROD two years after initial presentation. In the time between initial surgery in 2017 and definitive diagnosis, the patient continued to receive many courses of oral steroids and experienced adverse effects until steroids were no longer tolerable. As a relatively new pathology, it is expected that more cases of IgG4-ROD will be diagnosed after several therapies have been initiated. Understanding the role that radiotherapy can play in these cases provides a valuable addition to the literature and provides treatment experience that may apply to patients diagnosed under similar circumstances.

Without available prospective data, case reports are an important way to prompt our colleagues to consider IgG4-ROD when evaluating patients with inflammatory orbital disease. As with all newly described entities, given a tool to assess for IgG4 staining, the number of patients who can be assessed as having IgG4-ROD will rise and, with it, a desire for data related to treatment options. This case report provides an important perspective in that the diagnosis of IgG4-ROD was made several years after initial evaluation and attempted disease management with steroids that were not well tolerated. Consideration of low-dose radiotherapy may be reasonable in the right clinical circumstance.

Abbreviations

(IgG4-ROD):	IgG4-related ophthalmic disease
(IG-IMRT):	Image-guided intensity-modulated radiation therapy
(CT):	Computerized tomography
(MRI):	Magnetic resonance imaging
(MALT):	Mucosa-associated lymphoid tissue
(Gy):	Gray.

Authors' Contributions

RS carried out the literature search and image and data collection and drafted the manuscript. KH collected important background information and made substantial contributions to the manuscript, including revising it for relevant content. KM provided pathology images and additional edits to the manuscript. Additional edits were provided by VB, SH, AD, KF, AT, and CB. All authors read and approved the final manuscript.

Acknowledgments

We acknowledge the work of our colleagues in the pathology and radiology department in offering original images and data used in this article.

References

[1] Japanese Study Group for IgG4-Related Ophthalmic Disease, H. Goto, M. Takahira, and A. Azumi, "Diagnostic criteria for IgG_4-related ophthalmic disease," *Japanese Journal of Ophthalmology*, vol. 59, no. 1, pp. 1-7, 2015.

[2] N. H. Andrew, N. Sladden, D. J. Kearney, and D. Selva, "An analysis of IgG4-related disease (IgG4-RD) among idiopathic orbital inflammations and benign lymphoid hyperplasias using two consensus-based diagnostic criteria for IgG4-RD," *The British Journal of Ophthalmology*, vol. 99, no. 3, pp. 376–381, 2015.

[3] J. H. Stone, Y. Zen, and V. Deshpande, "IgG4-related disease," *The New England Journal of Medicine*, vol. 366, no. 6, pp. 539–551, 2012.

[4] K. Ohno, Y. Sato, K. I. Ohshima et al., "IgG_4-related disease involving the sclera," *Modern Rheumatology*, vol. 24, no. 1, pp. 195–198, 2014.

[5] C. S. Lee, G. J. Harocopos, C. L. Kraus et al., "IgG4-associated orbital and ocular inflammation," *Journal of Ophthalmic Inflammation and Infection*, vol. 5, no. 1, 2015.

[6] R. Deschamps, L. Deschamps, R. Depaz et al., "High prevalence of IgG4-related lymphoplasmacytic infiltrative disorder in 25 patients with orbital inflammation: a retrospective case series," *The British Journal of Ophthalmology*, vol. 97, no. 8, pp. 999–1004, 2013.

[7] T. G. Hardy, A. A. McNab, and G. E. Rose, "Enlargement of the infraorbital nerve: an important sign associated with orbital reactive lymphoid hyperplasia or immunoglobulin g4-related disease," *Ophthalmology*, vol. 121, no. 6, pp. 1297–1303, 2014.

[8] J. A. Ferry, V. Klepeis, A. R. Sohani et al., "IgG4-related orbital disease and its mimics in a Western population," *The American Journal of Surgical Pathology*, vol. 39, no. 12, pp. 1688–1700, 2015.

[9] A. Wu, N. H. Andrew, A. A. McNab, and D. Selva, "IgG_4-related ophthalmic disease: pooling of published cases and literature review," *Current Allergy and Asthma Reports*, vol. 15, no. 6, 2015.

[10] Z. S. Wallace, V. Deshpande, and J. H. Stone, "Ophthalmic manifestations of IgG4-related disease: single-center experience and literature review," *Seminars in Arthritis and Rheumatism*, vol. 43, no. 6, pp. 806–817, 2014.

[11] C. E. Rutter, B. R. Mancini, and K. B. Roberts, "A report of metachronous orbital involvement by IgG4 disease treated successfully with low-dose radiation therapy," *Practical Radiation Oncology*, vol. 6, no. 2, pp. 74–77, 2016.

[12] W. K. Yu, S. C. Kao, C. F. Yang, F. L. Lee, and C. C. Tsai, "Ocular adnexal IgG_4-related disease: clinical features, outcome, and factors associated with response to systemic steroids," *Japanese Journal of Ophthalmology*, vol. 59, no. 1, pp. 8–13, 2015.

[13] Y. H. Lin, S. H. Yen, C. C. Tsai, S. C. Kao, and F. L. Lee, "Adjunctive orbital radiotherapy for ocular adnexal IgG4-related disease: preliminary experience in patients refractory or intolerant to corticosteroid therapy," *Ocular Immunology and Inflammation*, vol. 23, no. 2, pp. 162–167, 2015.

[14] J. A. Plaza, J. A. Garrity, A. Dogan, A. Ananthamurthy, T. E. Witzig, and D. R. Salomão, "Orbital inflammation with IgG4-positive plasma Cells," *Archives of Ophthalmology*, vol. 129, no. 4, pp. 421–428, 2011.

[15] A. L. Buchman, "Side effects of corticosteroid therapy," *Journal of Clinical Gastroenterology*, vol. 33, no. 4, pp. 289–294, 2001.

[16] T. S. Chen, E. Figueira, O. C. F. Lau et al., "Successful "medical" orbital decompression with adjunctive rituximab for severe visual loss in IgG4-related orbital inflammatory disease with orbital myositis," *Ophthalmic Plastic & Reconstructive Surgery*, vol. 30, no. 5, pp. e122–e125, 2014.

25

Nocardia Subretinal Abscess: A Rare and Challenging Case Report

Ana Maria Cunha,[1] **Marta Silva,**[1] **Ana Catarina Pedrosa,**[1] **Fernando Falcão-Reis,**[1,2] **and Luís Figueira**[1,3,4]

[1]*Department of Ophthalmology, Centro Hospitalar Universitário de São João, Porto, Portugal*
[2]*Department of Surgery and Physiology, Faculty of Medicine, University of Porto, Porto, Portugal*
[3]*Department of Pharmacology and Therapeutics, Faculty of Medicine of the University of Porto, Porto, Portugal*
[4]*Center for Drug Discovery and Innovative Medicines (MedInUP), University of Porto, Porto, Portugal*

Correspondence should be addressed to Ana Maria Cunha; ana.cunha.18@gmail.com

Academic Editor: Kevin J. Blinder

Purpose. To describe a positive clinical response of a patient with submacular *Nocardia* abscess due to a rapid and efficient treatment. *Case report.* We describe a case of a 50-year-old man with a painless visual decline of the left eye. Four years later, he had been diagnosed with systemic nocardiosis. Examination of the left eye revealed a submacular white mass with fluffy borders and another smaller white lesion, with well-defined borders, in the inferior temporal vascular arch. A systemic antibiotic treatment with SMX-TMP and intravenous imipenem and a single intravitreal injection of bevacizumab was performed. *Conclusion.* Prompt diagnosis and treatment ensured an expeditious resolution of the abscess and significant improvement of visual acuity. The diagnostic approach of a high index of suspicion coupled with directed treatment is required when dealing with subretinal inflammatory lesions.

1. Introduction

Nocardia is an aerobic, gram-positive, Actinomycetales bacteria, which is ubiquitous in soil [1]. It usually manifests as an opportunistic infection in immunocompromised individuals [2].

Typically, systemic involvement includes the lungs, brain, kidneys, skin, and joints [3]. Initial clinical manifestations comprise mainly of pulmonary symptoms. Hematogenous spread to other organs is observed in approximately one-third of patients [4].

The ocular manifestations can be classified by mechanism of inoculation as exogenous, when occurs posttraumatically and endogenous, secondary to hematogenous spread [5, 6].

Ocular infection can manifest in various forms including keratitis, conjunctivitis, scleritis, periorbital infections, subretinal or choroidal abscess, and endophthalmitis [4, 7–9]. Only a few reports have posterior segment involvement. Choroidal and retina involvement mostly leads to loss of vision and, in some cases, to evisceration or enucleation [8, 10].

We describe a positive clinical response of a patient with submacular Nocardia abscess due to a rapid and efficient treatment.

2. Case Report

We describe a case of a 50-year-old man with a 3-day history of painless visual decline in the left eye. His past medical history included a diagnosis of pulmonary silicosis with progressive pulmonary fibrosis. In February 2016, he had been diagnosed with systemic nocardiosis with lung, cerebral, and skin abscess and had received sulfamethoxazole-trimethoprim (SMX-TMP) oral monotherapy until December 2017.

In October 2019, he presented, in the ophthalmic emergency room, with a visual acuity of 10/10 in the right eye and 4/10 in the left eye. The anterior examination in both eyes was unremarkable and intraocular pressure normal.

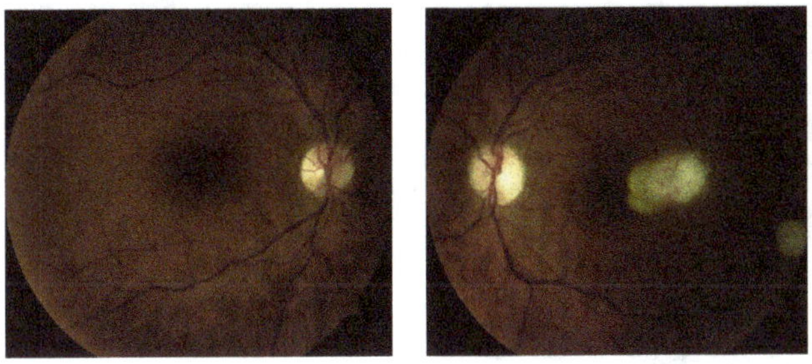

(a) (b)

FIGURE 1: (a) Normal fundus-photography of the right eye. (b) Fundus-photography of the left eye picturing a whitish, fluffy subretinal macular mass and another smaller white lesion, with well-defined limits, in the inferior temporal vascular arch.

Posterior segment examination of the right eye was normal (Figure 1(a)), and the left eye revealed absence of vitritis and a one disk diameter submacular white mass with fluffy borders and some intraretinal hemorrhages and another smaller white lesion, with well-defined borders, in the inferior temporal vascular arch (Figure 1(b)). The SD-OCT of the main macular lesion showed a subretinal mass with disorganization of retinal structures in association with subretinal fluid (Figure 2). The SD-OCT scan of the smaller white lesion in the inferior temporal vascular arch revealed a well define mass in the choroidal space (Figure 3). Fluorescein angiography (FA) revealed an area of early hypofluorescence, which progressed to a hyperfluorescence lesion with fluorescein leakage in late stages and a hyperfluorescence of the smaller lesion in the inferior temporal vascular arch without diffusion. Indocyanine Green Angiography (ICG) revealed a hypofluorescence in all stages (Figure 4).

Due to clinical chorioretinal lesion presentation, medical record, and additional symptoms (fever and dry cough), the patient began empiric systemic antibiotic treatment with SMX-TMP and intravenous imipenem.

After 3 days, the left eye visual acuity decreased to counting fingers. Although, in the ophthalmological exam of the anterior examination remains unremarkable and without vitritis in the posterior segment, the macular lesion enlarges had more intraretinal hemorrhages, neurosensorial detachment, and a pseudohypopyon aspect (Figures 5(a) and 5(b)).

Initial systemic study presented with an increased C-Reactive Protein (CRP) (84.8), but unremarkable virologic study (HIV, HCV, toxoplasmosis, *Treponema pallidum*, CMV, EBV, VHS1, and VHS2 negative). Further systemic workup with cranial MRI and thoraco abdominopelvic CT scan revealed no signs of active infection. Although the anterior chamber tap for aqueous humour CRP microbiological analysis was negative for *Mycobacterium tuberculosis*, Herpes virus, *Toxoplasma*, Syphilis, and *Nocardia*, the analysis of the bronchial secretion's specimen identified *Nocardia abscessus*.

After 6 days of treatment, the macular lesion began to decrease in size and decrease the subretinal fluid (Figures 5(c)–5(e)). The patient was treated with TMP-SMX and intravenous imipenem for three weeks, and later, with oral TMP-SMX and cefixime.

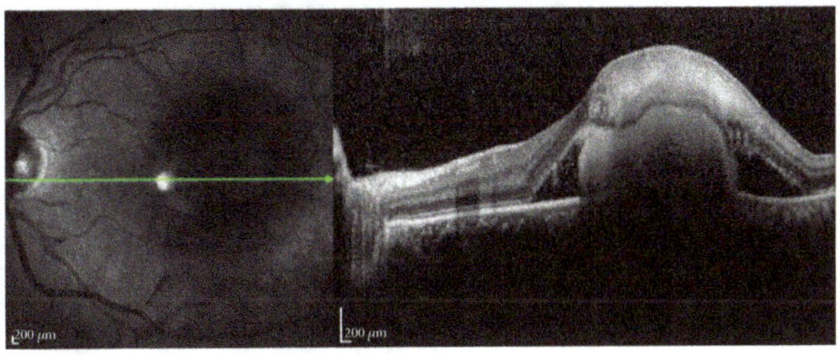

FIGURE 2: SD-OCT scan of the subretinal mass with disorganization of retinal structures with subretinal fluid.

He was discharged after 44 days of treatment. At this time, the left eye visual acuity was 0.008, and the macular lesion was smaller, but intraretinal hemorrhages had increased, and it kept intraretinal and subretinal fluid (Figure 5(e)). For this reason, it was performed one intravitreal injection of bevacizumab 1.25 mg. One month after the intravitreal injection, while continuing systemic treatment with oral TMP-SMX and cefixime, the ophthalmic examination revealed visual acuity of 10/10 in the right eye and 5/10 in the left eye. Slit lamp examination was quiet and intraocular pressure normal. Posterior segment exam revealed subretinal fibrosis in macula. The SD-OCT revealed fibrotic scarring lesion without subretinal and intraretinal fluid (Figures 6(a) and 6(b)). FA revealed an hyperfluorescence staining of the macular and peripheric lesions, without signs of activity. ICG revealed a hypofluorescence in all stages (Figure 7).

The patient will continue systemic treatment with oral TMP-SMX and cefixime until perform 12 months.

3. Discussion

Ocular nocardiosis usually presents with insidious and painless vision loss [11]. Most commonly, it appears in association with immunodeficiency causes such as AIDS or pharmacological immunosuppression in cases of stem cell transplantation [12], organ transplant [13], or malignancy [14]. Nevertheless, a few cases of the infection have also been reported in immunocompetent patients [15].

When ocular manifestations were present, 70% had pulmonary disease and 50% had central nervous system diseases [11]. For this reason, a pulmonary examination is warranted in all cases of *Nocardia* choroidal abscesses, with further evaluation of other organ systems guided by individual patient symptoms [8]. In our case, we identified pulmonary and ocular manifestations of *Nocardia*.

Severity of the ocular manifestations can be highly variable, which makes diagnosis difficult. Ocular *Nocardia* presentation can range from minimal inflammation to significant vitritis [16]. The fundoscopic findings are usually subretinal abscess, chorioretinal exudate, or inflammatory mass with associated superficial or intraretinal hemorrhages. In some cases, it is reported retinal detachment [8, 11]. Scleral thickening, choroidal edema, and panophthalmitis have been also described [10]. MRI may be helpful for quantifying the ocular involvement [11].

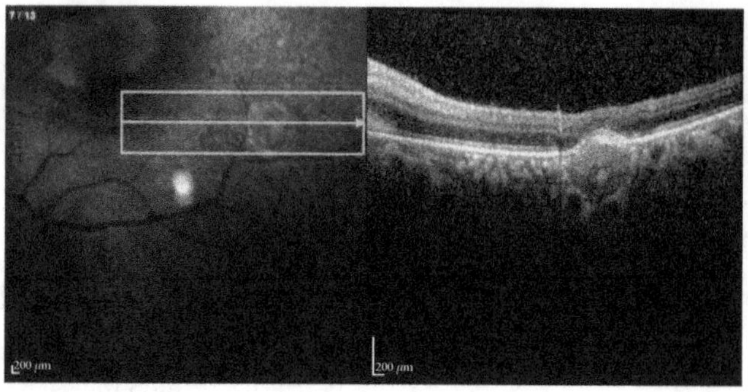

Figure 3: SD-OCT scan of the lesion in the inferior temporal vascular arch showing a well define mass in the choroidal space.

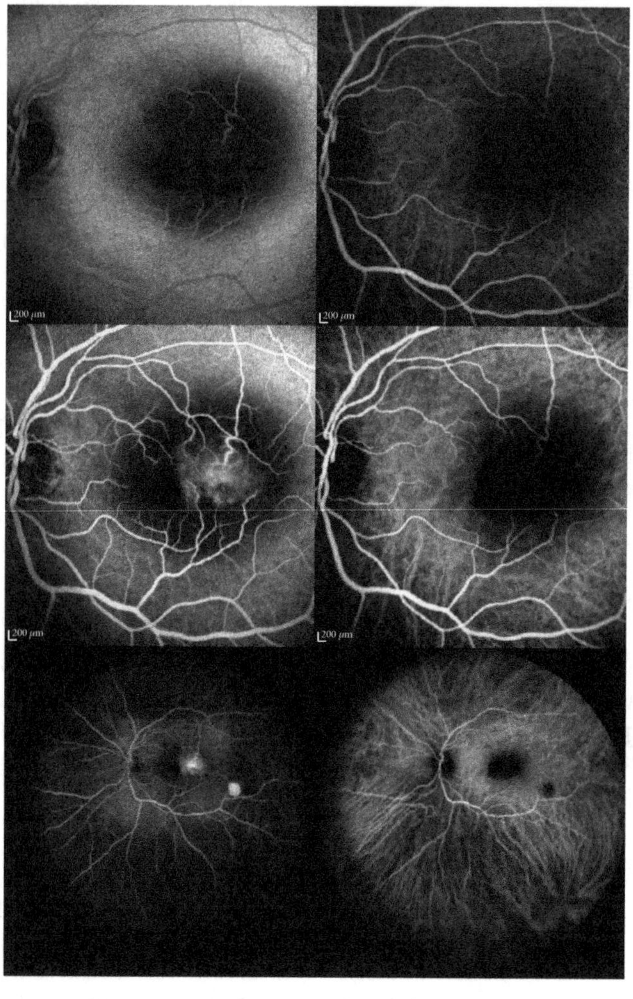

Figure 4: FA and ICG in the initial presentation at 0 : 56 min, 2 : 41 min, 4 : 01 min.

Consonant to our case, the unilateral and poor visual acuity at presentation and the location at the posterior pole are common [8]. The predisposition for the posterior pole may be associated with the higher choroidal blood flow in this region [8, 17].

The early diagnostic and specific treatment of *Nocardia* can be difficult by the unspecific manifestations and the broad differential diagnosis encompassing viral retinitis, toxoplasmosis, fungal endophthalmitis, and neoplasia [11]. In previous reported clinical cases, diagnosis delay could be 2 to 6 weeks, which can lead to a pathogen proliferates rapidly [8]. Viral retinitis generally can be distinguished from *Nocardia* choroidal abscesses as the former develops retinal necrosis accompanied by anterior and/or intermediate uveitis (i.e., in acute retinal necrosis) [8]. Ocular toxoplasmosis usually manifests as retinal necrosis, vitritis, inactive scars, and vasculitis [11, 18]. Fungal infections can have different presentations, like *Candida* endophthalmitis which usually presents as a small cream-coloured peripheral choroid lesion and flocculent fungal balls in vitreous [19] or

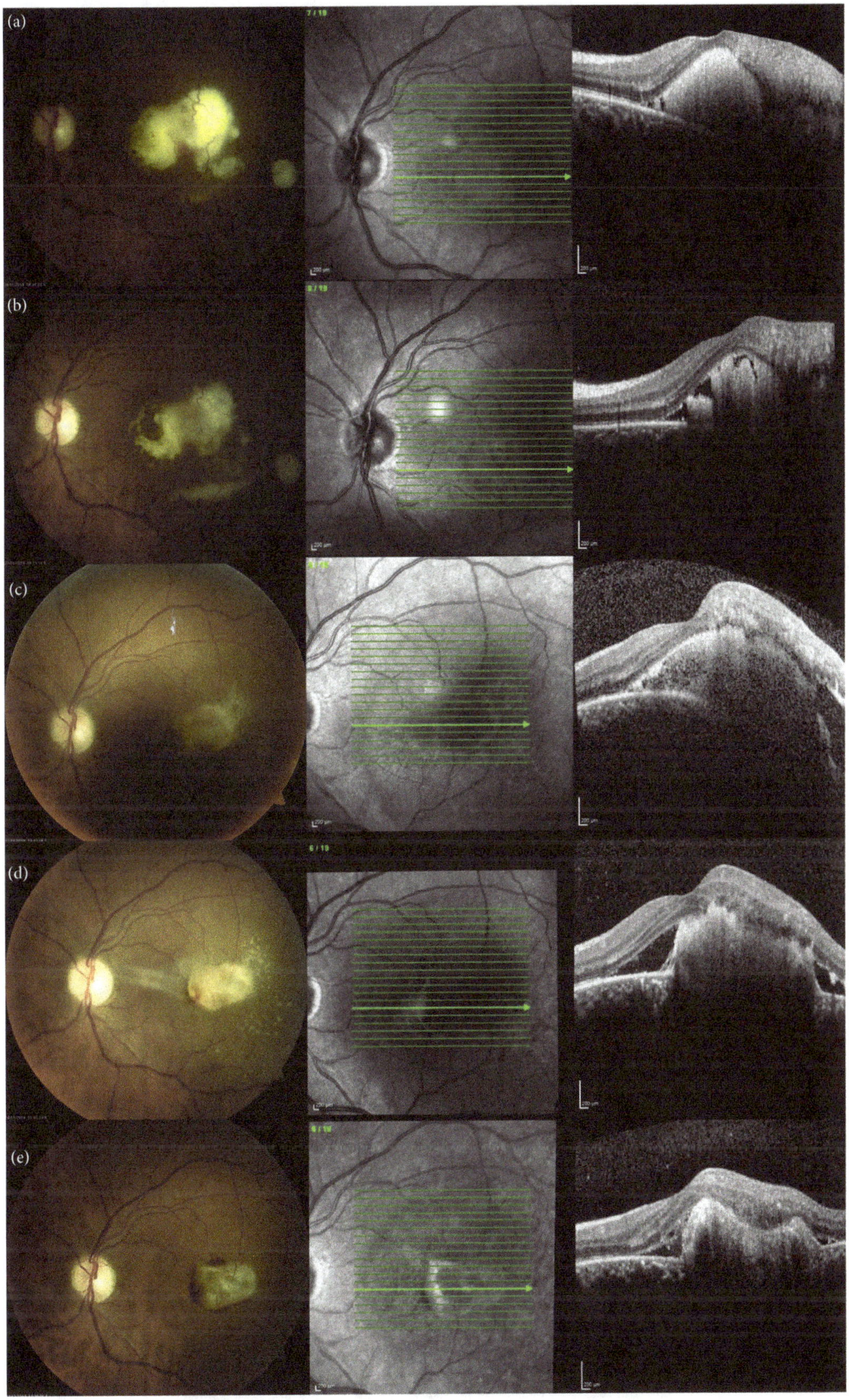

FIGURE 5: Chronological evolution of the macula lesion during treatment. (a) Macular lesion enlargement with neurosensorial detachment and a pseudohypopyon aspect at D3 of treatment. (b–e) Macular lesion regression and decreased subretinal fluid.

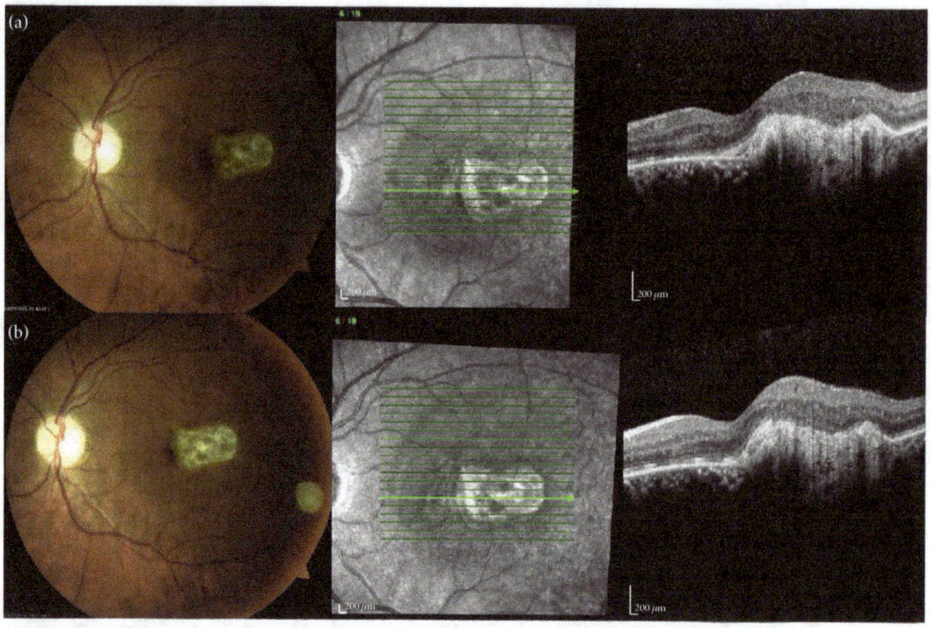

FIGURE 6: Chronological evolution of the macula lesion during treatment. One months (a) and two months (b) after the intravitreal injection, fibrotic scarring lesion without subretinal and intraretinal fluid and decreased intraretinal hemorrhages were identified.

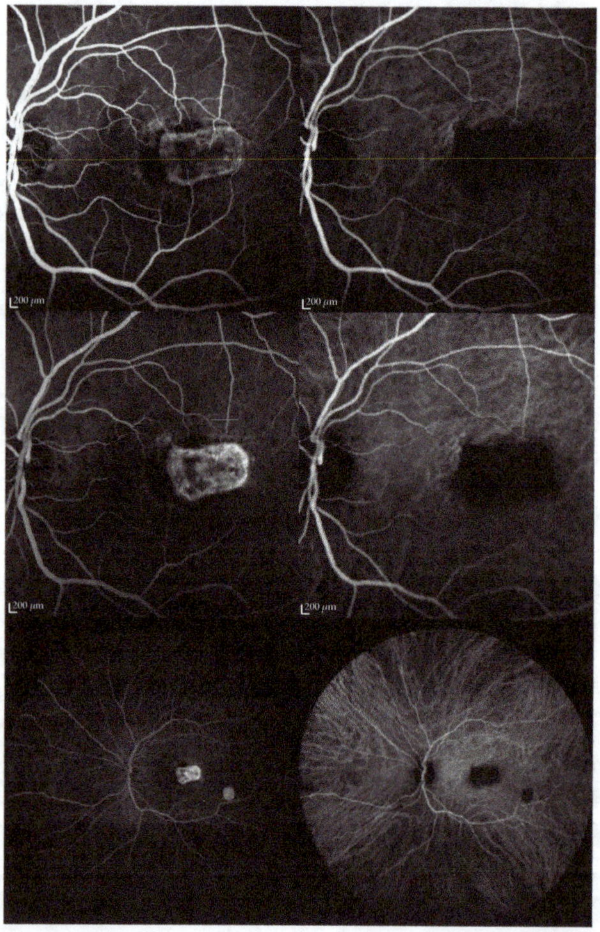

FIGURE 7: FA revealed a hyperfluorescence staining in macular and peripheric lesion. ICG revealed a hypofluorescence in all stages. (0 : 52 min; 2 : 16 min; 3 : 36 min).

endogenous *Aspergillus* endophthalmitis that has a more rapid progression and larger areas of infarcted haemorrhagic chorioretinitis [20]. Only a few other bacterial species are mentioned in literature, such as *Pseudomonas aeruginosa*, *Streptococcus viridans*, or *Klebsiella pneumoniae*, that cause subretinal abscess formation [11]. Neoplastic diseases, mainly choroidal metastases, are usually multifocal and occur in patients with a history of malignancy [21].

Therefore, the clinical presentation of a subretinal white fluffy abscess, which can progress to pseudohypopyon aspect, the superficial or intraretinal hemorrhages and the absence of vitritis in a patient with pulmonary disease or medical record of pulmonary disease, should lead to suspicion of nocardial aetiology. In the case of our patient, pulmonary nocardiosis had indeed been diagnosed in the past, rendering this specific diagnosis more likely.

Some reported cases have been treated with intravitreal injection of amikacin, due to the antibiotic sensitivity profile, but with minimal guidance on the frequency of injections [8]. However, macular ischemia following intravitreal amikacin is a serious risk to consider with individualized discussions [22]. In our case, due to the good response to systemic treatment and the aforementioned risk of macular ischemia, we decided to postpone intravitreal injection. Intravitreal injections of bevacizumab have been used to treat neovascular membranes or macular edema. In this case, the lesion had exudation, intraretinal and subretinal fluid caused by vascular component. Intravitreal injection of bevacizumab was cooperative in the regression of the vascular component and the resolution of the fluid.

4. Conclusion

The visual prognosis is variable and depends on the location of the abscess, as well as the tissue destruction, which limits establishing prognosis. Our patient had severely reduced vision in the setting of a large submacular abscess. Nevertheless, a quick diagnosis hypothesis and prompt systemic treatment ensured a marked resolution of the abscess and significant improvement of visual acuity. This case highlights that a diagnostic approach and a high index of suspicion (even if sometimes purely clinical one) coupled with directed treatment is required when dealing with subretinal inflammatory lesions.

References

[1] J. W. Wilson, "Nocardiosis: updates and clinical overview," *Mayo Clinic Proceedings*, vol. 87, no. 4, pp. 403–407, 2012.

[2] R. Kumar and M. G. Ison, "Opportunistic infections in transplant patients," *Infectious Disease Clinics of North America*, vol. 33, no. 4, pp. 1143–1157, 2019.

[3] R. J. Wallace Jr., L. C. Steele, G. Sumter, and J. M. Smith, "Antimicrobial susceptibility patterns of Nocardia asteroides," *Antimicrobial Agents and Chemotherapy*, vol. 32, no. 12, pp. 1776–1779, 1988.

[4] R. J. Gregor, C. A. Chong, J. J. Augsburger et al., "Endogenous Nocardia asteroides subretinal abscess diagnosed by transvitreal fine-needle aspiration biopsy," *Retina*, vol. 9, no. 2, pp. 118–121, 1989.

[5] B. L. Beaman and L. Beaman, "Nocardia species: host-parasite relationships," *Clinical Microbiology Reviews*, vol. 7, no. 2, pp. 213–264, 1994.

[6] H. Lakosha, C. J. Pavlin, and J. Lipton, "Subretinal abscess due to Nocardia farcinica infection," *Retina*, vol. 20, no. 3, 2000.

[7] J. F. Murray, S. M. Finegold, S. Froman, and D. W. Will, "The changing spectrum of nocardiosis. A review and presentation of nine cases," *The American Review of Respiratory Disease*, vol. 83, pp. 315–330, 1961.

[8] R. A. Silva, R. Young, J. Sridhar, and Nocardia Study Group, "Nocardia choroidal abscess: risk factors, treatment strategies, and visual outcomes," *Retina*, vol. 35, no. 10, pp. 2137–2146, 2015.

[9] A. Verner, A. Durrani, R. P. Kowalski, and V. Jhanji, "A case of Nocardia farcinica keratitis in a pediatric contact lens wearer," *Eye & Contact Lens*, vol. 46, no. 2, pp. e11–e12, 2020.

[10] E. Yu, S. Laughlin, E. E. Kassel, H. A. Messner, and Y. H. Yucel, "Nocardial endophthalmitis and subretinal abscess: CT and MR imaging features with pathologic correlation: a case report," *AJNR. American Journal of Neuroradiology*, vol. 26, no. 5, pp. 1220-1222, 2005.

[11] M. E. Eschle-Meniconi, Y. Guex-Crosier, and T. J. Wolfensberger, "Endogenous ocular nocardiosis: an interventional case report with a review of the literature," *Survey of Ophthalmology*, vol. 56, no. 5, pp. 383–415, 2011.

[12] E. W. Ng, I. E. Zimmer-Galler, and W. R. Green, "Endogenous Nocardia asteroides endophthalmitis," *Archives of Ophthalmology*, vol. 120, no. 2, pp. 210–213, 2002.

[13] W. B. Phillips, C. L. Shields, J. A. Shields, R. C. Eagle Jr., L. Masciulli, and D. L. Yarian, "Nocardia choroidal abscess," *British Journal of Ophthalmology*, vol. 76, pp. 694–696, 1992.

[14] R. Angermann, M. Stattin, and C. Zehetner, "Ocular nocardiosis: a case report," *Ocular Immunology and Inflammation*, vol. 27, no. 7, pp. 1114–1116, 2018.

[15] K. J. Kennedy, K. H. C. Chung, F. J. Bowden et al., "A cluster of nocardial brain abscesses," *Surgical Neurology*, vol. 68, no. 1, pp. 43–49, 2007.

[16] S. Puri, A. Hadayer, A. Breaux, and C. C. Barr, "Disseminated Nocardiosis with retinal abscess in a patient treated for bullous pemphigoid," *American Journal of Ophthalmology Case Reports*, vol. 10, pp. 145–147, 2018.

[17] R. Margolis and R. F. Spaide, "A pilot study of enhanced depth imaging optical coherence tomography of the choroid in normal eyes," *American Journal of Ophthalmology*, vol. 147, no. 5, pp. 811–815, 2009.

[18] R. B. Nussenblatt and R. Belfort Jr., "Ocular toxoplasmosis. An old disease revisited," *JAMA*, vol. 271, no. 4, pp. 304–307, 1994.

[19] N. A. Rao and A. A. Hidayat, "Endogenous mycotic endophthalmitis: variations in clinical and histopathologic changes in candidiasis compared with aspergillosis," *American Journal of Ophthalmology*, vol. 132, no. 2, pp. 244–251, 2001.

[20] P. D. Weishaar, H. W. Flynn Jr., T. G. Murray et al., "Endogenous Aspergillus endophthalmitis. Clinical features and treatment outcomes," *Ophthalmology*, vol. 105, no. 1, pp. 57–65, 1998.

[21] C. L. Shields, J. A. Shields, N. E. Gross, G. P. Schwartz, and S. E. Lally, "Survey of 520 eyes with uveal metastases," *Ophthalmology*, vol. 104, no. 8, pp. 1265–1276, 1997.

[22] G. Galloway, A. Ramsay, K. Jordan, and A. Vivian, "Macular infarction after intravitreal amikacin: mounting evidence against amikacin," *The British Journal of Ophthalmology*, vol. 86, no. 3, pp. 359-360, 2002.

26

Recurrent Self-Induced Nontraumatic Orbital Emphysema Causing Orbital Compartment Syndrome with Optic Nerve Dysfunction

S. Cutting,[1] C. Davies-Husband,[2] and C. Poitelea[3]

[1]*East Kent University Hospitals NHS Trust, UK*
[2]*Brighton and Sussex University Hospitals NHS Trust, UK*
[3]*Western Sussex Hospitals NHS Trust, UK*

Correspondence should be addressed to S. Cutting; scutting91@gmail.com

Academic Editor: Cristiano Giusti

The majority of cases of orbital emphysema are due to trauma. Complications are rare, and therefore, the need for surgical intervention is uncommon. We present the first case of which we are aware in which nontraumatic orbital emphysema led to orbital compartment syndrome and subsequent optic nerve dysfunction. The patient underwent emergency needle decompression. A 51-year-old man presented to the Emergency Department with right-sided unilateral proptosis, reduced visual acuity, and binocular diplopia. This occurred after performing a Valsalva manoeuvre with no history of head trauma. He also mentioned that over the past year he had experienced multiple episodes of transient proptosis occurring after Valsalva manoeuvres. Visual acuity in the right eye was reduced to 6/21. A relative afferent pupillary defect was present and intraocular pressure (IOP) was 12 mmHg. The CT scan showed significant orbital emphysema in the medial aspect of the right orbit. Needle decompression was performed resulting in immediate resolution of his symptoms. This case demonstrates that, in cases of orbital emphysema, a lack of a history of trauma and a normal IOP cannot always be used to rule out serious pathology.

1. Introduction

The majority of cases of orbital emphysema are due to trauma causing orbital wall fractures [1, 2]. Signs and symptoms suggestive of orbital emphysema are enophthalmos or proptosis, crepitus, diplopia, and protrusion on nose-blowing [1, 3]. Complications are uncommon and so is the need for intervention, but if severe enough to cause orbital compartment syndrome, it can have disastrous effects on vision through central retinal artery occlusion (CRAO) or compressive optic neuropathy [2, 4]. The acute presentation of orbital emphysema may not occur immediately after trauma. Instead, it may present days or weeks later after a Valsalva manoeuvre increases intranasal pressure. This can cause air to become trapped in the orbit via a one-way valve mechanism where it is likely that structures such as orbital fat prevent air leaving the orbit through the bony defect. Smaller fractures may be particularly prone to this phenomenon [2]. There have been case reports of rare, nontraumatic causes of orbital emphysema. These include surgery, infection, compressed air, osteomas or pneumocoeles of the paranasal sinuses and barotrauma [5]. Orbital emphysema due to pressure changes during air travel in a young man with recent traumatic orbital floor fracture has also been described [6]. Rarely, Valsalva manoeuvres have resulted in orbital emphysema without a history of prior trauma. Orbital wall fractures have been identified in a proportion of these cases, thought to be a result of the rise in intranasal pressure sneezing or nose-blowing confers [5]. Studies have quantified elevated intranasal pressures of 8 mmHg in the former but strikingly in excess of 70 mmHg in the latter [7, 8]. Cases of nontraumatic orbital emphysema tend to be mild and can be managed conservatively. We present an unusual case with recurrent self-induced, nontraumatic orbital emphysema which ultimately

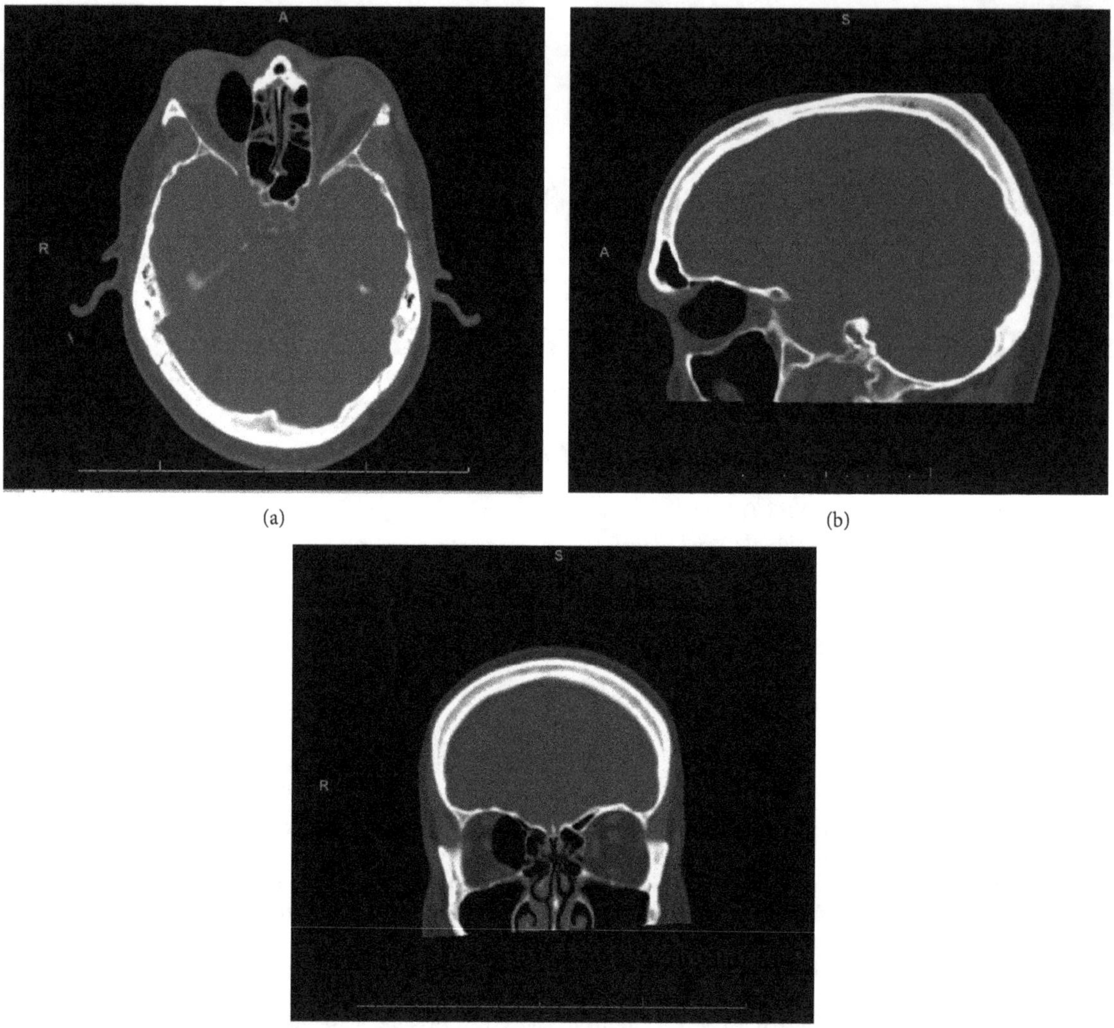

(a) (b) (c)

Figure 1: CT scan of patient with (a) axial, (b) sagittal, and (c) coronal views showing a 36 × 26 × 16 mm collection of gas in the medial aspect of right orbit causing displacement of intraorbital structures and resultant.

resulted in orbital compartment syndrome requiring urgent decompression.

2. Case Presentation

A 51-year-old man presented to the Emergency Department late at night complaining of proptosis of his right eye with accompanying diplopia. He provided a history of attempting to "unblock his ears" by performing a Valsalva manoeuvre. He stated he performed this Valsalva manoeuvre habitually on a daily basis, which often resulted in proptosis of the right eye that he was able to manually push back into place. He had not previously sought medical advice for this. His past medical history included Meniere's disease for which he performs Valsalva manoeuvres in an attempt to relieve his symptoms. His remaining past medical history was a radical mastoidectomy 22 years previously for cholesteatoma. There was no prior history of trauma.

Examination showed nonaxial proptosis of the right eye with infero-lateral displacement of the globe. Visual acuity in this eye was reduced to 6/21 (compared to 6/12 in the left eye). Binocular diplopia was apparent. He retained a good range of eye movement, and visual fields were normal to confrontation. Pupillary examination confirmed a relative afferent pupillary defect (RAPD); intraocular pressure (IOP) measure by Goldmann applanation was within the normal range at 12 mmHg, and fundoscopy demonstrated no optic nerve changes.

Accordingly, an urgent CT of the orbit was arranged, which showed significant orbital emphysema in the medial aspect of the orbit (Figure 1). There was a suggestion of a small bony defect in the superior aspect of the medial orbital wall. After a multidisciplinary discussion jointly between ophthalmology and otolaryngology consultants, preparations were provisionally made for urgent surgical decompression via endoscopic approach. However, on detailed review of the cross-sectional images, needle decompression was proposed in the first instance.

Sterile preparation was administered using aqueous chlorhexidine, followed by 2 ml lignospan with 1/80,000

TABLE 1: Intraocular pressure in cases of orbital emphysema in which patients underwent emergency decompression.

Reference	Cases which underwent emergency decompression	IOP prior to decompression
Fleishman et al. 1984 [30]	2	(i) "Over 100" (ii) Not stated
Dobler et al. 1993 [31]	1	45
Hunts et al. 1994 [2]	7	(i) 20 (ii) 37 (iii) 35 (iv) 28 (v) Not stated (vi) "Normal" (vii) 21
Wearne et al. 1998 [32]	1	20
Monaghan and Millar 2002 [6]	1	Not stated
Lee et al. 2006 [33]	1	80
Chaudry et al. 2007 [34]	1	25
Singh et al. 2007 [9]	1	37
Furlani et al. 2009 [35]	1	23*
Chak et al. 2012 [36]	1	46
Rowh et al. 2015 [37]	1	79
Lin et al. 2016 [38]	1	29

*Measured at 23 initially but only underwent emergency decompression when situation progressed after more sneezing (no remeasurement of IOP stated).

adrenaline infiltration into the right conjunctival mucosa. Using a syringe attached to a 16G cannula inserted adjacent to the carcuncle, 7 ml of air was subsequently aspirated from the orbit resulting in immediate resolution of his proptosis and diplopia, with concurrent improvement in visual acuity. IOP after the procedure was 17 mmHg in the right eye. As both pupils had been dilated to perform fundoscopy, assessment for resolution of the RAPD was not possible. A prophylactic dose of 375 mg coamoxiclav TDS was provided for five days. Ophthalmology follow-up was arranged for the next day, and the patient provided with information to avoid further nose-blowing/Valsalva manoeuvres, with strict instruction to return to casualty urgently if he experienced deterioration in vision. The patient subsequently declined follow-up and stated by telephone that this was not required due to lasting resolution in proptosis and diplopia, with concurrent normal visual acuity.

3. Discussion

Most reported cases of orbital emphysema follow a history of trauma, though not necessarily immediately [1, 2]. Patients with a preceding episode of trauma days or weeks before may present acutely with orbital emphysema after an episode of increased intranasal pressure provoked by sneezing or nose-blowing. However, in this case, there was no preceding injury noted. From a review of the literature, we have identified only 21 cases of orbital emphysema where no history of trauma or periocular surgery was evident [8–28]. Cases of orbital emphysema are usually mild and do not affect visual function, with approximately 12% of patients requiring decompression [5]. Of the 21 cases found with no history of trauma [8–28], one had nonurgent surgery due to persistent diplopia lasting more than a week [17]. In this case, fractures of the orbital floor were apparent, with fat entrapment. Two of the 21 cases reported emergency needle decompression [9, 12]. In the first, there was proptosis, restriction of eye movements, raised intraocular pressure (IOP), and a hazy cornea. However, it was noted that there was no RAPD or dyschromatopsia and therefore no evidence of optic nerve compromise. In the second, decompression was performed due to the extent of eyelid swelling precluding assessment of the eye. As such, our case is the first to document clear evidence of optic nerve dysfunction after nontraumatic orbital emphysema.

In addition, recurrent orbital emphysema is relatively rare and in our case contributed to by the patient's lack of desire to seek medical attention. Two posttraumatic cases describe short-term recurrence of symptoms due to increases in intranasal pressure: Valsalva manoeuvres while crying in one case and sneezing in the other [5, 29]. In our case, while the patient was not trying to cause proptosis of his eye, he was aware this was a consequence of him performing Valsalva manoeuvres. However, this practice was continued for a year and only led him to seek medical attention once it had become so severe as to cause optic nerve dysfunction. Given that he performed Valsalva manoeuvres on a daily basis, it may be that he already had a small pocket of intraorbital air prior to this acute episode which may be responsible for the severe and acute nature of optic nerve compromise.

Finally, the IOP was 12 mmHg prior to decompression despite significant intraorbital air, proptosis, and RAPD. This emphasises the fact that a normal IOP cannot exclude orbital compartment syndrome. Intraocular pressure is often used as a surrogate for intraorbital pressure. Documented IOP in all previously reported cases of orbital emphysema (both traumatic and nontraumatic) requiring emergency decompression ranged from 20 to over 100 mmHg (Table 1) [2, 6, 9,

30–38]. As such, our case highlights that while raised IOP can act as a surrogate measure to inform the decision for urgent orbital decompression, a normal measurement does not exclude optic nerve compromise.

In summary, we present the first documented case in which nontraumatic orbital emphysema resulted directly in orbital compartment syndrome with optic nerve dysfunction. The authors stress that the absence of a history of trauma and a normal IOP cannot definitively exclude the necessity for urgent orbital decompression.

References

[1] R. B. Birrer, T. Robinson, and P. Papachristos, "Orbital emphysema: how common, how significant?," *Annals of Emergency Medicine*, vol. 24, no. 6, pp. 1115–1118, 1994.

[2] J. H. Hunts, J. R. Patrinely, J. B. Holds, and R. L. Anderson, "Orbital emphysema: staging and acute management," *Ophthalmology*, vol. 101, no. 5, pp. 960–966, 1994.

[3] C. C. O'Malley, "Orbital emphysema simulating cellulitis," *The British Journal of Ophthalmology*, vol. 27, no. 5, pp. 222–226, 1943.

[4] I. E. Zimmer-Galler and G. B. Bartley, "Orbital emphysema: case reports and review of the literature," *Mayo Clinic Proceedings*, vol. 69, no. 2, pp. 115–121, 1994.

[5] K. A. Roelofs, V. Starks, and M. K. Yoon, "Orbital emphysema: a case report and comprehensive review of the literature," *Ophthalmic Plastic & Reconstructive Surgery*, vol. 35, no. 1, pp. 1–6, 2019.

[6] A. M. Monaghan and B. G. Millar, "Orbital emphysema during air travel: a case report," *Journal of Cranio-Maxillo-Facial Surgery*, vol. 30, no. 6, pp. 367-368, 2002.

[7] P. Clement and H. Chovanova, "Pressures generated during nose blowing in patients with nasal complaints and normal test subjects," *Rhinology*, vol. 41, no. 3, pp. 152–158, 2003.

[8] D. Halpenny, C. Corbally, and W. Torreggiani, "Blowout fracture of the orbital floor secondary to vigorous nose blowing," *Irish Medical Journal*, vol. 105, no. 7, pp. 245-246, 2012.

[9] M. Singh, V. M. Phua, and G. Sundar, "Sight-threatening orbital emphysema treated with needle decompression," *Clinical & Experimental Ophthalmology*, vol. 35, no. 4, pp. 386-387, 2007.

[10] B. Mohan and K. P. Singh, "Bilateral subcutaneous emphysema of the orbits following nose blowing," *The Journal of Laryngology and Otology*, vol. 115, no. 4, pp. 319-320, 2001.

[11] S. K. Singhai, A. Dass, G. B. Singh, and R. D. Virk, "Orbital pneumatocele," *Indian Journal of Otolaryngology and Head & Neck Surgery*, vol. 55, no. 4, pp. 292-293, 2003.

[12] J. J. García-Medina, M. García-Medina, and M. D. Pinazo-Durán, "Severe orbitopalpebral emphysema after nose blowing requiring emergency decompression," *European Journal of Ophthalmology*, vol. 16, no. 2, pp. 339–342, 2018.

[13] W. C. Chiu, T. Y. Huang, W. C. Ku, M. Lih, and W. Wang, "Spontaneous orbital subcutaneous emphysema after sneezing," *The American Journal of Emergency Medicine*, vol. 26, no. 3, article 381-e1, 2008.

[14] F. Di Lella, A. Bacciu, V. Vincenti, E. Pasanisi, and S. Bacciu, "Orbital and infratemporal fossa emphysema following nose blowing," *Clinical Otolaryngology*, vol. 33, no. 2, pp. 181-182, 2008.

[15] A. J. Rosh and R. Sharma, "Orbital emphysema after nose blowing," *The Journal of Emergency Medicine*, vol. 34, no. 3, pp. 327–329, 2008.

[16] J. A. Garcia De Marcos, J. L. del Castillo-Pardo de Vera, and J. Calderón-Polanco, "Orbital floor fracture and emphysema after nose blowing," *Oral and Maxillofacial Surgery*, vol. 12, no. 3, pp. 163–165, 2008.

[17] B. B. Rahmel, C. R. Scott, and A. J. Lynham, "Comminuted orbital blowout fracture after vigorous nose blowing that required repair," *The British Journal of Oral & Maxillofacial Surgery*, vol. 48, no. 4, pp. e21–e22, 2010.

[18] Q. A. Khader and K. J. Abdul-Baqi, "Orbital emphysema after a protracted episode of sneezing in a patient with no history of trauma or sinus surgery," *Ear, Nose, & Throat Journal*, vol. 89, no. 11, pp. E12–E13, 2010.

[19] D. Sen and P. K. Chaturvedi, "Orbital emphysema after sneezing: a case report," *Medical Journal, Armed Forces India*, vol. 67, no. 3, pp. 282–284, 2011.

[20] T. Watanabe, T. Kawano, S. Kodama, and M. Suzuki, "Orbital blowout fracture caused by nose blowing," *Ear, Nose, & Throat Journal*, vol. 91, no. 1, pp. 24-25, 2019.

[21] N. C. Pausch, A. Neff, K. Dhanuthai, N. Sirintawat, C. Vorakulpipat, and P. Pitak-Arnnop, "Grand rounds: eyelid swelling after nose blowing," *American Journal of Otolaryngology*, vol. 35, no. 3, pp. 456–459, 2014.

[22] O. Ozdemir, "Orbital emphysema occurring during weight lifting," *Seminars in ophthalmology*, vol. 30, no. 5-6, pp. 426–428, 2015.

[23] M. S. Jawaid, "Orbital emphysema: nose blowing leading to a blown orbit," *BMJ Case Reports*, vol. 2015, article bcr2015212554, 2015.

[24] R. F. Betances, E. C. Chiesa, and V. A. Osorio, "Orbital emphysema after blowing the nose," *Acta Otorrinolaringológica Española*, vol. 67, no. 4, article e28, 2016.

[25] H. C. Hu, A. Chang, and Y. H. Chiu, "Orbital emphysema after nose blowing," *QJM*, vol. 110, no. 1, p. 41, 2017.

[26] S. Ali, M. L. Ranney, and A. F. Jarman, "Transient orbital compartment syndrome caused by spontaneous lamina papyracea dehiscence," *R.I. Medical Journal*, vol. 101, no. 1, pp. 30–32, 2018.

[27] S. Myers and D. Bell, "Orbital blowout fracture from nose blowing," *BMJ Case Reports*, vol. 2018, article bcr-2018, 2018.

[28] C. Aubin-Lemay, P. Acar, N. Alnaif, A. Alamri, A. J. Azzi, and S. Cugno, "Orbital subcutaneous emphysema in a child," *The Journal of Craniofacial Surgery*, vol. 29, no. 4, pp. 1020–1022, 2018.

[29] P. Marzuillo, F. Aliberti, and V. Tipo, "Pneumo-orbita mimicking hordeolum," *Archives of Disease in Childhood*, vol. 101, no. 2, p. 183, 2016.

[30] J. A. Fleishman, R. W. Beck, and R. O. Hoffman, "Orbital emphysema as an ophthalmologic emergency," *Ophthalmology*, vol. 91, no. 11, pp. 1389–1391, 1984.

[31] A. A. Dobler, A. L. Nathenson, J. D. Cameron, E. T. Carpel, A. M. Janda, and J. E. Pederson, "A case of orbital emphysema as an ocular emergency," *Retina*, vol. 13, no. 2, pp. 166–168, 1993.

[32] M. J. Wearne, J. Frank, and S. Bryan, "Management of orbital emphysema," *Eye (London, England)*, vol. 12, no. 6, pp. 1016-1017, 1998.

[33] S. L. Lee, D. M. Mills, D. R. Meyer, and S. M. Silver, "Orbital

emphysema," *Ophthalmology*, vol. 113, no. 11, article 2113.e1, 2006.

[34] I. A. Chaudhry, A. Al-Amri, F. A. Shamsi, and W. Al-Rashed, "Visual recovery after evacuation of orbital emphysema," *Orbit*, vol. 26, no. 4, pp. 283–285, 2009.

[35] A. B. Furlani, B. Diniz, L. G. Bitelli, and E. N. Martins, "Enfisema orbitário compressivo após asseio nasal: relato de caso," *Arquivos Brasileiros de Oftalmologia*, vol. 72, no. 2, pp. 251–253, 2009.

[36] G. Chak, J. M. Joseph, and J. P. Tao, "Needle decompression of acute orbital emphysema: case report with video," *The British Journal of Ophthalmology*, vol. 96, no. 10, pp. 1346-1347, 2012.

[37] A. D. Rowh, J. W. Ufberg, T. C. Chan, G. M. Vilke, and R. A. Harrigan, "Lateral canthotomy and cantholysis: emergency management of orbital compartment syndrome," *The Journal of Emergency Medicine*, vol. 48, no. 3, pp. 325–330, 2015.

[38] C. Y. Lin, C. C. Tsai, S. C. Kao, H. C. Kau, and F. L. Lee, "Needle decompression in a patient with vision-threatening orbital emphysema," *Taiwan Journal of Ophthalmology*, vol. 6, no. 2, pp. 93–95, 2016.

27

Intravitreal Aflibercept as a Rescue Therapy for Retinal Neovascularization and Macular Edema due to Eales Disease

Ning-Yi Hsia,[1] Chun-Ju Lin,[1,2,3] Chun-Ting Lai,[1] Henry Bair,[1,4] Cheng-Hsien Chang,[1,2,3] Jane-Ming Lin,[1,2,3] and Yi-Yu Tsai[1,2,3]

[1]*Department of Ophthalmology, China Medical University Hospital, China Medical University, Taichung, Taiwan*
[2]*School of Medicine, College of Medicine, China Medical University, Taichung, Taiwan*
[3]*Department of Optometry, Asia University, Taichung, Taiwan*
[4]*Stanford University School of Medicine, Stanford, CA, USA*

Correspondence should be addressed to Chun-Ju Lin; doctoraga@gmail.com

Academic Editor: Stephen G. Schwartz

We report the rescue effect of intravitreal aflibercept injections on retinal neovascularization and macular edema due to Eales disease. Case 1 was a 36-year-old female. Intravitreal aflibercept was administered as rescue therapy after persistent retinal neovascularization following retinal photocoagulation, periocular triamcinolone, and intravitreal ranibizumab injection. Retinal neovascularization initially regressed, but recurred after 5 months along with macular edema. Two more intravitreal aflibercept injections were given, and retinal neovascularization with macular edema regressed. Her vision improved to 20/25 and remained stable after 43 months. Case 2 was a 27-year-old female. Intravitreal aflibercept was administered after persistent retinal neovascularization and macular edema following periocular triamcinolone injection. The macular edema initially subsided but recurred after 3 months. Intravitreal aflibercept injections were then administered once every three months to maintain her vision 20/20. The patient has been followed up for 28 months. Intravitreal aflibercept was effective as a rescue therapy in the treatment of Eales disease to regress retinal neovascularization, though repeated injections were necessary in cases of recurrence.

1. Introduction

Eales disease is a potentially blinding idiopathic retinal vasculopathy, involving inflammatory venous occlusion that primarily affects the peripheral retina of healthy young adults. Retinal changes include periphlebitis, peripheral nonperfusion, and neovascularization. In addition, visual loss is characteristically caused by recurrent vitreous hemorrhage [1–3].

The presence of inflammatory cytokines (interleukin-6, interleukin-8, and monocyte chemoattractant protein-1) and vascular endothelial growth factor (VEGF) in the vitreous has previously been observed in Eales disease [4, 5]. Angiogenesis is a highly complex and coordinated process in which VEGF plays a pivotal role, under both normal and pathological conditions. Since VEGF is upregulated during retinal hypoxia, anti-VEGF agents are now being used for treatment of pathological ocular angiogenesis and macular edema.

We report the rescue effects of intravitreal aflibercept (EYLEA, Regeneron Pharmaceuticals, Tarrytown, NY) injections in two cases of retinal neovascularization and macular edema in Eales disease. These two cases had persistent retinal neovascularization with macular edema after focal retinal photocoagulation, periocular depot triamcinolone, or intravitreal ranibizumab treatment. To our knowledge, this is the first report describing the use of intravitreal aflibercept in a relatively advanced stage of Eales disease.

2. Case Presentation

We retrospectively reviewed two patients with retinal neovascularization (NV) and macular edema (ME) due to Eales disease, who were treated with intravitreal 2.0 mg/0.05 mL aflibercept injections as rescue therapy. Diagnosis and assessment of Eales disease were based on the findings of fluorescein angiography (FA) and negative interferon-gamma

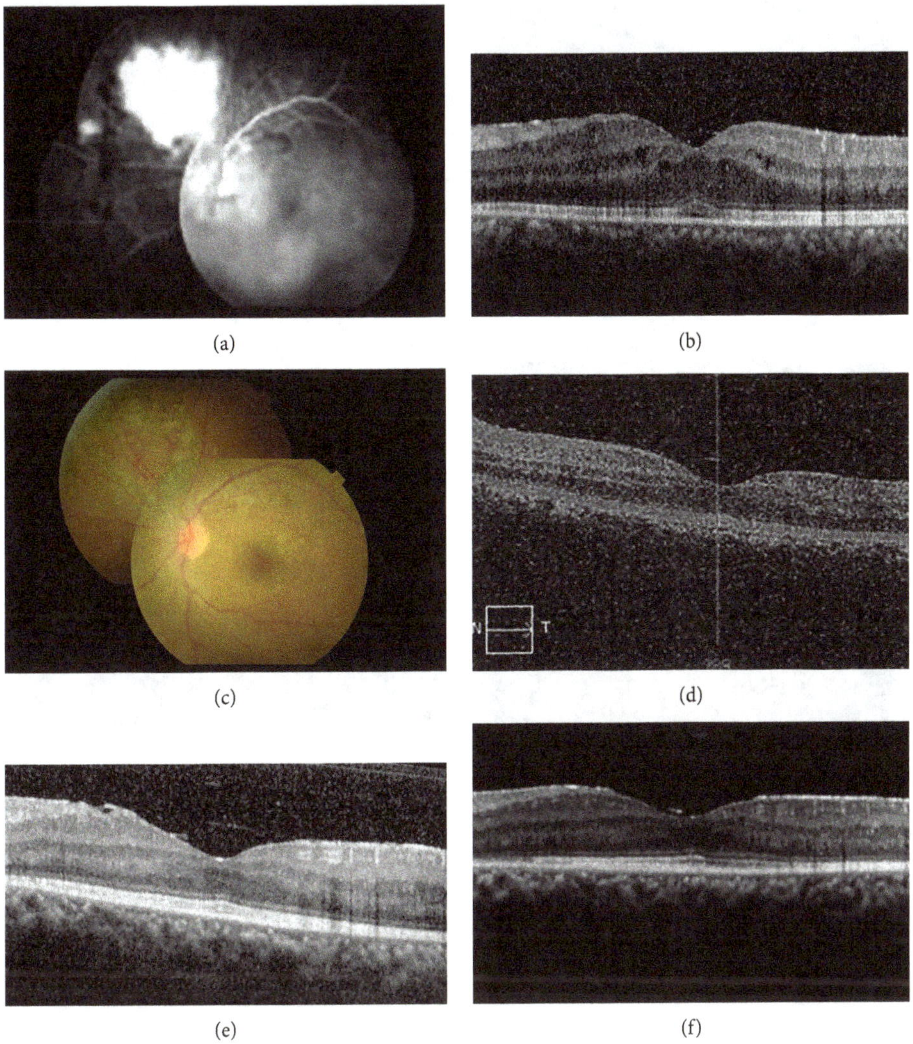

Figure 1: (a) FA showed vascular tortuosity, peripheral retinal neovascularization (NV), and macular edema (ME). (b) OCT revealed ME (central foveal thickness 376 μm). (c) After the first intravitreal aflibercept injection, the retinal NV regressed. (d) ME also decreased (central foveal thickness 293 μm). (e) ME recurred 5 months after the first intravitreal aflibercept injection (central foveal thickness 305 μm). (f) No recurrent ME 15 months after the third intravitreal aflibercept injection (central foveal thickness 295 μm).

release assays (QuantiFERON®-TB test). Magnetic resonance imaging (MRI) was also performed to differentiate optic neuritis-induced retinal NV. They had no significant past medical history either physical signs of mucosal ulceration or arthritis. Their laboratory study for ruling out infection and autoimmune disease, such as complete blood counts, HLA-B27, HLA-B51, antiphospholipid antibodies, antinuclear autoantibodies, antineutrophil cytoplasmic autoantibodies, anti-dsDNA, anti-Sm, or rheumatoid factor, was all negative results.

Case 1 was a 36-year-old female with presenting BCVA counting fingers OS due to vitreous hemorrhage (VH). Oral transamin and topical steroid treatment were given. FA showed vascular tortuosity, peripheral retinal NV, and ME (Figure 1(a)). OCT also revealed ME (Figure 1(b)). Intravitreal aflibercept was used as rescue therapy due to persistent retinal NV and ME after administration of focal retinal photocoagulation, periocular depot triamcinolone acetonide, and intravitreal ranibizumab injections. After the first intravitreal aflibercept injection, the retinal NV regressed (Figure 1(c)) and ME decreased (Figure 1(d)). ME recurred after 5 months (Figure 1(e)). Supplemental retinal photocoagulation was performed, and the second intravitreal aflibercept injection was given. The retinal NV regressed again and ME resolved. Recurrent VH was noted after 15 months, and a third intravitreal aflibercept injection was given. VH and ME were then resolved (Figure 1(f)). The patient's BCVA improved to 20/25 and was followed up for 43 months. Her intraocular pressure was within normal limits during the whole course.

Case 2 was a 27-year-old female with presenting BCVA 20/30 OD due to VH. Oral transamin and topical steroid treatment were given. FA showed vascular tortuosity, peripheral retinal NV, and cystoid macular edema (CME) (Figure 2(a)). Intravitreal aflibercept was used as rescue therapy due to persistent CME and retinal NV after administration of periocular depot triamcinolone acetonide injection and topical nepafenac (Figure 2(b)). After the first intravitreal aflibercept injection, the retinal NV regressed

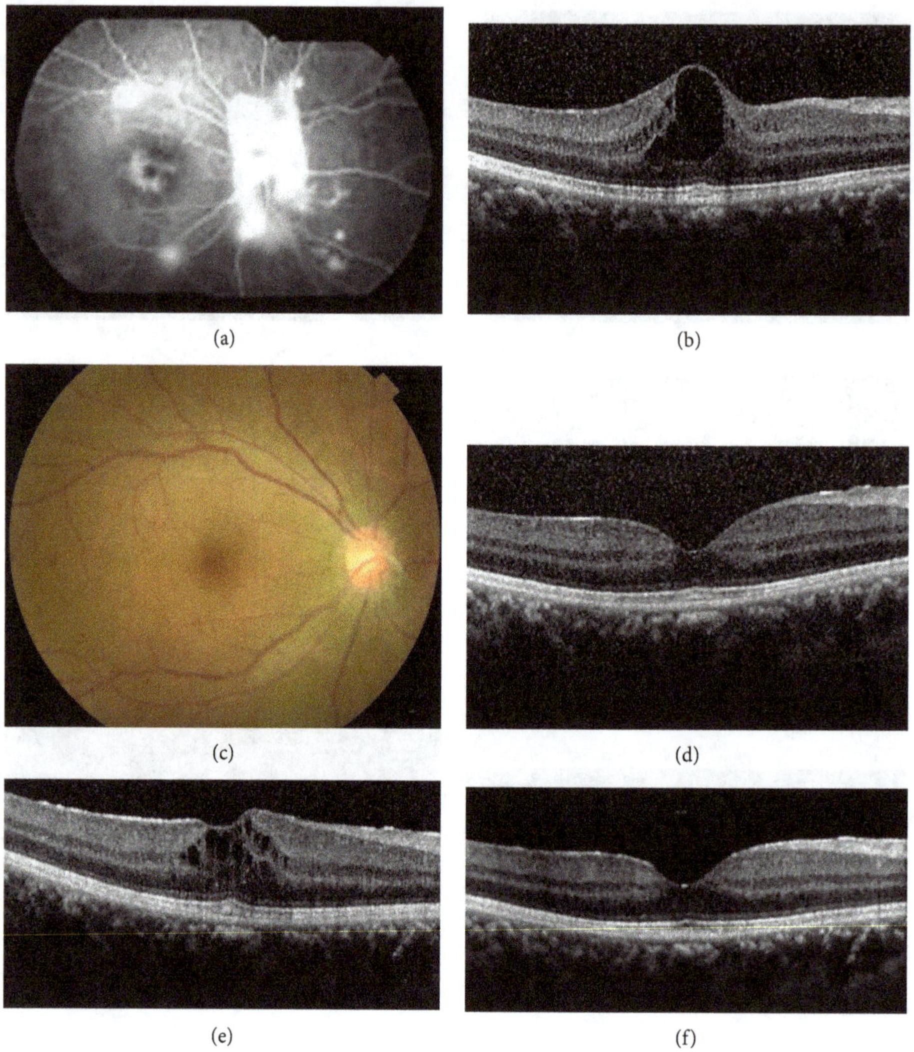

FIGURE 2: (a) FA showed vascular tortuosity, peripheral retinal NV, and ME. (b) Persistent ME after periocular depot triamcinolone acetonide injection (central foveal thickness 538 μm). (c) After the first intravitreal aflibercept injection, the retinal NV regressed. (d) ME also subsided (central foveal thickness 309 μm). (e) ME recurred after 3 months (central foveal thickness 438 μm). (f) Intravitreal aflibercept injections had to be performed every three months to keep macula free from edema (central foveal thickness 295 μm).

(Figure 2(c)) and CME subsided (Figure 2(d)). The patient's BCVA improved to 20/25. However, ME recurred after 3 months (Figure 2(e)). Thereafter, intravitreal aflibercept injections were administered once every three months to keep her BCVA 20/20 (Figure 2(f)). The patient has been followed up for 28 months. Her intraocular pressure was within normal limits during the whole course. The treatment was well tolerated by both patients without significant adverse events.

3. Discussion

Eales disease was first described in 1880, and idiopathic inflammatory disorder of the retinal vessels (primarily veins) was presumed thereafter [1–3]. Recurrent vitreous and retinal hemorrhages resulted in sudden visual impairment. It is thought to be related to tuberculosis and is predisposed in certain geographic areas and age groups (15 to 40 years) [6].

Currently, the most favored etiologies of Eales disease are tuberculosis and hypersensitivity to tuberculoprotein [6]. 50-70% of epiretinal membrane samples were found positive for *Mycobacterium* species by polymerase chain reaction (PCR) analysis. MPB64 gene of *M. tuberculosis* has been found in a significant number of well-documented Eales disease patients. However, cultures of vitreous specimen did not show growth of *M. tuberculosis* in any of the vitreous aspirates. Thus, although Eales disease patients may not carry viable organisms, they may harbor nonviable organisms or deoxyribonucleic acid (DNA) of *M. tuberculosis* [7].

No recent studies have been able to definitively differentiate Eales disease from tuberculous vasculitis, though some association exists between this type of occlusive vasculitis and tuberculosis. Negative results of QuantiFERON®-TB tests ruled out ocular tuberculosis in the two patients reported here. Moreover, a negative workup, including the use of MRI to differentiate optic neuritis-induced retinal

NV, in such cases, could indicate idiopathic occlusive vasculitis [8–10].

The management of Eales disease includes medical therapy, intravitreal injections, photocoagulation, and surgery [7, 11–13]. Corticosteroids are the mainstay of therapies used in the active perivasculitis stage to control inflammation. In patients with hypersensitivity to tuberculoproteins (positive Mantoux test), antitubercular treatment should also been given for 9 months. Panretinal photocoagulation can be performed for ischemic retina.

In cases of macular involvement, periocular depot triamcinolone acetonide injections can be attempted first. If ME or VH persists, treatment with intravitreal anti-VEGF agent such as bevacizumab (Avastin, Genentech Inc., South San Francisco, CA) has been reported [11, 12]. Massive VEGF expression observed in Eales disease might be due to retinal ischemia and chronic low-grade inflammation [4, 5]. Intravitreal bevacizumab has been effective in regressing NV, hastening the resolution of VH, or reducing the need for vitrectomy. Intravitreal bevacizumab as an adjunct to vitrectomy in advanced Eales disease has also been advocated [10]. However, it might increase the risk of tractional retinal detachment.

To the best of our knowledge, aflibercept has not been previously used in the treatment of Eales disease. In case 1, intravitreal ranibizumab was first administered but showed no obvious response. Therefore, aflibercept was used and showed effects in regressing retinal NV. In case 2, only aflibercept was used and showed favorable results. Our explanation for the better response of intravitreal aflibercept treatment was that aflibercept binds not only all isoforms of VEGF-A, and VEGF-B, but also placental growth factor (PGF). In addition, aflibercept had faster association rate and higher binding affinity for VEGF than ranibizumab. Aflibercept thus may neutralize intravitreal VEGF level more effectively and had further positive effect on reduced inflammation [14, 15].

Intravitreal aflibercept appeared effective in regressing retinal NV in Eales disease. Because there may be bleeding or ME on more than one occasion in these patients, repeated injections were necessary in cases of recurrence. This study demonstrated the rescue effects of intravitreal aflibercept in the treatment of persistent retinal NV and ME in Eales disease. More cases and long-term follow-up are mandatory to further elucidate the mechanisms involved and quantitate the therapeutic potential.

Consent

The study was performed with informed consent.

References

[1] H. Eales, "Retinal haemorrhages associated with epistaxis and constipation," *Brim Med*, vol. 9, p. 262, 1880.

[2] T. Das, J. Biswas, A. Kumar, P. N. Nagpal, P. Namperumalsamy, and H. K. Tewari, "Eales disease," *Indian Journal of Ophthalmology*, vol. 42, no. 1, pp. 3–18, 1994.

[3] L. S. Atmaca, F. Batioglu, and S. P. Atmaca, "A long-term follow-up of Eales disease," *Ocular Immunology and Inflammation*, vol. 10, pp. 213–221, 2009.

[4] P. Murugeswari, D. Shukla, A. Rajendran, R. Kim, P. Namperumalsamy, and V. Muthukkaruppan, "Proinflammatory cytokines and angiogenic and anti-angiogenic factors in vitreous of patients with proliferative diabetic retinopathy and Eales disease," *Retina*, vol. 28, no. 6, pp. 817–824, 2008.

[5] P. Murugeswari, D. Shukla, R. Kim, P. Namperumalsamy, A. W. Stitt, and V. Muthukkaruppan, "Angiogenic potential of vitreous from proliferative diabetic retinopathy and Eales disease patients," *PLoS One*, vol. 9, no. 10, article e107551, 2014.

[6] U. B. Singh, S. Mohapatra, V. K. Wagh, C. Porwal, A. Kaushik, and Rajpal, "Association of *Mycobacterium tuberculosis* in the causation of Eales disease: an institutional experience," *Indian Journal of Medical Microbiology*, vol. 33, no. 5, p. 43, 2015.

[7] J. Biswas, R. K. Ravi, A. Naryanasamy, L. T. Kulandai, and H. N. Madhavan, "Eales' disease - current concepts in diagnosis and management," *Journal of Ophthalmic Inflammation and Infection*, vol. 3, no. 1, p. 11, 2013.

[8] C.-w. Su, C.-j. Lin, Y.-y. Lo, and Y.-Y. Tsai, "Pediatric optic neuritis complicated with vitreous hemorrhage from retinal neovascularization," *Retinal Physician*, vol. 13, pp. 54–57, 2016.

[9] J. M. Katsimpris, J. K. Petropoulos, and N. M. Pharmakakis, "Bilateral peripheral retinal neovascularization in a patient with multiple sclerosis," *Journal Français d Ophtalmologie*, vol. 25, no. 8, pp. 813–816, 2002.

[10] J. Lee and S. Ferrucci, "Peripapillary subretinal neovascular membranes: a review," *Optometry - Journal of the American Optometric Association.*, vol. 82, no. 11, pp. 681–688, 2011.

[11] A. Kumar and S. Sinha, "Rapid regression of disc and retinal neovascularization in a case of Eales disease after intravitreal bevacizumab," *Canadian Journal of Ophthalmology*, vol. 42, no. 2, pp. 335-336, 2007.

[12] S. D. Patwardhan, R. Azad, B. M. Shah, and Y. Sharma, "Role of intravitreal bevacizumab in Eales disease with dense vitreous hemorrhage: a prospective randomized control study," *Retina*, vol. 31, no. 5, pp. 866–870, 2011.

[13] M. Thakar, N. R. Bamrolia, U. K. Raina, and B. Ghosh, "Intravitreal bevacizumab as an adjunct to vitrectomy in advanced Eales disease," *Journal of Ophthalmic Inflammation and Infection*, vol. 2, no. 2, pp. 105–108, 2012.

[14] N. Kumar, M. Marsiglia, S. Mrejen et al., "Visual and anatomical outcomes of intravitreal aflibercept in eyes with persistent subfoveal fluid despite previous treatments with ranibizumab in patients with neovascular age-related macular degeneration," *Retina*, vol. 33, no. 8, pp. 1605–1612, 2013.

[15] Y. Liu, J. Cheng, Y. Gao, L. Qin, X. Min, and M. Zhang, "Efficacy of switching therapy to aflibercept for patients with persistent diabetic macular edema: a systematic review and meta-analysis," *Annals of Translational Medicine*, vol. 8, no. 6, p. 382, 2020.

28

Central Serous Chorioretinopathy: Multimodal Imaging and Management Options

Prashanth G. Iyer, Stephen G. Schwartz, Jonathan F. Russell, and Harry W. Flynn Jr.

Department of Ophthalmology, Bascom Palmer Eye Institute, University of Miami Miller School of Medicine, Miami, Florida, USA

Correspondence should be addressed to Stephen G. Schwartz; sschwartz2@med.miami.edu

Academic Editor: Shigeki Machida

Central serous chorioretinopathy (CSCR) is an idiopathic maculopathy characterized by thickened choroid, retinal pigment epithelial detachment, and variable subretinal fluid. CSCR predominantly affects young men, with risk factors including corticosteroid use, the type A behavior pattern, and psychological stress. While usually self-limited with a good visual prognosis, recurrent and persistent CSCR can lead to outer retinal and/or retinal pigment epithelial atrophy, choroidal neovascularization, and visual loss. This article reviews current multimodal imaging and treatment options, which include observation, mineralocorticoid receptor antagonists, thermal laser photocoagulation, and off-label photodynamic therapy with verteporfin.

1. Introduction

Central serous chorioretinopathy (CSCR) is a macular disorder thought to be due to alterations of the choroidal vasculature that overwhelm the ability of the retinal pigment epithelial (RPE) to dehydrate the subretinal space, with consequent accumulation of subretinal fluid. [1–3] Thickened choroid, RPE detachments, and variable subretinal fluid are cardinal features of CSCR. Patients may be asymptomatic or may complain of central scotoma, metamorphopsia, dyschromatopsia, and micropsia [4–6].

CSCR generally affects individuals between ages 30 and 50 years, with a predominance for men [7–11]. CSCR is most commonly seen in Asian and Caucasian patients [8]. Other risk factors include corticosteroid exposure, the type A behavior pattern (including a preponderance of a competitive drive, a sense of urgency, an aggressive nature, and a hostile temperament), psychological stress, *Helicobacter pylori* infection, use of phosphodiesterase 5 inhibitors, exogenous testosterone supplementation, obstructive sleep apnea, pregnancy, and some endocrine disorders [6, 11–19].

2. Clinical Features

Patients with acute CSCR typically present with clear and well-demarcated subretinal fluid. There is typically a smooth pigment epithelial detachment (PED) underlying the subretinal fluid, although the PED can be small and challenging to identify with biomicroscopy alone. The clinical course of CSCR is usually self-limited, with spontaneous resolution of subretinal fluid and restoration of visual acuity by three months [20]. The presence of turbid subretinal fluid and/or blood should alert the physician to the possibility of another diagnosis, including idiopathic choroidal neovascularization (CNV), exudative age-related macular degeneration, or polypoidal choroidal vasculopathy.

Some patients with CSCR will have a persistent or recurrent course beyond three months. Chronic CSCR can involve multifocal or diffuse RPE disruption and atrophy throughout the posterior pole, potentially causing severe visual loss [8]. RPE atrophy, along with outer retinal atrophy, secondary CNV, cystoid macular edema (CME), and choriocapillaris atrophy are causes of permanent visual loss [20] [21].

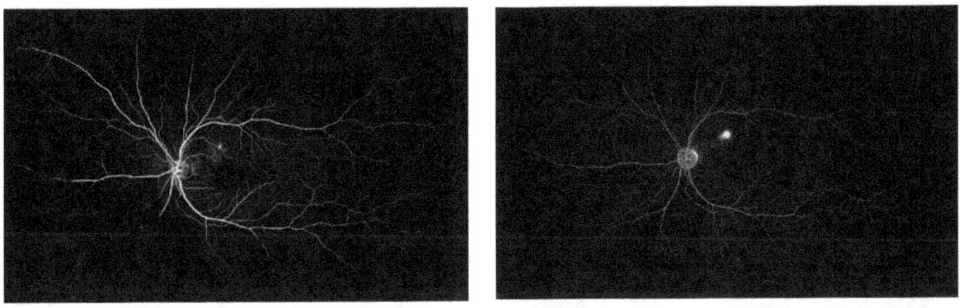

(a) (b)

FIGURE 1: Fluorescein angiography with focal leakage, sometimes called an expansile dot. (a) Early phase. (b) Late phase.

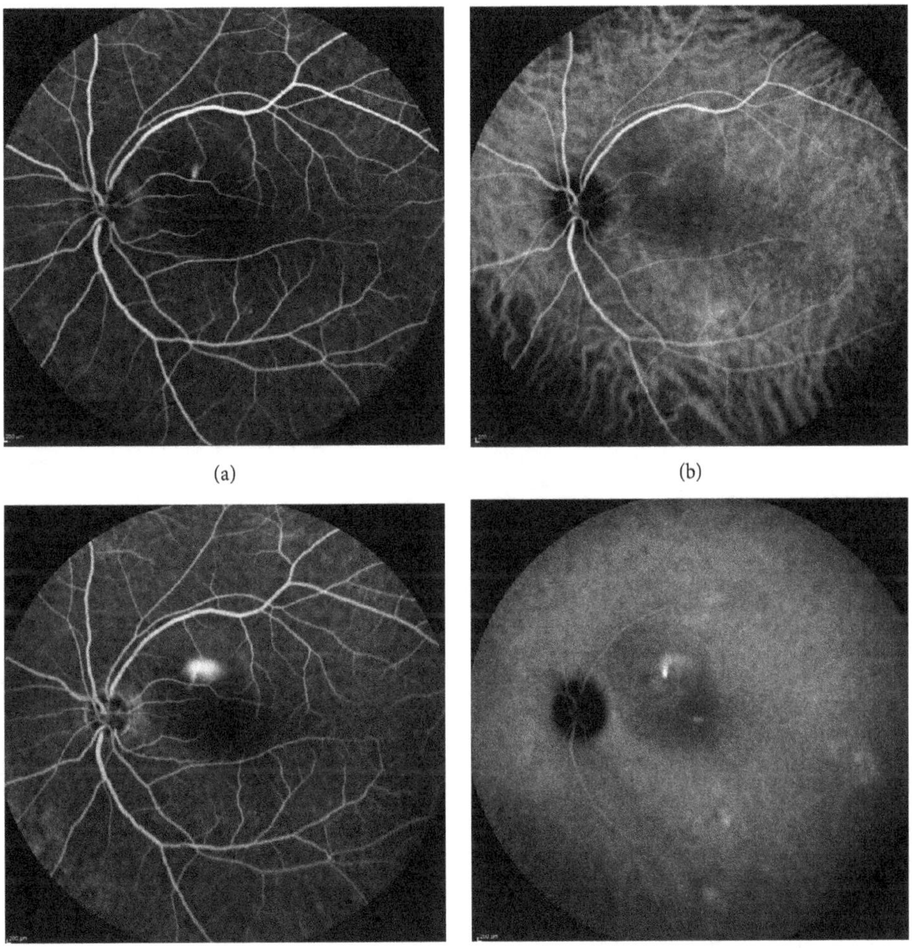

(a) (b) (c) (d)

FIGURE 2: Simultaneous fluorescein angiography and indocyanine green angiography with a smokestack pattern. Early (a, b) and late (c, d) phase images are shown.

3. Imaging Modalities

3.1. Fluorescein Angiography. Fluorescein angiography (FA) can reveal various patterns in acute CSCR including focal leakage (sometimes called expansile dot) in the majority of cases (Figure 1) and a smokestack pattern in 10-20% of patients (Figure 2) [22].

Chronic CSCR may show multiple areas of mottled hyperfluorescence, indicating widespread patchy RPE dysfunction and/or atrophy [23]. FA can also detect the presence of secondary CNV.

3.2. Indocyanine Green Angiography. Indocyanine green angiography (ICGA) is another dye-based test that can detect

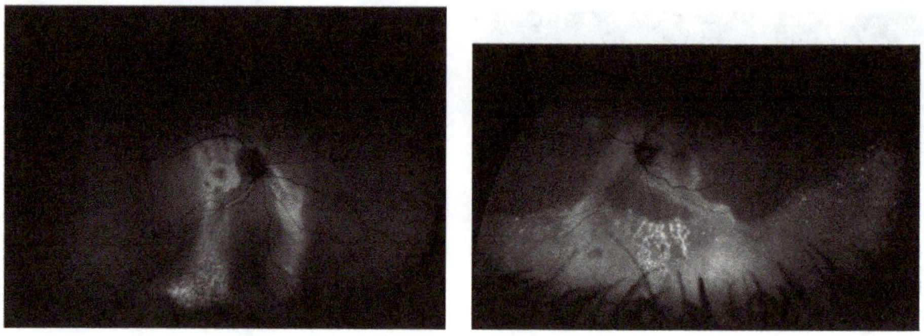

(a) (b)

FIGURE 3: Fundus autofluorescence of two different patients with chronic central serous chorioretinopathy with descending tracts or "guttering".

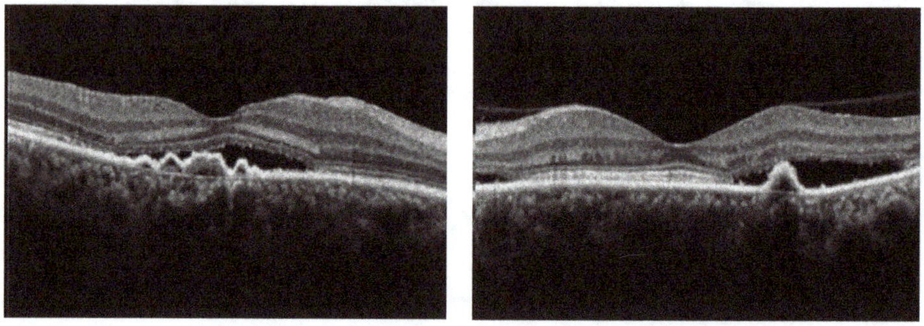

(a) (b)

FIGURE 4: Optical coherence tomography in central serous chorioretinopathy. Note multiple pigment epithelial detachments, subretinal fluid, and "shaggy" photoreceptors.

impaired choroidal circulation in CSCR, including choroidal hypoperfusion, delays in choroidal circulation, and hyperfluorescence corresponding to areas of choroidal hyperpermeability [24, 25].

3.3. Fundus Autofluorescence. Fundus autofluorescence (FAF) detects the endogenous fluorophores found in lipofuscin of the RPE cells, providing information regarding the health of the RPE [26, 27]. FAF patterns in acute CSCR may include confluent or granular hypoautofluorescence signifying loss of RPE cells and hyperautofluorescence representing accumulation of unphagocytized photoreceptor outer segments [28]. In chronic CSCR, there is multifocal or diffuse mottled hypoautofluorescence representing atrophy of the RPE. There can be areas of hyperautofluorescence. Descending tracts, also known as "guttering", (Figure 3) with increased and decreased autofluorescence may be seen [28, 29].

3.4. Optical Coherence Tomography. Optical coherence tomography (OCT) allows for rapid noninvasive identification of PED, CME, subretinal fluid, and other structural abnormalities (Figure 4). In addition, enhanced depth imaging OCT can detect increased choroidal thickness, which is characteristic of CSCR [30] (Figure 5). CSCR

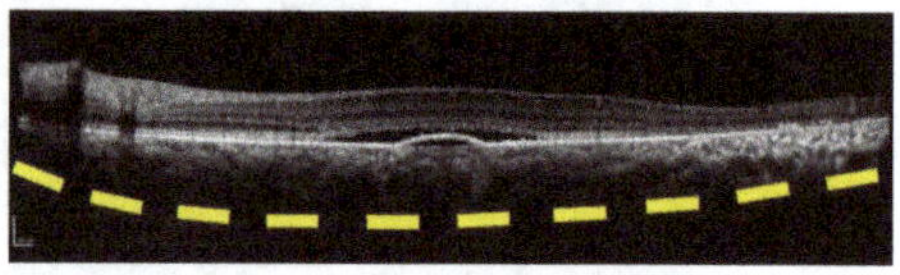

FIGURE 5: Optical coherence tomography in central serous chorioretinopathy. Note the pigment epithelial detachment and subretinal fluid. Enhanced depth imaging shows a thickened choroid (yellow dashes indicate the sclerochoroidal junction).

can be described in the spectrum of pachychoroid diseases, which share similar features of choroidal thickening and retinal pigment epithelial changes. [21, 31–33] The exact clinical significance of the different pachychoroid disorders with respect to treatment outcomes is uncertain and still under investigation [34].

3.5. Optical Coherence Tomography Angiography. Optical coherence tomography angiography (OCT-A) is a noninvasive, non-dye-based technique of angiography that can identify vascular flow in the different layers of the retina and choroid. OCT-A in CSCR can detect choroidal and choriocapillaris deficits, underlying CNV, and simultaneously

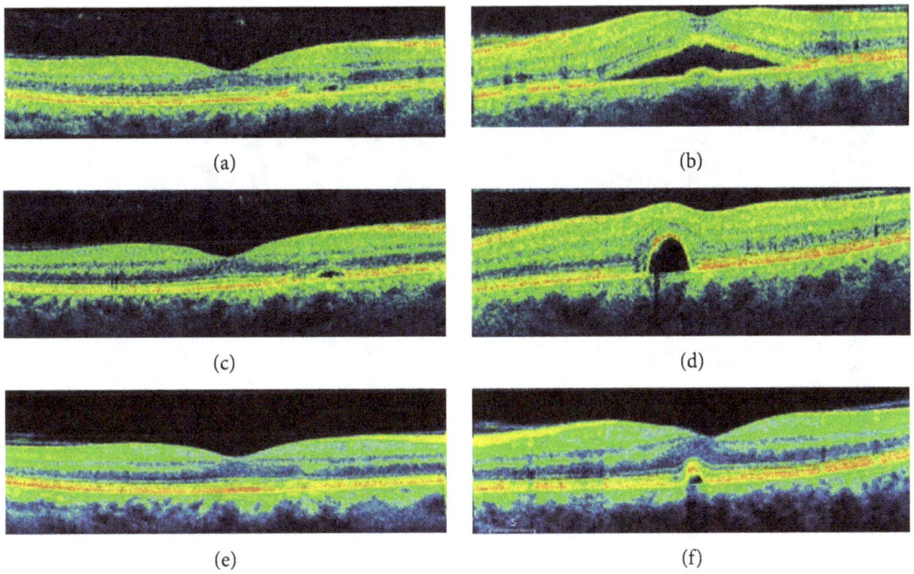

Figure 6: Observation of a patient with bilateral central serous chorioretinopathy. A 52-year-old male with a history of oral corticosteroid use presented with many months of blurred vision, left eye worse than the right eye. The patient was observed every few months without therapy. (a, b) Right and left eye (respectively) optical coherence tomography scans at baseline revealed subretinal fluid and pigment epithelial disruptions. (c, d) One year later, the left eye subretinal fluid had resolved but the pigment epithelial detachment was more elevated. (e, f) Two years later, the subretinal fluid had resolved in both eyes with mild pigment epithelial disruptions. Visual acuity remained stable at 20/20 in each eye throughout this timeframe.

includes B-scans that may feature PED, subretinal fluid, CME, and outer retinal and/or RPE atrophy [35–37].

4. Management

4.1. Observation. The majority of patients with CSCR will have spontaneous resolution of subretinal fluid with recovery of vision. Observation is the first-line therapy for most patients who have had symptoms for less than about three months [5, 21] (Figures 6 and 7). The use of exogenous corticosteroids should be reduced or discontinued if possible. Occasionally, treatment can be initiated sooner for patients requiring more rapid improvement in vision for occupational or other needs.

4.2. Thermal Laser Photocoagulation. Thermal laser photocoagulation is a well-established option for treating CSCR by directly applying argon laser to a leaking site seen on FA and/or ICGA (Figures 8 and 9). Thermal laser photocoagulation has been reported to decrease subretinal fluid and improve visual acuity [38]. However, long-term visual outcomes have not been reported to improve significantly with argon laser treatment [39, 40]. While most studies reported no differences in recurrence rates associated with laser photocoagulation, there are a few studies that reported lower rates of recurrence in laser-treated patients [41–44]. Complications of thermal laser photocoagulation include scar formation and secondary CNV. Given the potential for scarring, argon laser is most appropriate for extrafoveal leaking sites [42].

Subthreshold micropulse laser was initially described by Bandello and colleagues. In their pilot study, five patients with chronic CSCR were treated and had complete subretinal fluid resorption without recurrence; follow-up data and subsequent case studies have been promising [45–47].

4.3. Photodynamic Therapy. Off-label photodynamic therapy (PDT) with verteporfin (Visudyne, Bausch + Lomb, Bridgewater, NJ) was first described in a case series of 15 patients with chronic CSCR. Complete resolution of subretinal fluid occurred in 12 of the 15 patients [48]. PDT has been reported effective in resolving subretinal fluid and improving visual acuity [48–50]. Complications associated with PDT include secondary CNV, choriocapillaris hypoperfusion, and RPE damage [51]. In an effort to reduce complications, low dose verteporfin and lower fluence PDT have been reported effective with lower risks of adverse effects [52, 53]. Half-dose PDT has been reported to reduce subretinal fluid compared to argon laser in CSCR; however, visual acuity outcomes were similar in both groups [40] (Figures 10–12). The authors are anecdotally aware of, but have no personal experience with, the use of PDT in pediatric patients.

4.4. Eplerenone and Spironolactone. Eplerenone and spironolactone are two mineralocorticoid receptor (MR) antagonists that are increasingly used in the off-label treatment of CSCR. One hypothesis for the etiology of CSCR is inappropriate activation of MR by glucocorticoids; of note, corticosterone induces choroidal dilation,

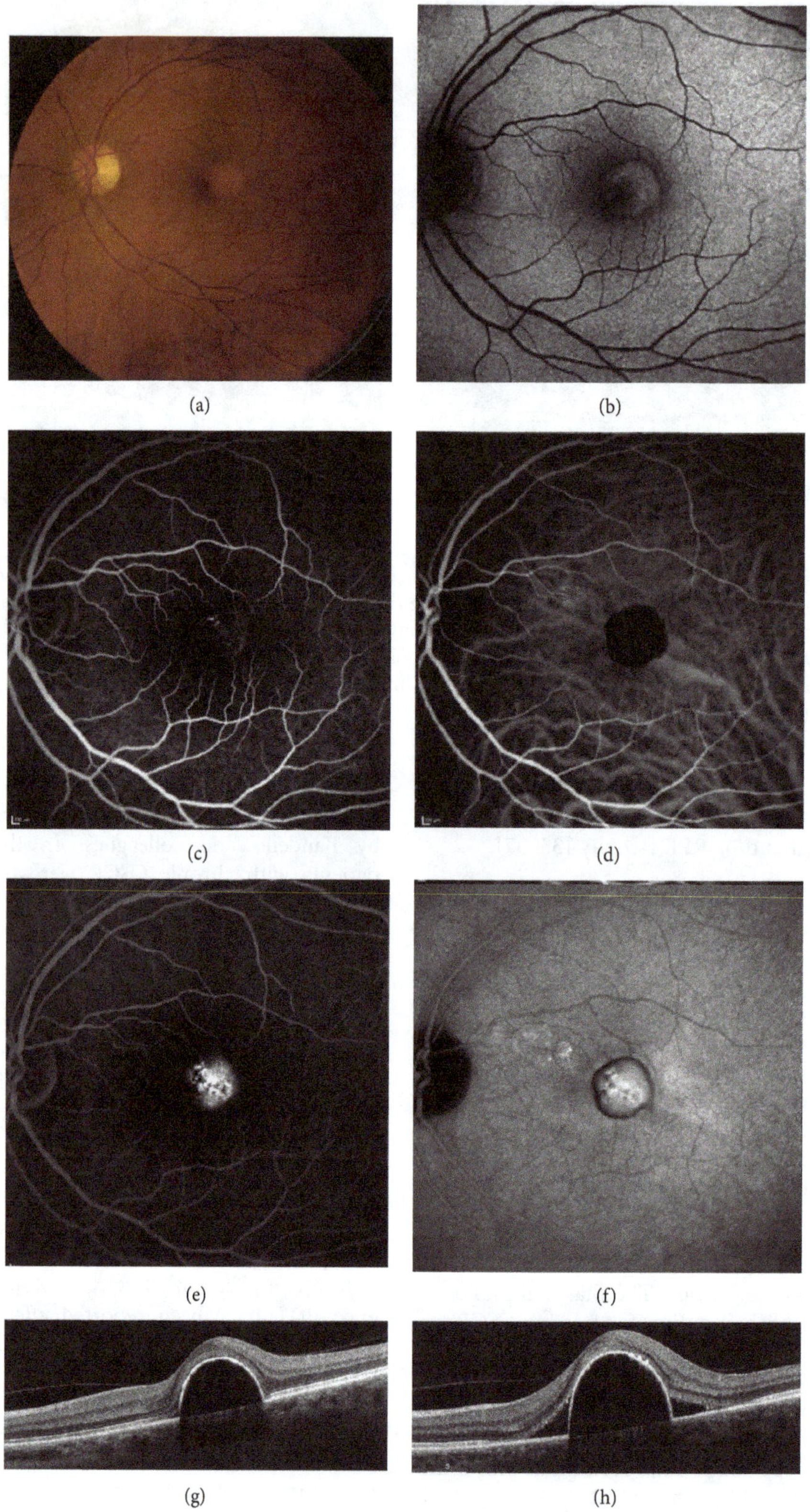

FIGURE 7: Central serous chorioretinopathy of the left eye. A 56-year-old male was observed for 3 years with worsening of metamorphopsia. (a) Fundus photography showed pigment irregularities and clumping over a pigment epithelial detachment (PED). (b) Fundus autofluorescence showed hypoautofluorescent changes surrounding the PED with granular hyperautofluorescence centrally. (c) Early-phase fluorescein angiography (FA) revealed faint pinpoint leakage and staining of the PED. (d) Early-phase indocyanine green angiography (ICGA) showed blockage due to the PED. (e, f) Late-phase FA and ICGA showed macular leakage. (g) Optical coherence tomography (OCT) showed a PED but no subretinal fluid. (h) One year later, OCT showed worsening of the PED and new subretinal fluid.

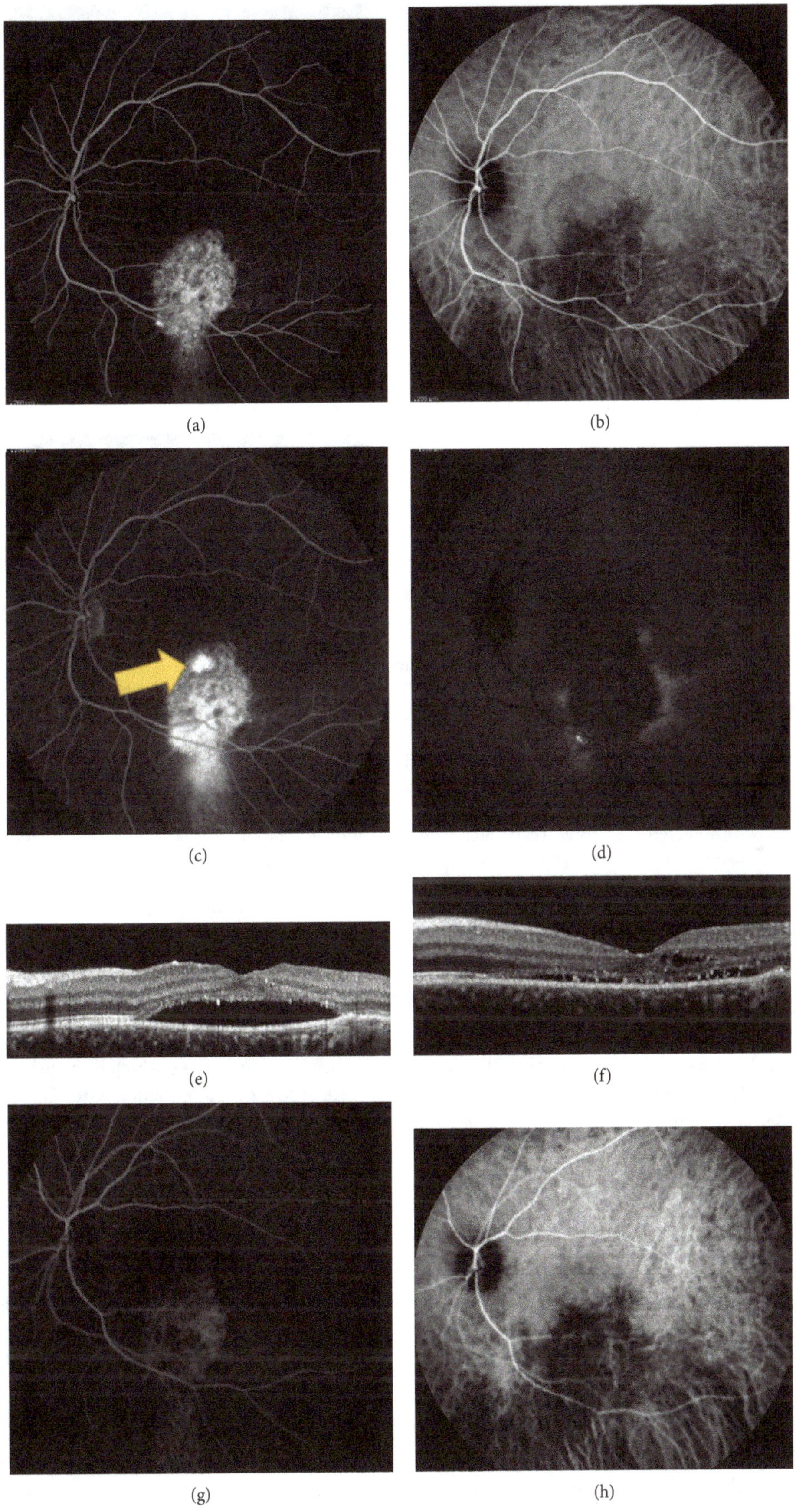

(a) (b) (c) (d) (e) (f) (g) (h)

Figure 8: Continued.

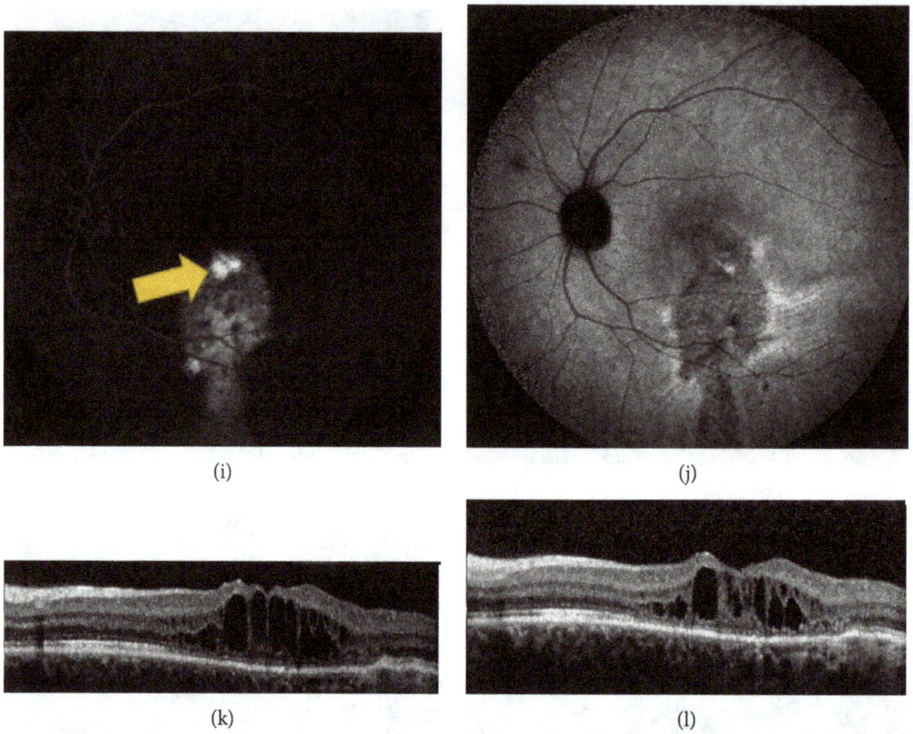

FIGURE 8: Chronic central serous chorioretinopathy treated with thermal laser photocoagulation. A 21-year-old female presented with visual distortion for over one year. Visual acuity in the left eye was 20/150 at presentation. (a–f) Images at baseline. (a) Early-phase fluorescein angiography (FA) showed a broad area of hyperfluorescence. (b) Early-phase indocyanine green angiography (ICGA) showed areas of hypofluorescence corresponding to the hyperfluorescence on FA. (c) Late-phase FA showed extrafoveal focal leakage, noted by the yellow arrow. (d) Late-phase ICGA showed hyperfluorescence corresponding to the focal leak on FA. Thermal laser was applied to the area corresponding to the leakage on FA and ICGA. Visual acuity improved to 20/100. (e) Optical coherence tomography (OCT) prior to thermal laser showed subretinal fluid and "shaggy" photoreceptors. (f) Post thermal laser, there was improvement in subretinal fluid. The patient was lost to follow-up but returned three years later with worsening symptoms. Visual acuity was 20/800. (g) Early-phase FA showed broad hyperfluorescence. (h) Early-phase ICGA showed hypofluorescence. (i) Late-phase FA showed two small areas of extrafoveal focal leakage, noted by the yellow arrow. (j) Late-phase ICGA showed one area of focal hyperfluorescence corresponding to the leakage on FA. (k) OCT prior to repeat thermal laser treatment showed loss of outer retinal layers with recurrent intraretinal fluid. (l) OCT following the second argon photocoagulation (yellow arrow in (i)) showed improvement in fluid as well as macular thickness. Visual acuity returned to 20/150 after treatment.

hyperpermeability, and egress of fluid across the RPE into the subretinal space [54]. Spironolactone is a nonselective antagonist of the aldosterone receptor. Its effects of blocking the aldosterone receptor are hypothesized to decrease choroidal hyperpermeability from off-target binding of corticosteroids. Spironolactone has multiple effects on estrogens and androgens that can result in unwanted side effects in male patients such as gynecomastia, decreased libido, and erectile dysfunction [55–57].

Eplerenone is a newer, more selective aldosterone antagonist that binds to the MR and less to the other steroid receptors. Eplerenone has a 10- to 20-fold lower affinity to MR, and a 100- to 1000-fold lower affinity to the other steroid receptors than spironolactone, resulting in fewer side effects [57, 58]. In general, both MR antagonists are prone to hyperkalemia and potassium levels should be monitored [55]. The authors have no personal experience with the use of MR antagonists in pregnancy or in pediatric patients.

Bousquet et al. conducted a prospective, nonrandomized study of 13 patients with CSCR symptomatic for at least four months. These patients were treated with 25 mg of oral eplerenone daily for one week, followed by 50 mg daily for 1-3 months. Treatment with eplerenone was associated with significant improvements in central macular thickness, subretinal fluid, and visual acuity [59]. The authors followed up with a prospective, randomized, double-masked, placebo-controlled study of 16 patients randomized to receive 50 mg of spironolactone or placebo daily for 30 days. There was a significant reduction of subretinal fluid and subfoveal thickness in the treatment arm compared to placebo; however, no significant changes in best-corrected visual acuity were reported [60]. Herold et al. reported another prospective, nonrandomized study in 18 patients with chronic CSCR evaluating spironolactone 25 mg twice daily for 12 weeks. They reported improvements in subretinal fluid, central macular thickness, and visual acuity [61] (Figure 13).

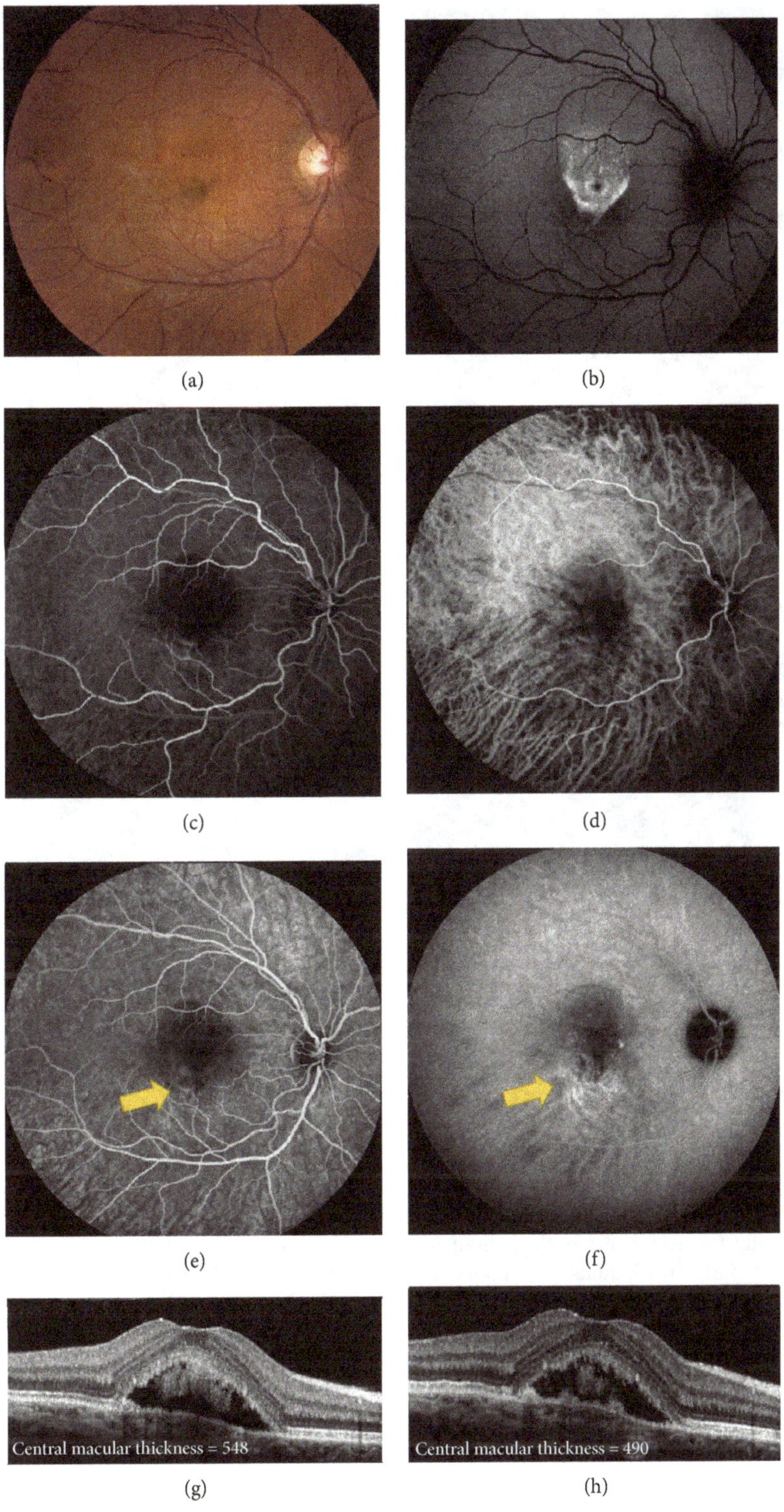

FIGURE 9: Chronic central serous chorioretinopathy treated with thermal photocoagulation. A 17-year old male presented with blurred vision of the right eye for nine months. Visual acuity was 20/50 in the right eye. (a) Fundus photography showed pigment changes and subretinal fluid in the right eye. (b) Fundus autofluorescence showed hyperautofluorescence of the macula, corresponding to the subretinal fluid seen clinically. (c, d) Early-phase fluorescein angiography (FA) and indocyanine green angiography (ICGA) showed focal hyperfluorescence corresponding to the inferior edge of the fluid seen clinically. (e) Late-phase FA showed leakage in the inferior macula, noted by the yellow arrow. (f) Late-phase ICGA confirmed the leakage, noted by the yellow arrow. Thermal photocoagulation was chosen because of the young age and extrafoveal focal leakage. Yellow arrows indicate where thermal laser was applied. (g, h) Optical coherence tomography before (g) and one month after (h) thermal photocoagulation showed decrease in subretinal fluid (measured in μm) and improvement in central macular thickness. Visual acuity improved to 20/40+. The patient was then lost to follow-up.

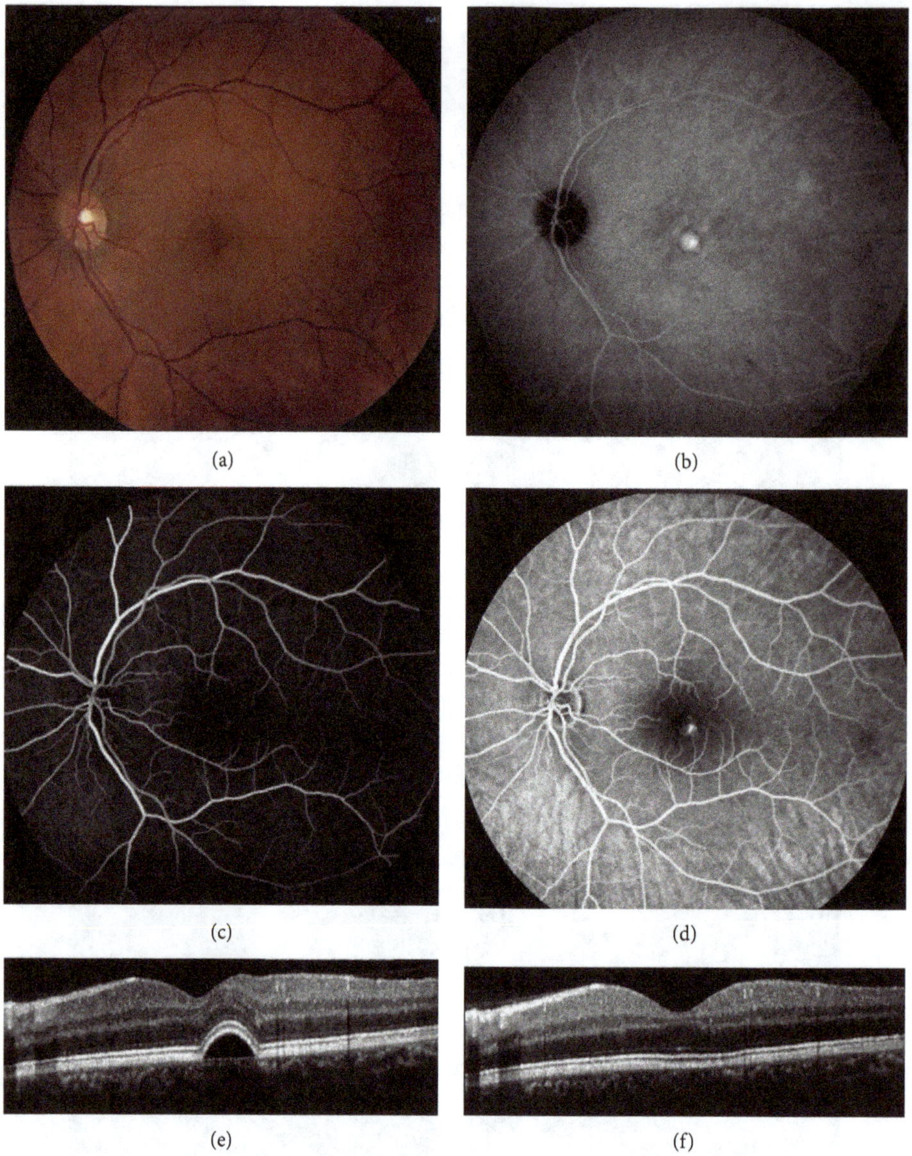

FIGURE 10: Chronic central serous chorioretinopathy treated with photodynamic therapy (PDT). A 35-year old male presented with 6 months of visual distortion in the left eye, although visual acuity was 20/20. (The amount of metamorphopsia was not formally measured.) He had tried 50 mg of eplerenone daily for over one month without improvement. (a) Fundus photography showed pigment changes and a pigment epithelial detachment (PED). (b) Fundus autofluorescence showed an area of hyperautofluorescence corresponding to the PED. (c) Early-phase fluorescein angiography (FA) showed a faint area of leakage in the macula. (d) Late-phase FA showed increased leakage in the macula. (e) Optical coherence tomography prior to and (f) after half-fluence PDT showed resolution of the PED. Visual acuity remained 20/20 and the patient reported subjective improvement.

4.5. Anti-vascular Endothelial Growth Factor Therapy. Anti-vascular endothelial growth factor (anti-VEGF) therapy is mainly used for chronic CSCR with secondary CNV (Figures 14 and 15). In cases without CNV, there is no evidence of elevated VEGF levels in plasma or aqueous, suggesting that anti-VEGF agents would be ineffective for the treatment of acute or chronic CSCR [62]. However, a few case series have reported variable efficacy using anti-VEGF agents for patients with chronic CSCR and no apparent CNV [63–65].

5. Conclusions

Acute CSCR is often self-limiting, so treatment of CSCR is generally not indicated except when symptoms persist for more than about 3 months. Some patients, especially monocular patients or patients with specific occupational needs, may benefit from earlier intervention. Chronic, nonresolving CSCR has no widely accepted and definitive treatment, due to the paucity of head-to-head clinical trials. In such cases, the authors prefer to use combined

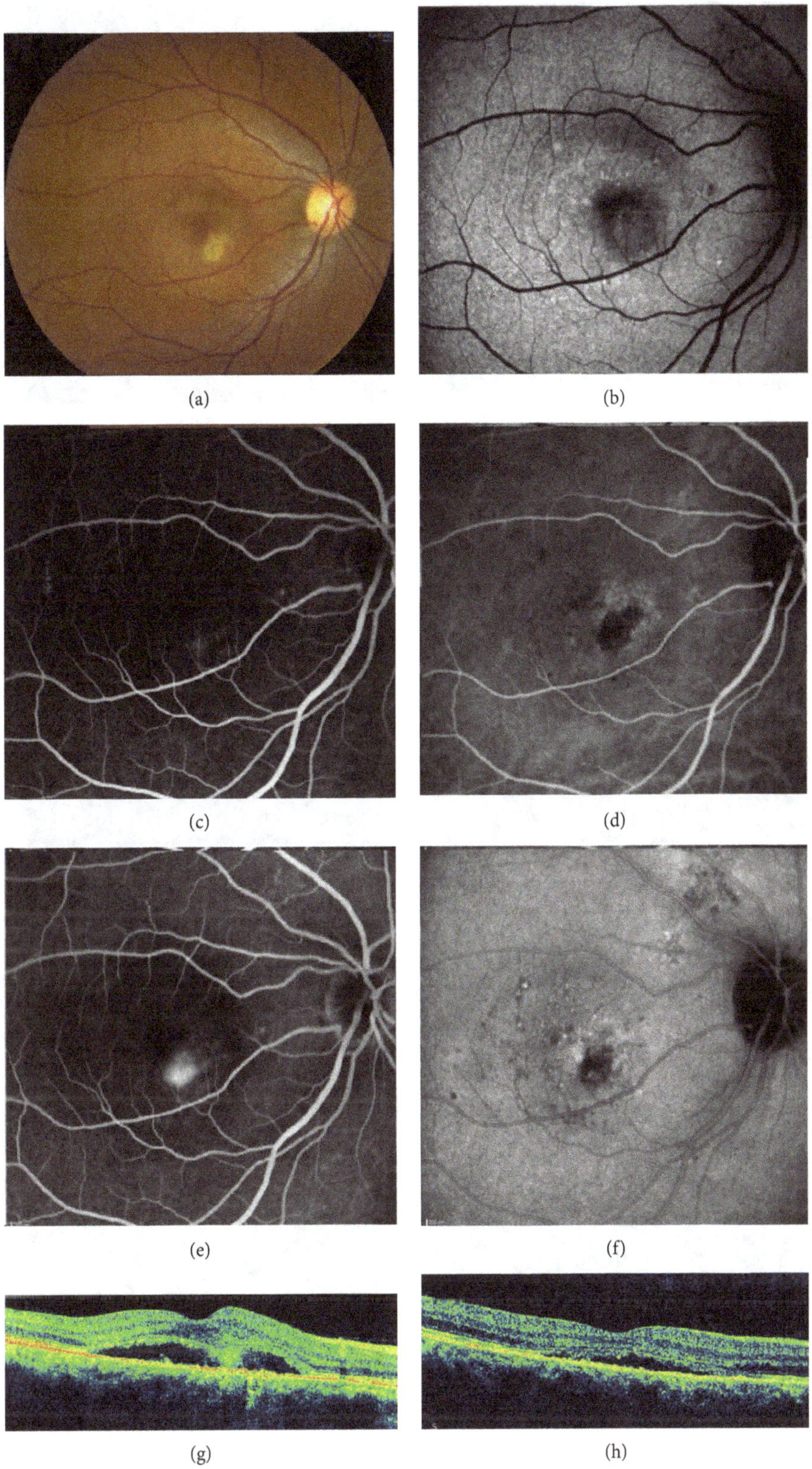

FIGURE 11: Chronic central serous chorioretinopathy of the right eye treated with reduced fluence photodynamic therapy (PDT). A 49-year old female presented with blurred vision in the right eye. Visual acuity was 20/50. (a) Fundus photography showed pigmentary changes of the right eye. (b) Fundus autofluorescence showed hypoautofluorescence at the macula. (c, d) Early-phase fluorescein angiography (FA) and indocyanine green angiography (ICGA) showed hyperfluorescence. (e, f) Late-phase FA and ICGA showed leakage in the inferior macula. (g) Optical coherence tomography prior to and (h) after half-fluence PDT showed improvement of subretinal fluid. Visual acuity improved to 20/25.

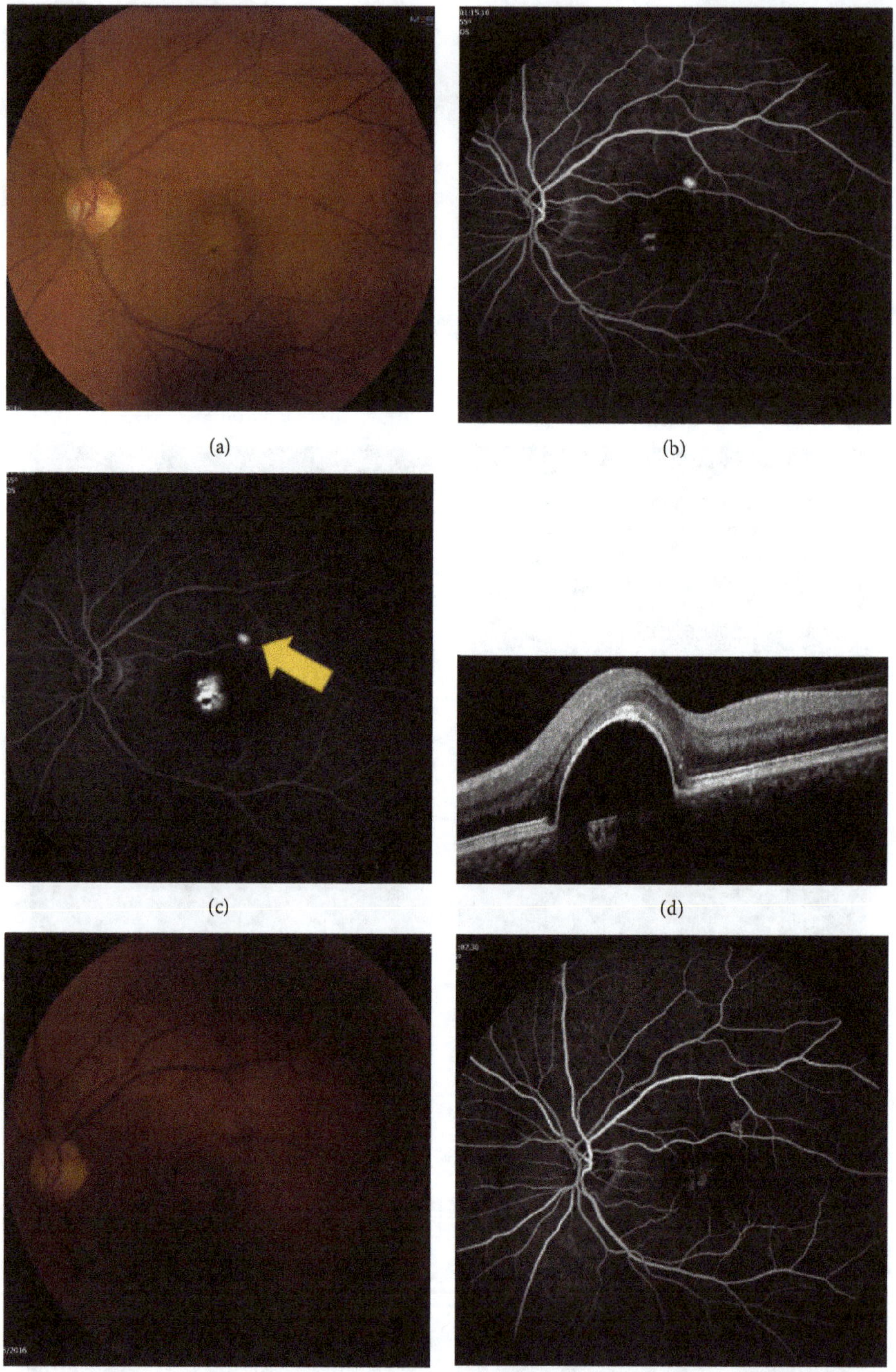

(a) (b) (c) (d) (e) (f)

Figure 12: Continued.

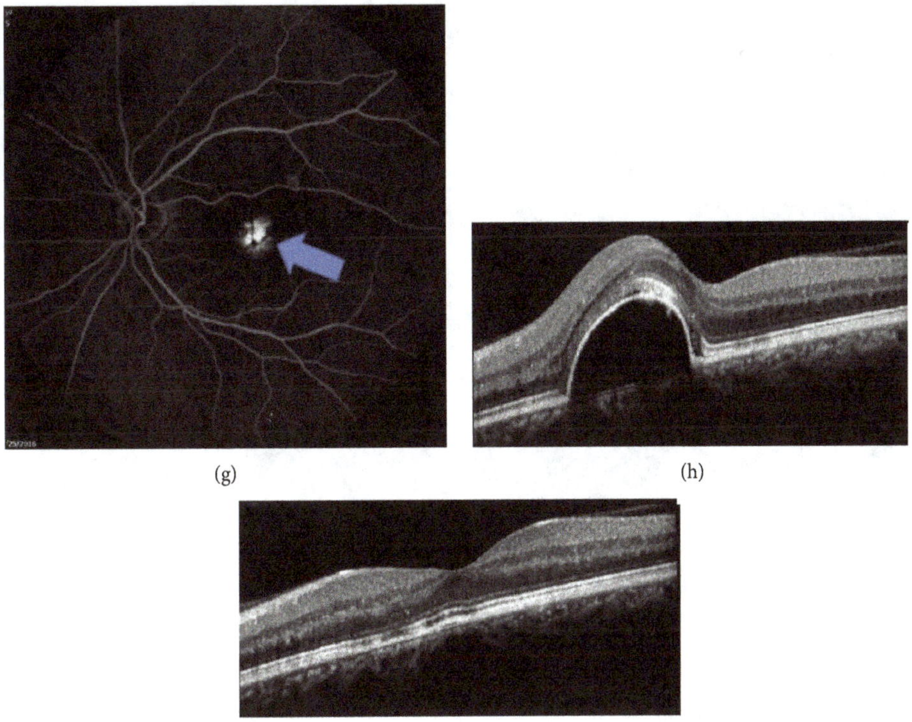

Figure 12: Chronic central serous chorioretinopathy of the left eye treated with both thermal laser photocoagulation and half fluence photodynamic therapy (PDT). A 42-year old female presented with blurred vision for two years. (a–d) Images at baseline. (a) Fundus photography showed pigmentary changes around a pigment epithelial detachment (PED). (b) Early-phase fluorescein angiography (FA) showed leakage in the fovea as well as slightly superotemporal. (c) Late-phase FA showed increased leakage; the superotemporal lesion is noted by the yellow arrow. (d) Optical coherence tomography (OCT) showed a large subfoveal PED. The patient was initially treated with thermal photocoagulation to the superotemporal lesion (yellow arrow in (c)), so as to spare the fovea. (e) Following thermal photocoagulation, the clinical appearance did not change. (f) Early-phase FA and (g) late-phase FA showed improvement of the treated superotemporal lesion but persistent leakage of the untreated subfoveal PED. (h) OCT showed no change in the subfoveal PED (noted by the blue arrow in (g)). The patient then underwent half-fluence PDT (blue arrow in (g)). (i) One month later, OCT showed resolution of the pigment epithelial defect. Visual acuity improved from 20/30 to 20/20.

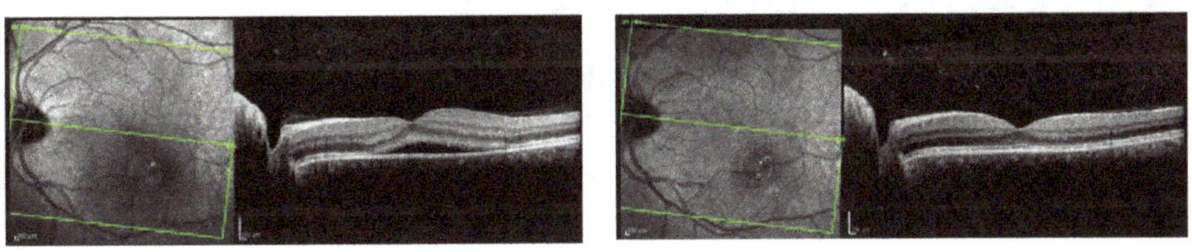

Figure 13: Central serous chorioretinopathy treated with eplerenone. A 44 year old Hispanic male presented with distortion in left eye although visual acuity was 20/20. He reported symptoms for three months. (a) Optical coherence tomography (OCT) confirmed subretinal fluid. The patient was started on eplerenone 25 mg daily. (b) One month after starting treatment, OCT showed resolution of the subretinal fluid. Subjectively, the patient reported improvement.

FA and ICGA to identify extrafoveal sites of leakage that might be amenable to thermal photocoagulation, which is safe to use in almost all patients, including pregnant patients and in pediatric patients.

If there is no focal extrafoveal leak on angiography, options other than thermal photocoagulation include reduced fluence PDT and/or MR antagonists. This is typically an individualized decision. Some patients may be more willing to take a long-term systemic medication rather than undergo PDT with its required period of sunlight avoidance; other patients may prefer the reverse. Figure 16 summarizes the treatment options in CSCR.

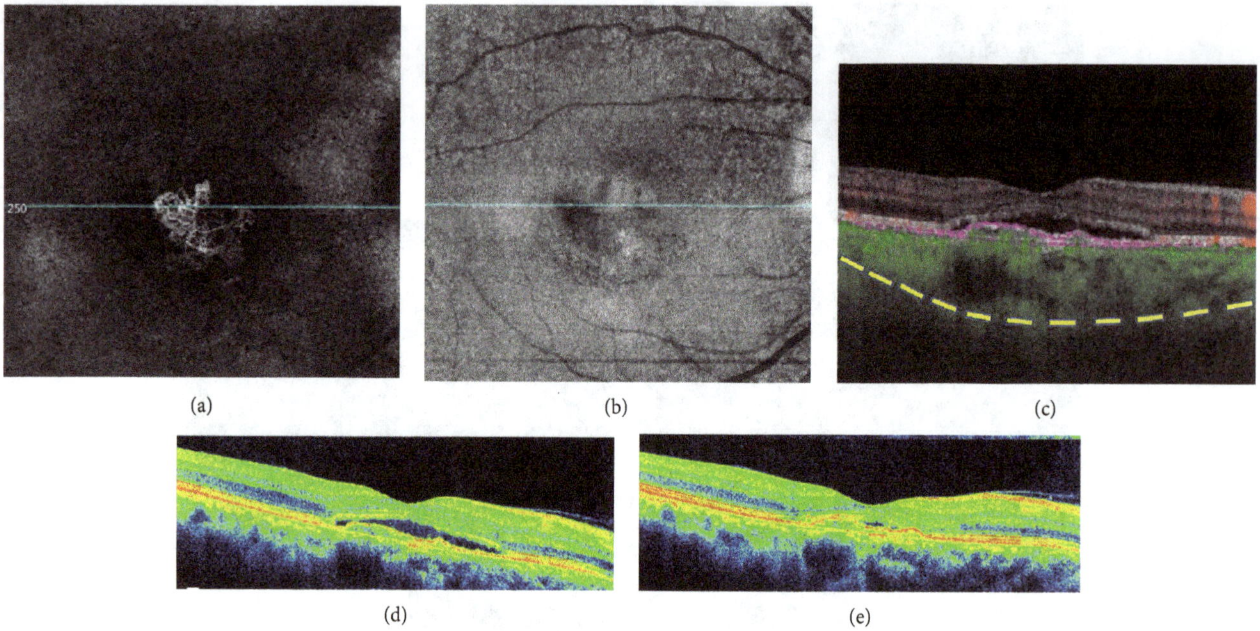

FIGURE 14: Chronic central serous chorioretinopathy of the right eye with secondary choroidal neovascularization (CNV). A 53-year old female with chronic central serous chorioretinopathy presented with worsening subretinal fluid. Using swept source optical coherence tomography angiography (SS-OCTA–PLEX Elite 9000, Carl Zeiss Meditec, Dublin, CA) 6 × 6 scans were performed; shown is the slab between the retinal pigment epithelium (RPE) and Bruch's membrane. (a) En face angiography showed the presence of type 1 choroidal neovascularization (CNV). (b) En face structural imaging showed the RPE elevation due to underlying CNV. (c) B-scan demonstrated subretinal fluid. The presence of a pigment epithelial detachment was seen, with increased flow (green) within the detachment indicating increased choroidal flow in the presence of CNV. The sclerochoroidal junction (yellow dashes) was highlighted to demonstrate the thick choroid. OCT prior to (d) and after (e) anti-vascular endothelial growth factor injections showed improvement of subretinal fluid.

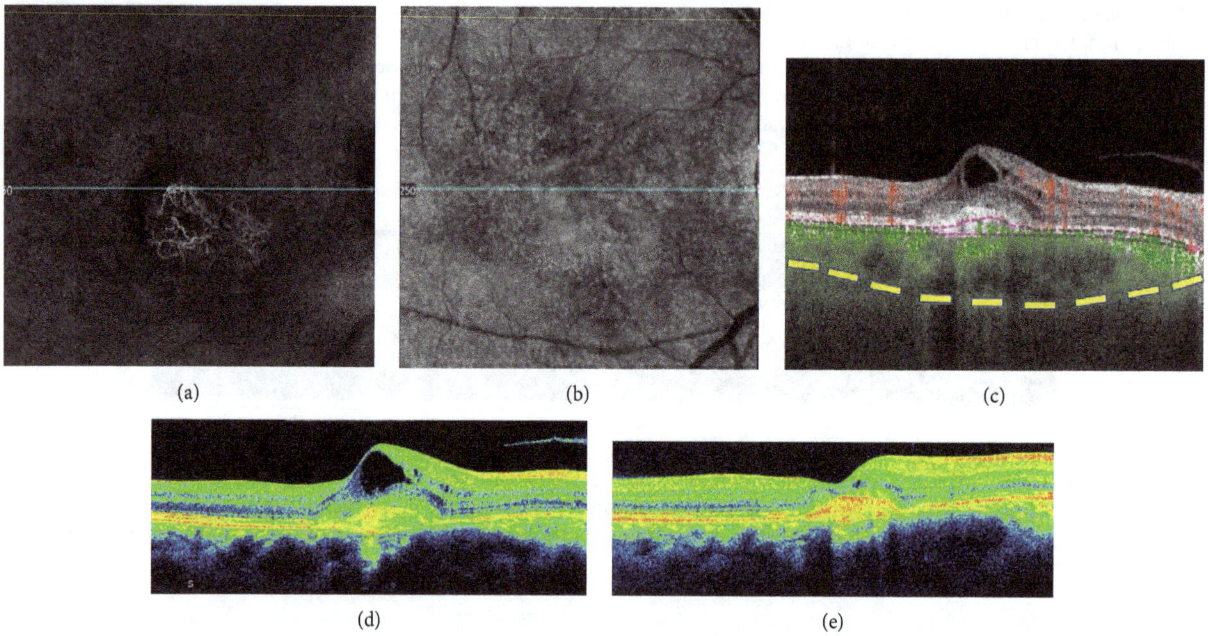

FIGURE 15: Chronic central serous chorioretinopathy of the right eye with secondary choroidal neovascularization (CNV). A 59-year old male with a history of inhaled triamcinolone use for asthma presented with worsening vision. Using swept source optical coherence tomography angiography (SS-OCTA – PLEX Elite 9000, Carl Zeiss Meditec, Dublin, CA), 6 × 6 scans were analyzed; shown is the slab between the retinal pigment epithelium (RPE) and Bruch's membrane. (a) En face angiography showed the presence of type 1 choroidal neovascularization. (b) En face structural imaging showed RPE elevation causing shadowing. (c) B-scan demonstrated cystoid macular edema, with increased flow (green) indicating increased choroidal flow in the presence of CNV. The sclerochoroidal junction (yellow dashes) was highlighted to demonstrate the thick choroid. (d, e) OCT prior to and after anti-vascular endothelial growth factor injections showed improvement of intraretinal fluid and hyperreflective material.

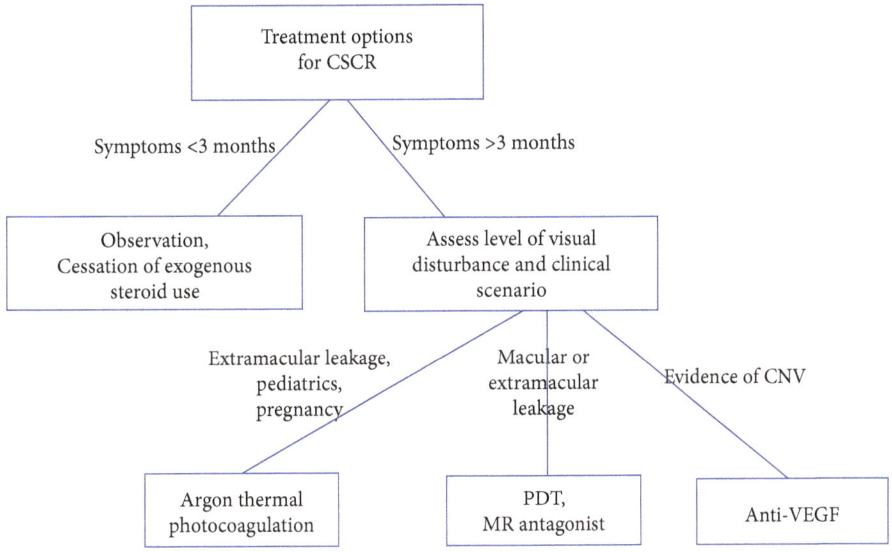

Figure 16: Review of treatment options in patients with central serous chorioretinopathy (CSCR). CNV: choroidal neovascularization; MR: mineralocorticoid; PDT: photodynamic therapy; VEGF: vascular endothelial growth factor.

Acknowledgments

This study is partly supported by the NIH Center Core Grant P30EY014801 and by an unrestricted grant from the Research to Prevent Blindness.

References

[1] A. Pryds, B. Sander, and M. Larsen, "Characterization of subretinal fluid leakage in central serous chorioretinopathy," *Investigative Ophthalmology & Visual Science*, vol. 51, no. 11, pp. 5853–5857, 2010.

[2] R. F. Spaide, M. Goldbaum, D. W. K. Wong, K. C. Tang, and T. Iida, "Serous detachment of the retina," *Retina*, vol. 23, no. 6, pp. 820–846, 2003, quiz 895-826.

[3] D. R. Guyer, L. A. Yannuzzi, J. S. Slakter, J. A. Sorenson, A. Ho, and D. Orlock, "Digital indocyanine green videoangiography of central serous chorioretinopathy," *Archives of Ophthalmology*, vol. 112, no. 8, pp. 1057–1062, 1994.

[4] J. D. Gass, "Pathogenesis of disciform detachment of the neuroepithelium," *American Journal of Ophthalmology*, vol. 63, no. 3, Supplement, pp. 1–139, 1967.

[5] A. Ross, A. H. Ross, and Q. Mohamed, "Review and update of central serous chorioretinopathy," *Current Opinion in Ophthalmology*, vol. 22, no. 3, pp. 166–173, 2011.

[6] R. Haimovici, S. Koh, D. R. Gagnon, T. Lehrfeld, and S. Wellik, "Risk factors for central serous chorioretinopathy: a case-control study," *Ophthalmology*, vol. 111, no. 2, pp. 244–249, 2004.

[7] A. S. Kitzmann, J. S. Pulido, N. N. Diehl, D. O. Hodge, and J. P. Burke, "The incidence of central serous chorioretinopathy in Olmsted County, Minnesota, 1980-2002," *Ophthalmology*, vol. 115, no. 1, pp. 169–173, 2008.

[8] R. F. Spaide, L. Campeas, A. Haas et al., "Central serous chorioretinopathy in younger and older adults," *Ophthalmology*, vol. 103, no. 12, pp. 2070–2080, 1996, discussion 2079-2080.

[9] J. Castro-Correia, M. F. Coutinho, V. Rosas, and J. Maia, "Long-term follow-up of central serous retinopathy in 150 patients," *Documenta Ophthalmologica*, vol. 81, no. 4, pp. 379–386, 1992.

[10] C. M. Gilbert, S. L. Owens, P. D. Smith, and S. L. Fine, "Long-term follow-up of central serous chorioretinopathy," *The British Journal of Ophthalmology*, vol. 68, no. 11, pp. 815–820, 1984.

[11] G. Bennett, "Central serous retinopathy," *The British Journal of Ophthalmology*, vol. 39, no. 10, pp. 605–618, 1955.

[12] R. Haimovici, E. S. Gragoudas, J. S. Duker, R. N. Sjaarda, and D. Eliott, "Central serous chorioretinopathy associated with inhaled or intranasal corticosteroids," *Ophthalmology*, vol. 104, no. 10, pp. 1653–1660, 1997.

[13] G. S. Gelber and H. Schatz, "Loss of vision due to central serous chorioretinopathy following psychological stress," *The American Journal of Psychiatry*, vol. 144, no. 1, pp. 46–50, 1987.

[14] L. A. Yannuzzi, "Type A behavior and central serous chorioretinopathy," *Retina*, vol. 32, Supplement 1, p. 709, 2012.

[15] L. C. Chumbley and R. N. Frank, "Central serous retinopathy and pregnancy," *American Journal of Ophthalmology*, vol. 77, no. 2, pp. 158–160, 1974.

[16] E. A. Bouzas, M. H. Scott, G. Mastorakos, G. P. Chrousos, and M. I. Kaiser-Kupfer, "Central serous chorioretinopathy in endogenous hypercortisolism," *Archives of Ophthalmology*, vol. 111, no. 9, pp. 1229–1233, 1993.

[17] F. W. Fraunfelder and F. T. Fraunfelder, "Central serous chorioretinopathy associated with sildenafil," *Retina*, vol. 28, no. 4, pp. 606–609, 2008.

[18] P. Kloos, I. Laube, and A. Thoelen, "Obstructive sleep apnea in patients with central serous chorioretinopathy," *Graefe's Archive for Clinical and Experimental Ophthalmology*, vol. 246, no. 9, pp. 1225–1228, 2008.

[19] L. Cotticelli, M. Borrelli, A. C. D'alessio et al., "Central serous chorioretinopathy and helicobacter pylori," *European Journal of Ophthalmology*, vol. 16, no. 2, pp. 274–278, 2018.

[20] H. Schatz, M. D. Osterloh, H. R. McDonald, and R. N. Johnson, "Development of retinal vascular leakage and cystoid macular oedema secondary to central serous chorioretinopathy," *The British Journal of Ophthalmology*, vol. 77, no. 11, pp. 744–746, 1993.

[21] F. B. Aggio, L. Roisman, G. B. Melo, D. Lavinsky, J. A. Cardillo, and M. E. Farah, "Clinical factors related to visual outcome in central serous chorioretinopathy," *Retina*, vol. 30, no. 7, pp. 1128–1134, 2010.

[22] K. Yamada, S. Hayasaka, and T. Setogawa, "Fluorescein-angiographic patterns in patients with central serous chorioretinopathy at the initial visit," *Ophthalmologica*, vol. 205, no. 2, pp. 69–76, 1992.

[23] M. Wang, I. C. Munch, P. W. Hasler, C. Prunte, and M. Larsen, "Central serous chorioretinopathy," *Acta Ophthalmologica*, vol. 86, no. 2, pp. 126–145, 2008.

[24] N. Kitaya, T. Nagaoka, T. Hikichi et al., "Features of abnormal choroidal circulation in central serous chorioretinopathy," *The British Journal of Ophthalmology*, vol. 87, no. 6, pp. 709–712, 2003.

[25] R. F. Spaide, L. Hall, A. Haas et al., "Indocyanine green videoangiography of older patients with central serous chorioretinopathy," *Retina*, vol. 16, no. 3, pp. 203–213, 1996.

[26] F. C. Delori, C. K. Dorey, G. Staurenghi, O. Arend, D. G. Goger, and J. J. Weiter, "In vivo fluorescence of the ocular fundus exhibits retinal pigment epithelium lipofuscin characteristics," *Investigative Ophthalmology & Visual Science*, vol. 36, no. 3, pp. 718–729, 1995.

[27] G. E. Eldred and M. L. Katz, "Fluorophores of the human retinal pigment epithelium: separation and spectral characterization," *Experimental Eye Research*, vol. 47, no. 1, pp. 71–86, 1988.

[28] R. F. Spaide and J. M. Klancnik Jr., "Fundus autofluorescence and central serous chorioretinopathy," *Ophthalmology*, vol. 112, no. 5, pp. 825–833, 2005.

[29] Y. Imamura, T. Fujiwara, and R. F. Spaide, "Fundus autofluorescence and visual acuity in central serous chorioretinopathy," *Ophthalmology*, vol. 118, no. 4, pp. 700–705, 2011.

[30] Y. Imamura, T. Fujiwara, R. Margolis, and R. F. Spaide, "Enhanced depth imaging optical coherence tomography of the choroid in central serous chorioretinopathy," *Retina*, vol. 29, no. 10, pp. 1469–1473, 2009.

[31] D. J. Warrow, Q. V. Hoang, and K. B. Freund, "Pachychoroid pigment epitheliopathy," *Retina*, vol. 33, no. 8, pp. 1659–1672, 2013.

[32] O. Gal-Or, K. K. Dansingani, D. Sebrow, R. Dolz-Marco, and K. B. Freund, "Inner choroidal flow signal attenuation in pachychoroid DISEASE," *Retina*, vol. 38, no. 10, pp. 1984–1992, 2018.

[33] S. Akkaya, "Spectrum of pachychoroid diseases," *International Ophthalmology*, vol. 38, no. 5, pp. 2239–2246, 2018.

[34] J. Siedlecki, B. Schworm, and S. G. Priglinger, "The pachychoroid disease spectrum-and the need for a uniform classification system," *Ophthalmol Retina.*, vol. 3, no. 12, pp. 1013–1015, 2019.

[35] Y. Jia, S. T. Bailey, D. J. Wilson et al., "Quantitative optical coherence tomography angiography of choroidal neovascularization in age-related macular degeneration," *Ophthalmology*, vol. 121, no. 7, pp. 1435–1444, 2014.

[36] M. Q.-E. Maftouhi, A. El Maftouhi, and C. M. Eandi, "Chronic central serous chorioretinopathy imaged by optical coherence tomographic angiography," *American Journal of Ophthalmology*, vol. 160, no. 3, pp. 581–587.e1, 2015.

[37] R. F. Spaide, J. M. Klancnik Jr., and M. J. Cooney, "Retinal vascular layers imaged by fluorescein angiography and optical coherence tomography angiography," *JAMA Ophthalmology*, vol. 133, no. 1, pp. 45–50, 2015.

[38] R. Brancato, A. Scialdone, A. Pece, G. Coscas, and M. Binaghi, "Eight-year follow-up of central serous chorioretinopathy with and without laser treatment," *Graefe's Archive for Clinical and Experimental Ophthalmology*, vol. 225, no. 3, pp. 166–168, 1987.

[39] L. Ficker, G. Vafidis, A. While, and P. Leaver, "Long-term follow-up of a prospective trial of argon laser photocoagulation in the treatment of central serous retinopathy," *The British Journal of Ophthalmology*, vol. 72, no. 11, pp. 829–834, 1988.

[40] J. W. Lim, S. W. Kang, Y. T. Kim, S. E. Chung, and S. W. Lee, "Comparative study of patients with central serous chorioretinopathy undergoing focal laser photocoagulation or photodynamic therapy," *The British Journal of Ophthalmology*, vol. 95, no. 4, pp. 514–517, 2011.

[41] G. Quin, G. Liew, I. V. Ho, M. Gillies, and S. Fraser-Bell, "Diagnosis and interventions for central serous chorioretinopathy: review and update," *Clinical & Experimental Ophthalmology*, vol. 41, no. 2, pp. 187–200, 2013.

[42] P. Iacono, M. B. Parodi, B. Falcomatà, and F. Bandello, "Central serous chorioretinopathy treatments: a mini review," *Ophthalmic Research*, vol. 55, no. 2, pp. 76–83, 2015.

[43] A. Negi and M. F. Marmor, "Experimental serous retinal detachment and focal pigment epithelial damage," *Archives of Ophthalmology*, vol. 102, no. 3, pp. 445–449, 1984.

[44] E. Burumcek, A. Mudun, S. Karacorlu, and M. O. Arslan, "Laser photocoagulation for persistent central serous retinopathy: results of long-term follow-up," *Ophthalmology*, vol. 104, no. 4, pp. 616–622, 1997.

[45] P. Scholz, L. Altay, and S. Fauser, "A review of subthreshold micropulse laser for treatment of macular disorders," *Advances in Therapy*, vol. 34, no. 7, pp. 1528–1555, 2017.

[46] P. Lanzetta, F. Furlan, L. Morgante, D. Veritti, and F. Bandello, "Nonvisible subthreshold micropulse diode laser (8_{10} nm) treatment of central serous chorioretinopathy. A pilot study," *European Journal of Ophthalmology*, vol. 18, no. 6, pp. 934–940, 2018.

[47] F. Bandello, P. Lanzetta, F. Furlan, and A. Polito, "Non-visible subthreshold micropulse diode laser treatment of idiopathic central serous chorioretinopathy. A pilot study," *Investigative Ophthalmology & Visual Science*, vol. 44, no. 5, p. 4858, 2003.

[48] L. A. Yannuzzi, J. S. Slakter, N. E. Gross et al., "Indocyanine green angiography-guided photodynamic therapy for treatment of chronic central serous chorioretinopathy: a pilot study," *Retina*, vol. 23, no. 3, pp. 288–298, 2003.

[49] M. D. Ober, L. A. Yannuzzi, D. V. Do et al., "Photodynamic therapy for focal retinal pigment epithelial leaks secondary to central serous chorioretinopathy," *Ophthalmology*, vol. 112, no. 12, pp. 2088–2094, 2005.

[50] J. I. Lim, A. R. Glassman, L. P. Aiello, U. Chakravarthy, C. J. Flaxel, and R. F. Spaide, "Collaborative retrospective macula society study of photodynamic therapy for chronic central

serous chorioretinopathy," *Ophthalmology*, vol. 121, no. 5, pp. 1073–1078, 2014.

[51] T. Y. Y. Lai, W.-M. Chan, H. Li, R. Y. K. Lai, D. T. L. Liu, and D. S. C. Lam, "Safety enhanced photodynamic therapy with half dose verteporfin for chronic central serous chorioretinopathy: a short term pilot study," *The British Journal of Ophthalmology*, vol. 90, no. 7, pp. 869–874, 2006.

[52] M.-W. Zhao, P. Zhou, H.-X. Xiao et al., "Photodynamic therapy for acute central serous chorioretinopathy: the safe effective lowest dose of verteporfin," *Retina*, vol. 29, no. 8, pp. 1155–1161, 2009.

[53] W.-M. Chan, T. Y. Y. Lai, R. Y. K. Lai, D. T. L. Liu, and D. S. C. Lam, "Half-Dose Verteporfin Photodynamic Therapy for Acute Central Serous Chorioretinopathy: One-Year Results of a Randomized Controlled Trial," *Ophthalmology*, vol. 115, no. 10, pp. 1756–1765, 2008.

[54] M. Zhao, I. Célérier, E. Bousquet et al., "Mineralocorticoid receptor is involved in rat and human ocular chorioretinopathy," *The Journal of Clinical Investigation*, vol. 122, no. 7, pp. 2672–2679, 2012.

[55] A. Struthers, H. Krum, and G. H. Williams, "A comparison of the aldosterone-blocking agents eplerenone and spironolactone," *Clinical Cardiology*, vol. 31, no. 4, pp. 153–158, 2008.

[56] A. Karim, "Spironolactone: disposition, metabolism, pharmacodynamics, and bioavailability," *Drug Metabolism Reviews*, vol. 8, no. 1, pp. 151–188, 2008.

[57] E. Rahimy, J. D. Pitcher III, M. S. Fineman, C. Prunte, and J. Hsu, "Oral mineralocorticoid receptor antagonists for the treatment of CSC," *Retinal Physicians*, vol. 13, pp. 22–27, 2016.

[58] M. de Gasparo, U. Joss, H. P. Ramjoué et al., "Three new epoxy-spirolactone derivatives: characterization in vivo and in vitro," *The Journal of Pharmacology and Experimental Therapeutics*, vol. 240, no. 2, pp. 650–656, 1987.

[59] E. Bousquet, T. Beydoun, M. Zhao, L. Hassan, O. Offret, and F. Behar-Cohen, "Mineralocorticoid receptor antagonism in the treatment of chronic central serous chorioretinopathy: a pilot study," *Retina*, vol. 33, no. 10, pp. 2096–2102, 2013.

[60] E. Bousquet, T. Beydoun, P. R. Rothschild et al., "Spironolactone for nonresolving central serous chorioretinopathy: a randomized controlled crossover study," *Retina*, vol. 35, no. 12, pp. 2505–2515, 2015.

[61] T. R. Herold, K. Prause, A. Wolf, W. J. Mayer, and M. W. Ulbig, "Spironolactone in the treatment of central serous chorioretinopathy - a case series," *Graefe's Archive for Clinical and Experimental Ophthalmology*, vol. 252, no. 12, pp. 1985–1991, 2014.

[62] J. W. Lim, M. U. Kim, and M. C. Shin, "Aqueous humor and plasma levels of vascular endothelial growth factor and interleukin-8 in patients with central serous chorioretinopathy," *Retina*, vol. 30, no. 9, pp. 1465–1471, 2010.

[63] O. Artunay, E. Yuzbasioglu, R. Rasier, A. Sengul, and H. Bahcecioglu, "Intravitreal bevacizumab in treatment of idiopathic persistent central serous chorioretinopathy: a prospective, controlled clinical study," *Current Eye Research*, vol. 35, no. 2, pp. 91–98, 2010.

[64] Y. R. Chung, E. J. Seo, H. M. Lew, and K. H. Lee, "Lack of positive effect of intravitreal bevacizumab in central serous chorioretinopathy: meta-analysis and review," *Eye*, vol. 27, no. 12, pp. 1339–1346, 2013.

[65] S. J. Lim, M. I. Roh, and O. W. Kwon, "Intravitreal bevacizumab injection for central serous chorioretinopathy," *Retina*, vol. 30, no. 1, pp. 100–106, 2010.

29

Multimodal Imaging in AIDS-Related Ocular Cryptococcosis

Maria Fernanda Flores Herrera[1] **Nicolas Dauby**[2] **Evelyne Maillart,**[3] **Agnes Libois**[2] **Alberto Papaleo**[3] **Hind El Ouardighi,**[1] **Laurence Postelmans,**[4] **François Willermain,**[1] **and Dorine Makhoul**[1]

[1]*Department of Ophthalmology, CHU Saint-Pierre, Université Libre de Bruxelles (ULB), Brussels, Belgium*
[2]*Department of Infectious Diseases, CHU Brugmann, Université Libre de Bruxelles (ULB), Brussels, Belgium*
[3]*Department of Infectious Diseases, CHU Saint-Pierre, Université Libre de Bruxelles (ULB), Brussels, Belgium*
[4]*Department of Ophthalmology, CHU Brugmann, Université Libre de Bruxelles (ULB), Brussels, Belgium*

Correspondence should be addressed to Maria Fernanda Flores Herrera; flores.herrera.mf@gmail.com

Academic Editor: Alexander A. Bialasiewicz

Purpose. To report multimodal imaging findings in two cases of AIDS-related cryptococcal chorioretinitis associated with uveitis and vasculitis. *Methods.* Findings on clinical examination, color fundus photography, fluorescein and indocyanine green angiographies, and optical coherence tomography. *Patients.* Both patients were diagnosed with *Cryptococcus neoformans* meningitis in the setting of untreated HIV infection with CD4+ T cell count < 100/mm^3. Ocular manifestations occurred during the course of the antifungal therapy for meningitis. *Results.* In both cases, fundus showed vitritis. Fluorescein angiography allowed the characterization of vasculitis lesions, and indocyanine green angiography indicated choroidal involvement. In combination with optical coherence tomography, ICG and FA allowed the assessment of treatment response. *Conclusion.* These two cases reveal the potential of *C. neoformans* to infect almost all ocular structures and the critical role of multimodal imaging in baseline evaluation and in the follow-up of patients.

1. Introduction

Cryptococcosis is an invasive mycosis mainly caused by two species: *Cryptococcus neoformans* and *Cryptococcus gattii* that can affect both immunocompromised and immunocompetent subjects. *C. neoformans* is a major cause of meningitis in HIV-infected patients with advanced immunosuppression and is associated with high morbidity and mortality in resource-limited settings [1]. *C. neoformans* spreads hematogenously from the lungs to the central nervous system causing fungal meningitis. Ocular manifestations are frequently observed during cryptococcal meningitis in AIDS patients. Papilledema, visual loss, and cranial nerve palsy are the most frequent ocular findings [2]. Intraocular involvement, due to hematogenous dissemination or extension through the leptomeninges, is unusual and includes choroiditis and chorioretinitis [3].

We report two cases of cryptococcal intraocular involvement in two AIDS patients with concomitant cryptococcal meningitis. Fluorescein (FA) and indocyanine green (ICG) angiographies as well as optical coherence tomography (OCT) findings are discussed.

2. Case 1

A 25-year-old man from Sub-Saharan Africa presented at our ophthalmology department for itchy red right eye since 3 weeks. The patient was infected with HIV following vertical transmission and diagnosed with HIV infection at the age of 7. The nadir CD4 count was 67/mm^3. He was diagnosed with cryptococcal meningitis 9 months before. He received a treatment with liposomal amphotericin B and flucytosine followed by fluconazole secondary prophylaxis. After two months, he suffered from a relapse after voluntarily stopping his prophylaxis and the same treatment was given.

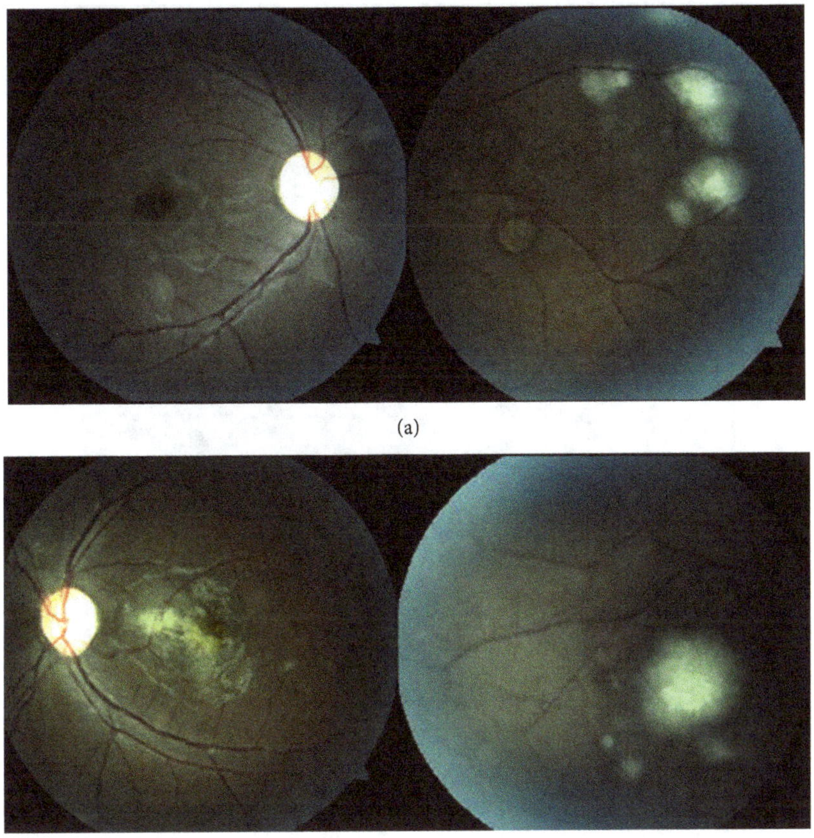

(a)

(b)

Figure 1: Fundus photograph of the (a) right and (b) left eyes displayed multiple yellowish subretinal lesions through the posterior pole and midperiphery in both eyes with a well-demarcated large deep macular lesion on the left eye.

At presentation day in our clinic, the patient had again voluntarily stopped both antiretroviral treatment (elvitegravir/cobicistat/emtricitabine/tenofovir) and fluconazole 2 months before.

Visual acuity was 1/10 in the right eye and counting fingers in the left eye (LE); intraocular pressure was normal. Anterior chamber examination revealed bilateral conjunctival hyperemia, along with granulomatous keratic precipitates. Both eyes' fundus displayed mild vitritis along with multiple yellowish subretinal lesions through the posterior pole and midperiphery, with a well-demarcated large deep macular lesion on the LE (Figure 1). Late-phase fluorescein angiography (FA) of the LE showed vasculitis of large venous vessels, hot disc, some macular hypofluorescent lesions, and with a mild staining of some lesions (Figure 2(a)). ICG angiography demonstrated numerous hypocyanescent spots, more numerous than the lesions seen on eye fundus and FA, suggesting associated widespread choroidal lesions (Figure 2(b)). Macular spectral domain optical coherence tomography (SD-OCT) demonstrated retinal infiltration in the inferior part of the macula with a diffuse thickening (Figure 2(c)). Multimodal imaging findings were consistent with infectious bilateral panuveitis with multifocal chorioretinitis, vasculitis, and papillitis.

The patient was admitted, and laboratory investigations were performed. *C. neoformans* grew on multiples blood cultures with positive cryptococcal antigen (CRAG). A lumbar puncture demonstrated cerebrospinal fluid (CSF) lymphocytosis, hypoglycorrhachia, a positive CRAG, and *C. neoformans* culture. Vitreal culture was not performed. Computed tomography of the brain did not reveal any abnormalities, including signs of cerebral toxoplasmosis. Pulmonary tuberculosis was ruled out: both sputum and bronchoalveolar lavage direct examination, PCR, and culture were negative for *M. tuberculosis*. Blood culture was also negative for *Mycobacteria* sp. Physical examination was notable for papular verrucous skin lesions on the face. A skin biopsy was performed and PAS, Mucicarmine, and Grocott stainings revealed also the presence of *Cryptococcus*. Peripheral blood HIV viral load was 36400 copies/ml, and CD4+ T cells count was 61/mm^3 (4% of total T cells).

A diagnosis of systemic and ocular cryptococcal infection was thus made, and combination therapy with liposomal amphotericin B (250 mg/24 h) and flucytosine (1750 mg/6 h) was restarted for a total of 14 days. The patient was discharged with fluconazole 800 mg along with antiretroviral therapy. At 10-month follow-up, peripheral blood HIV viral load was undetectable (<20 copies/ml) and CD4 count was 144/mm^3. The patient was still taking fluconazole secondary prophylaxis. Visual acuity was, respectively, 10/10 and 4/10 and there was no sign of inflammation on the slit lamp. The eye fundus

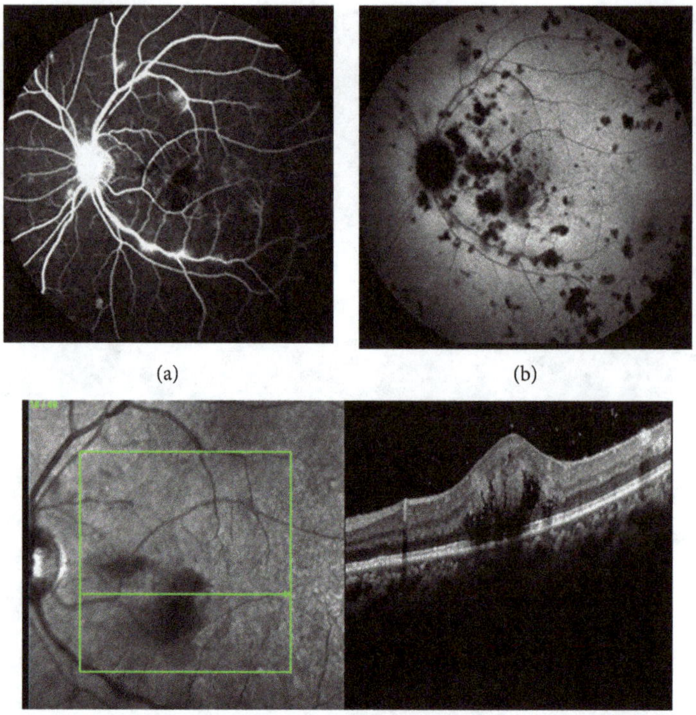

(a) (b)

(c)

FIGURE 2: Case 1: left eye at presentation. (a) Late-phase fluorescein angiogram (FA) showed vasculitis of large venous vessels, hot disc, some macular hypofluorescent lesions, and mild diffusion at the level of some central lesion and midperipheral probably retinal lesions. (b) Indocyanine green angiography demonstrated numerous hypofluorescent spots, more numerous than the lesions seen on eye fundus and FA, suggesting associated widespread choroidal lesions. (c) Macular spectral domain optical coherence tomography demonstrated retinal infiltration in the inferior part of the macula with a diffuse thickening.

examination demonstrated multiple bilateral peripheral inactive lesions and a macular scar on the LE.

Late-phase FA showed regression of the vasculitis, remaining late diffusion of the optic nerve, and staining of the macular and peripheral cicatricial retinal lesions (Figure 3(a)). Late-phase ICGA demonstrated a drastic improvement with persistence of some discrete hypocyanescent spots probably corresponding to the cicatricial lesions seen on eye fundus and FA (Figure 3(b)).

SD-OCT in the left eye showed a retrofoveolar scar with disruption of the retinal pigment epithelium and a loss of macular inner retinal structure (Figure 3(c)).

3. Case 2

A 32-year-old man was admitted for confusion and loss of consciousness. HIV-1 testing was positive. CSF examination revealed positive CRAG and Indian ink examination. Both CSF culture and blood cultures grew for *C. neoformans*. Brain MRI did not reveal signs of cerebral toxoplasmosis. Pulmonary tuberculosis was ruled out: both sputum and bronchoalveolar lavage direct examination, PCR, and culture were negative for *M. tuberculosis*. Peripheral blood HIV-1 viral load was 800,000 copies/ml, and CD4+ T cell count was $12/\text{mm}^3$. On the third day of hospitalization, combination therapy by liposomal amphotericin B (350 mg/24 h) and flucytosine (100 mg/kg/24 h) was initiated and was stopped after 18 days because of acute kidney failure possibly related to liposomal amphotericin B and thrombocytopenia possibly related to flucytosine. Secondary prophylaxis by fluconazole 400 mg was initiated. Nevertheless, on the 30th day of hospitalization, fever relapsed accompanied with headaches. Lumbar puncture analysis revealed positive Indian ink examination but negative *C. neoformans* culture. Consequently, liposomal amphotericin B treatment was reinitiated for probable relapse of cryptococcal meningitis. On the fifth day of hospitalization, the patient, complaining of floaters, was referred to the ophthalmology department. The visual acuity was 10/10 on both eyes. Slit lamp examination revealed few cells in the anterior chamber with no keratic precipitates or synechia. Fundus examination showed mild vitritis in both eyes associated to bilaterally multiple dot and blot hemorrhages, cotton wool spots, multiples deep yellowish lesions, and large whitish peripheral retinal areas (Figure 4). Vitreal culture was not performed. FA showed asymmetric papillitis and occlusive vasculitis in both eyes (Figure 5). ICGA demonstrated multiple hypocyanescent spots throughout the posterior pole and the midperiphery (Figure 6(a)). Enhanced Depth Imaging-OCT (EDI-OCT) performed on a superotemporal hypocyanescent spot in the left eye revealed a well-delineated lesion occupying all the choroidal space and considered as a cryptococcal granuloma, associated with a small serous retinal detachment which could be related to a secondary inflammatory response to the underlying choroidal lesion (Figure 6(b)).

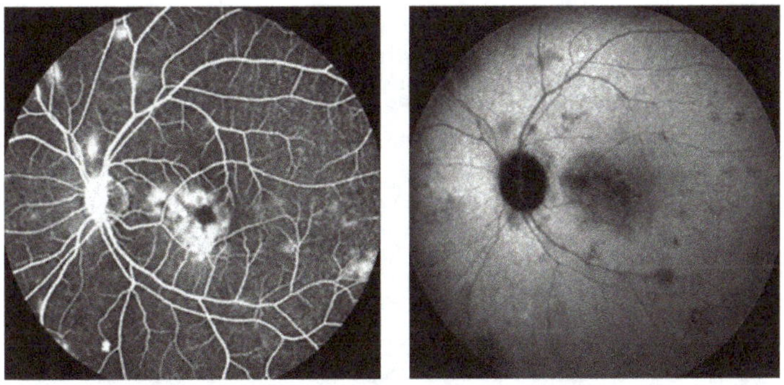

(a) (b)

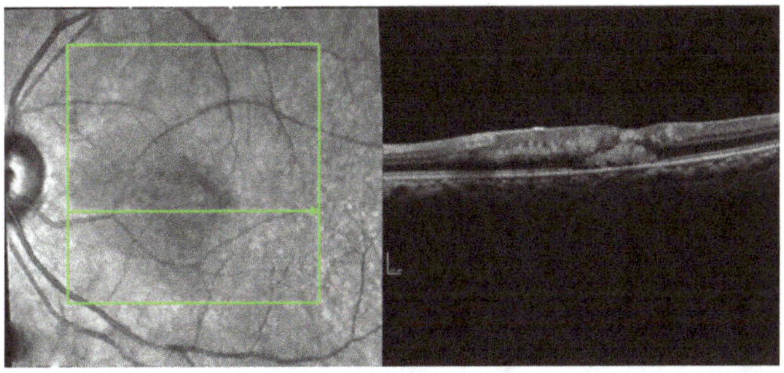

(c)

Figure 3: Case 1: left eye at 10-month follow-up. (a) Late-phase fluorescein angiogram showed regression of the vasculitis, remaining late diffusion of the optic nerve, and staining of the macular and peripheral scarring retinal lesions. (b) Late-phase ICGA demonstrated a drastic improvement with persistence of some discrete hypofluorescent spots probably corresponding to the scarring lesions seen on eye fundus and FA. (c) Spectral domain optical coherence tomography in the left eye showed a retrofoveolar scar with disruption of the retinal pigment epithelium and a loss of macular inner retinal structure.

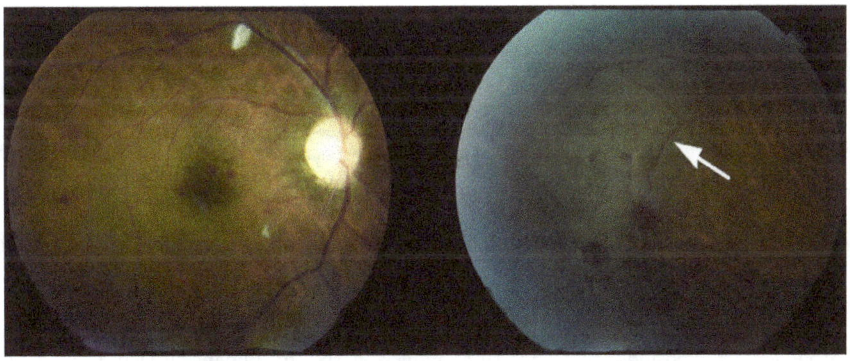

(a)

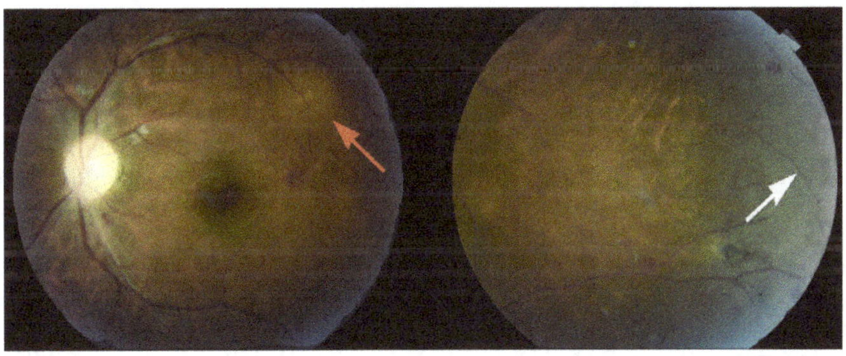

(b)

Figure 4: Case 2: fundus examination at presentation. Fundus photographs of the (a) right eye and the (b) left eye displaying multiple dot and blot hemorrhages, cotton wool spots, bilateral multiple deep yellowish lesions (red arrow), and large whitish peripheral retinal areas (white arrow).

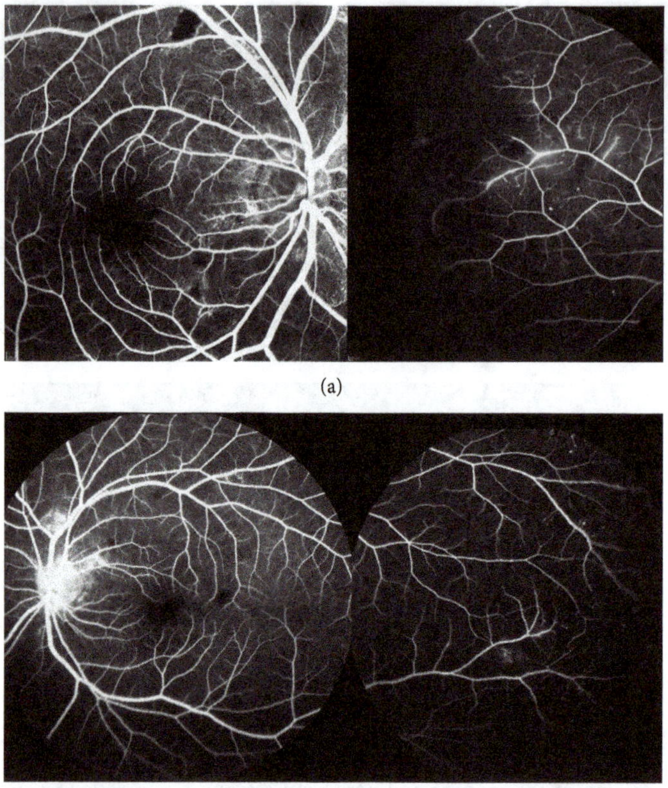

(a) (b)

FIGURE 5: Case 2: fluorescein angiography findings at presentation. Asymmetric papillitis and occlusive vasculitis are seen in the (a) right and (b) left eyes.

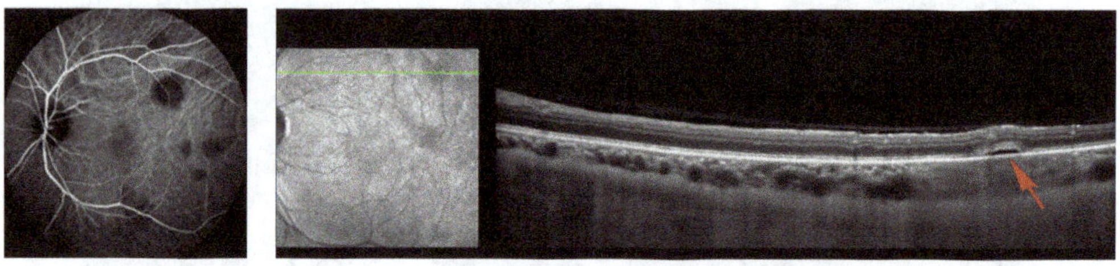

(a) (b)

FIGURE 6: Case 2: ICG angiography and EDI-OCT at presentation (left eye). (a) Indocyanine green angiography demonstrated multiple hypofluorescent spots throughout the posterior pole and the midperiphery. (b) Enhanced Depth Imaging-OCT performed on a superotemporal hypocyanescent spot revealed a well-delineated lesion occupying all the choroidal space and considered as a cryptococcal granuloma, associated with a small serous retinal detachment (red arrow).

All those findings were compatible with cryptococcal chorioretinitis associated with papillitis and occlusive vasculitis.

At 6-month follow-up, LE fundus indicated a significant regression of the initial lesions with also resorption of hemorrhages and retinal cotton wools (Figure 7(a)). Late-phase FA showed decreased papillary diffusion with a remaining mild vasculitis on the posterior pole (Figure 7(b)). On ICGA, the hypocyanescent lesions were still present but decreased in size, suggestive of a healing process (Figure 7(c)). EDI-OCT showed resorption of the serous retinal detachment, a decrease in hyperreflectivity of choroidal infiltration and resorption of serous retinal detachment (Figure 7(d)).

4. Discussion

We report 2 rare cases of cryptococcal chorioretinitis associated with uveitis and vasculitis in 2 untreated AIDS patients with profound immunosuppression and concomitant cryptococcal meningitis.

Cryptococcal choroiditis represents an uncommon OI of persons with advanced HIV/AIDS. Visual loss in the setting of AIDS entails a broad differential diagnosis. Putative etiologies include HIV retinopathy, CMV retinitis, acute or progressive outer retinal necrosis (i.e., herpes simplex or varicella zoster virus-mediated), toxoplasma chorioretinitis, syphilitic chorioretinitis, *Pneumocystis jirovecii* choroiditis,

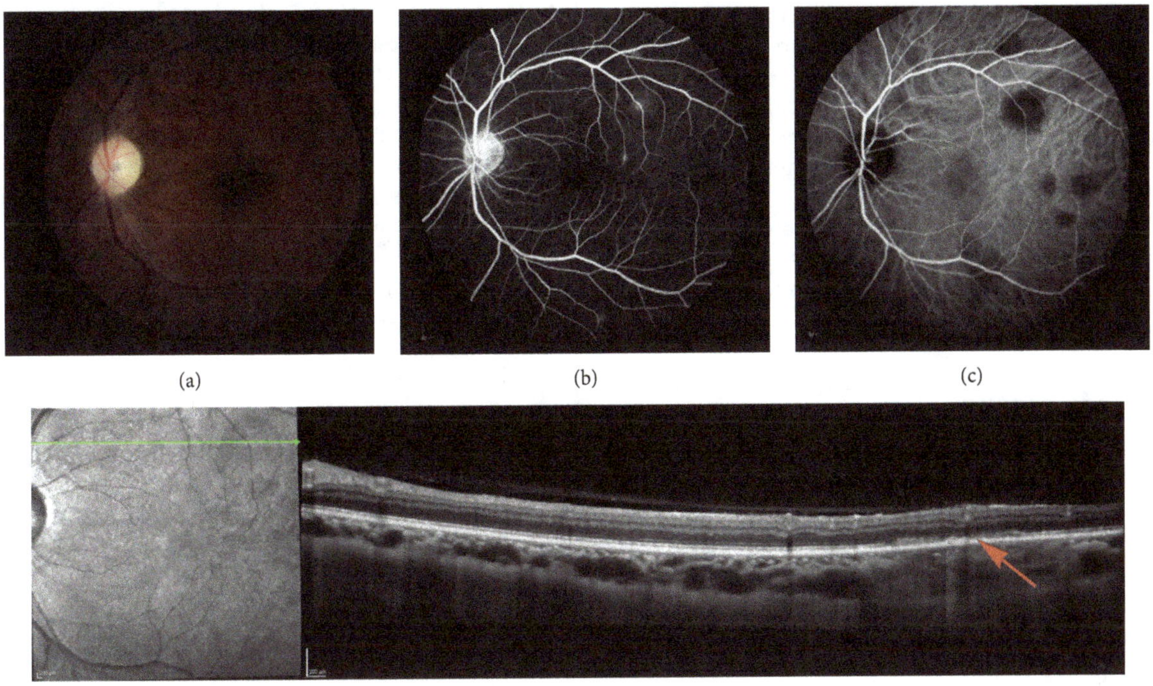

(a) (b) (c)

(d)

FIGURE 7: Case 2: left eye at 6-month follow-up. (a) Left eye fundus indicated a significant regression of the initial lesions with also resorption of hemorrhages and retinal cotton wools. (b) Late-phase FA showed decreased papillary diffusion with a remaining mild vasculitis on the posterior pole. (c) On ICGA, the hypocyanescent lesions are still present but decreased in size. (d) EDI-OCT showed resorption of the serous retinal detachment (red arrow).

ocular tuberculosis or Mycobacterium avium complex, candida, histoplasma or aspergillus endophthalmitis/vitritis, immune reconstitution uveitis, and lymphoma [4, 5]. Cryptococcal meningitis is frequently associated with ocular manifestations. In a study performed in Sub-Saharan Africa before the era of antiretroviral therapy on 80 patients with cryptococcal disease, papilledema was the most common ocular manifestation and was found in around 30% of the subjects [2]. Other frequent manifestations included cranial nerve palsy (9%) and loss of visual acuity (9%). Causes of bilateral visual loss included optic atrophy, optic neuropathy with abolishment of pupillary responses in one, and cortical blindness. Unilateral visual loss was caused by an occlusion of the central retinal vein with macular edema. Only two patients had signs of choroidal involvement: one with choroidal infiltrates and the other one with cryptococcoma. However, intraocular involvement following cryptococcal meningitis has rarely been reported [3–7]. The most common manifestation is choroiditis while anterior uveitis, vasculitis, and retinitis, as described in the present cases, are less common [6]. Previous reports indicate that the yeast can be directly isolated from intraocular tissues or fluids [6]. Dissemination likely occurs via the hematogenous route as illustrated in both cases with angiography exams that indicated both proximal and distal vessel lesions.

Interestingly, in both of our cases, chorioretinitis manifests during the course of treatment for cryptococcal meningitis. In the first case, the patient had already received months of treatment and chorioretinitis manifests in the context of a relapse. Similarly, in the second case, ocular inflammation occurs in the setting of a presumed relapse or clinical failure. Similar cases have been reported previously. Carney et al. reported cases of cryptococcal choroiditis in which choroiditis manifests 10 days after initiation of amphotericin B [7]. The authors proposed a scheme of progression of ocular infection following hematogenous dissemination: (1) cryptococcal choroiditis, (2) cryptococcal chorioretinitis, and (3) cryptococcal uveitis/vitritis/endophthalmitis [7].

Simultaneous involvement of all the different eye structures (anterior chamber, choroid, retina, and vessels) has rarely been reported in the course of disseminated *C. neoformans* infection, as well as reports describing multimodal imaging findings. Most cases were reported in patients with concomitant immunosuppression. Previous cases were reported in patients with advanced AIDS [8–10] or with T cell leukemia [11]. As described in the latter cases [8, 9], EDI-OCT and ICG have proven most useful in directing the diagnostic algorithm in panuveitis in immunosuppressed patients by defining the localization of lesions and assessing response to treatment. The two cases presented here highlight the potential of *C. neoformans* to infect all ocular structures including the optic nerve, retinal vessel, and choroidal stroma, leading, respectively, to papillitis, vasculitis, and choroiditis in immunocompromised patients. This involvement is found in some systemic granulomatous diseases, leading to the most frequent differential diagnoses of tuberculosis and sarcoidosis, but also syphilis, which remains the main masquerade syndrome in uveitis patients [12]. We excluded the possibility of intraocular cryptococcal/toxoplasma coinfection, because CT scan and MRI of the brain did not reveal signs of cerebral toxoplasmosis. Moreover, bilateral multifocal choroidal infiltrates are an uncommon presentation of ocular toxoplasmosis [13].

On the other hand, limited involvement of the eye presenting as uveitis with concomitant cryptococcal meningitis has been reported in nonimmunocompromised patients [14, 15].

In conclusion, these two cases reveal the potential of *C. neoformans* to infect all ocular structures mimicking other ocular diseases and this leads us to consider Cryptococcus as "a good masquerader" like syphilis and tuberculosis.

Acknowledgments

We thank Raphaël Polat for the excellent technical assistance.

References

[1] E. K. Maziarz and J. R. Perfect, "Cryptococcosis," *Infectious Disease Clinics of North America*, vol. 30, no. 1, pp. 179–206, 2016.

[2] P. Kestelyn, H. Taelman, J. Bogaerts et al., "Ophthalmic manifestations of infections with *Cryptococcus neoformans* in patients with the acquired immunodeficiency syndrome," *American Journal of Ophthalmology*, vol. 116, no. 6, pp. 721–727, 1993.

[3] S. A. Gandhi, A. A. McMeeking, D. Friedberg, and R. S. Holzman, "Cryptococcal choroiditis in a patient with AIDS: case report and review," *Clinical Infectious Diseases*, vol. 23, no. 5, pp. 1193-1194, 1996.

[4] A. S. Banker, "Posterior segment manifestations of human immunodeficiency virus/acquired immune deficiency syndrome," *Indian Journal of Ophthalmology*, vol. 56, no. 5, pp. 377–383, 2008.

[5] E. N. Morinelli, P. U. Dugel, R. Riffenburgh, and N. A. Rao, "Infectious multifocal choroiditis in patients with acquired immune deficiency syndrome," *Ophthalmology*, vol. 100, no. 7, pp. 1014–1021, 1993.

[6] J. R. C. Crump, S. G. Elner, V. M. Elner, and C. A. Kauffman, "Cryptococcal endophthalmitis: case report and review," *Clinical Infectious Diseases*, vol. 14, no. 5, pp. 1069–1073, 1992.

[7] M. D. Carney, J. L. Combs, and W. Waschler, "Cryptococcal choroiditis," *Retina*, vol. 10, no. 1, pp. 27–32, 1990.

[8] C. M. Aderman, I. R. Gorovoy, D. L. Chao, M. M. Bloomer, A. Obeid, and J. M. Stewart, "Cryptococcal choroiditis in advanced AIDS with clinicopathologic correlation," *American Journal of Ophthalmology Case Reports*, vol. 10, pp. 51–54, 2018.

[9] S. Baillif, J. Delas, A. Asrargis, and P. Gastaud, "Multimodal imaging of bilateral cryptococcal choroiditis," *Retina*, vol. 33, no. 1, pp. 249–251, 2013.

[10] G. S. Canfield, S. Reingold, A. Ho et al., "AIDS-related *Cryptococcus neoformans* choroiditis," *IDCases*, vol. 22, article e00931, 2020.

[11] W. Yamada, H. Yamada, K. Murata et al., "Case of cryptococcal choroiditis in adult with T-cell leukemia/lymphoma," *Journal of Infection and Chemotherapy*, vol. 25, no. 1, pp. 59–64, 2019.

[12] S. L. Woolston, S. Dhanireddy, and J. Marrazzo, "Ocular syphilis: a clinical review," *Current Infectious Disease Reports*, vol. 18, no. 11, p. 36, 2016.

[13] C. Ozgonul and C. G. Besirli, "Recent developments in the diagnosis and treatment of ocular toxoplasmosis," *Ophthalmic Research*, vol. 57, no. 1, pp. 1–12, 2017.

[14] S. Nakamura, K. Izumikawa, M. Seki et al., "Reversible visual disturbance due to cryptococcal uveitis in a non-HIV individual," *Medical Mycology*, vol. 46, no. 4, pp. 367–370, 2008.

[15] S. P. Stone, J. Bendig, J. Hakim, P. E. Kinnear, B. S. Azadian, and F. Clifford-Rose, "Cryptococcal meningitis presenting as uveitis," *British Journal of Ophthalmology*, vol. 72, no. 3, pp. 167–170, 1988.

30

OCT Angiography and En Face OCT Reflectance Aid in Monitoring Subclinical Inflammation in Serpiginous Choroidopathy

Carl S. Wilkins, Jorge S. Andrade Romo, Toco Y. P. Chui, Richard B. Rosen, and Stephanie Llop

Department of Ophthalmology, New York Eye and Ear Infirmary of Mount Sinai, 310 East 14th Street, New York, NY 10003, USA

Correspondence should be addressed to Carl S. Wilkins; cswilkins013@gmail.com

Academic Editor: Takaaki Hayashi

Introduction. We present a case of serpiginous choroidopathy (SC) with novel OCTA and en face OCT reflectance findings which help identify subclinical disease progression. *Case Presentation.* En face OCT reflectance images demonstrated outer retinal tubules (ORT) at the serpiginous lesion margins of affected and unaffected retina on multimodal imaging. OCTA findings demonstrate variable dropout of choriocapillaris in "normal" retina beyond lesion borders which was not visible on standard imaging and which demonstrated a clear transition zone beyond the ORT. *Discussion.* This is the first report of choriocapillaris atrophy identified on OCTA not identified on traditional multimodal imaging in serpiginous choroidopathy. Damage to vasculature only visible with OCTA may help characterize the distribution of inflammation, aiding in monitoring of suppression not illustrated by traditional imaging and which may threaten the central macula. ORT in SC suggest death and reorganization of outer segments from dysfunction of the choriocapillaris and RPE, as well as serve to demarcate the area of chronic or old inflammation, supporting the hypothesis that the choriocapillaris is the primary site of inflammation in SC. Based on these findings, we recommend OCTA on all patients with serpiginous choroidopathy to monitor underlying state of inflammation and help determine immunosuppressive threshold.

1. Introduction

The pathogenesis of SC is poorly understood, with clinical and histologic studies suggesting autoimmune, infectious, vasculopathic, and retinal degenerative etiologies [1, 2]. Recent advances in retinal imaging have ushered in a new era of new diagnostics in posterior uveitic diseases. Given the unclear cause from clinical and laboratory studies, much attention has shifted towards these new modalities. A patient presented with serpiginous choroidopathy (SC) and underwent OCTA and en face OCT reflectance imaging. We report novel OCTA and en face OCT reflectance imaging findings of outer retinal tubules (ORT) in SC.

2. Case Report

A 37-year-old female with no past medical or ocular history presented with 2 weeks of redness, pain, and photophobia of her right eye (OD). She was diagnosed with acute anterior uveitis by an outside provider and started on topical difluprednate four times daily (QID) and cyclopentolate once daily (QD) OD. Upon presentation to our facility, she reported slight improvement in her symptoms 2 weeks into treatment.

On initial examination, visual acuity was 20/20 in her right and 20/20 in her left eye (OS) with unremarkable pupillary exam and normal intraocular pressure. Anterior segment

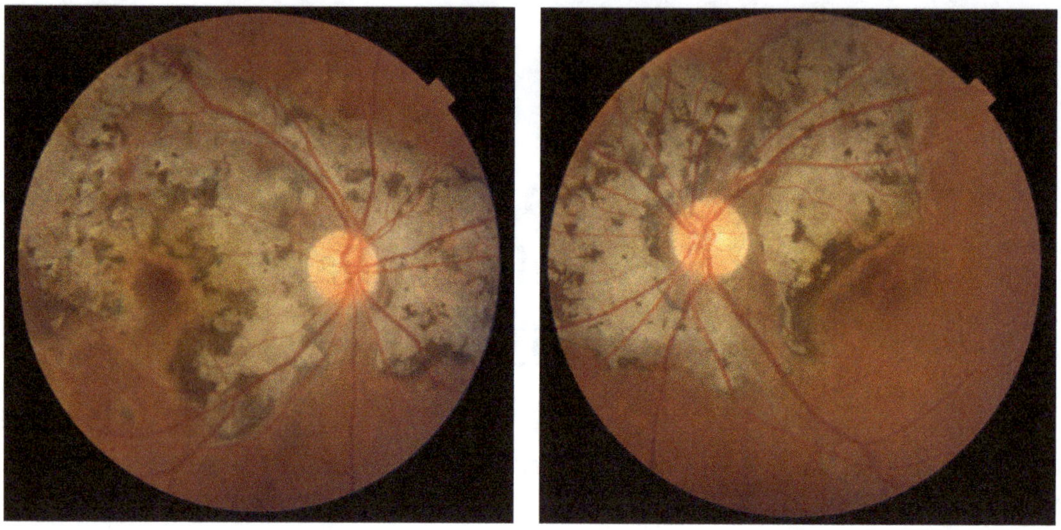

(a) (b)

FIGURE 1: Color fundus photo of the right eye (a) and left eye (b).

examination of the right eye (OD) revealed 2 areas of anterior corneal stromal scarring and 0.5+ anterior chamber cell without flare. One area of anterior stromal scarring and trace cell without flare was seen OS. Fundoscopy revealed 0.5+ vitreous cell without haze in both eyes (OU); healthy appearing optic nerves OU; and extensive, serpentine peripapillary chorioretinal scarring OU with extension into the macula (Figures 1(a) and 1(b)). There were no hemorrhages or vascular sheathing, and the peripheral retina was unremarkable. Fluorescein angiography (FA) was performed, which demonstrated hyperfluorescence at the lesion margins visible on gross funduscopy. Fundus autofluorescence (FAF) demonstrated hyperautofluoresence at lesion margins and hypoautofluorescence in areas of atrophic retina. Pertinent laboratory workup included negative QuantiFERON-TB Gold, fluorescent treponemal antibody (FTA), and Lyme IgM and IgG. A diagnosis of serpiginous choroidopathy was made, and the patient started on oral prednisone 60 mg daily, with a taper of the difluprednate OD by one drop per week.

The patient rapidly improved, and immunomodulatory therapy was initiated with a standard steroid taper. At one-month follow-up, en face OCT reflectance and OCTA imaging were obtained, which demonstrated severe atrophy with outer retinal tubules and patchy dropout of choriocapillaris in areas of otherwise normal-appearing retina, respectively (Figure 2). Over the next 2 months, the prednisone was slowly tapered and she continued mycophenolate mofetil 1 gram twice daily without recurrence of intraocular inflammation or activation of disease at the lesion margins. Repeat SD-OCT and OCTA imaging remained stable.

3. Discussion

We present a case of serpiginous choroidopathy (SC) imaged with OCTA and en face OCT reflectance imaging. Images were obtained and processed based upon previously described methodologies in the literature [3, 4].

OCTA imaging showed dropout of the choriocapillaris at lesion margins and discontinuously in adjacent areas centrally which appeared normal on traditional imaging such as FA (Figure 2(d)). Prior to obtaining OCTA, these areas closer to the fovea were presumed to be unaffected by SC based upon FA and examination. Fortunately, with high-dose oral steroids and immunomodulatory therapy, these subclinical areas remained stable and the patient did not experience further vision loss. Additionally, there was markedly increased visibility of the choriocapillaris between the outer retinal tubule and lesion borders, likely indicating some degree of reconstitution of choriocapillaris in affected retina and RPE atrophy improving visibility of underlying choroidal vasculature. This is consistent with prior reports [5].

OCT angiography allows a noninvasive assessment of choroidal and deep vasculature sometimes not evident on fluorescein angiography (FA). Recently, several small case series of OCTA in SC have suggested extensive inflammation in deep retinal vessels, RPE, and choriocapillaris. Desai et al. reported a series of 6 eyes of 3 patients with active and inactive SC. In this series, active patients demonstrated absence of choriocapillaris with thickening of overlying RPE and outer retinal layers on OCTA in areas of atrophic serpiginous lesions [5]. Inactive patients demonstrated partial reappearance of choriocapillaris at lesion margins with absence of outer retina, RPE, and choriocapillaris at inactive geographic regions [5]. Another case series of active and inactive SC lesions demonstrated disproportionate involvement of choriocapillaris compared to overlying RPE and deep retinal vasculature, suggesting that the choriocapillaris may be the primary pathologic site in SC [6]. In our patient, dropout of deep retinal vasculature was seen beyond lesion borders identified on photography and fluorescein angiography, indicating subclinical inflammation in areas not previously identifiable.

We analyzed en face OCT reflectance image slabs, as well as cross-sectional OCT images. En face OCT reflectance imaging demonstrated outer retinal tubules at the quiescent

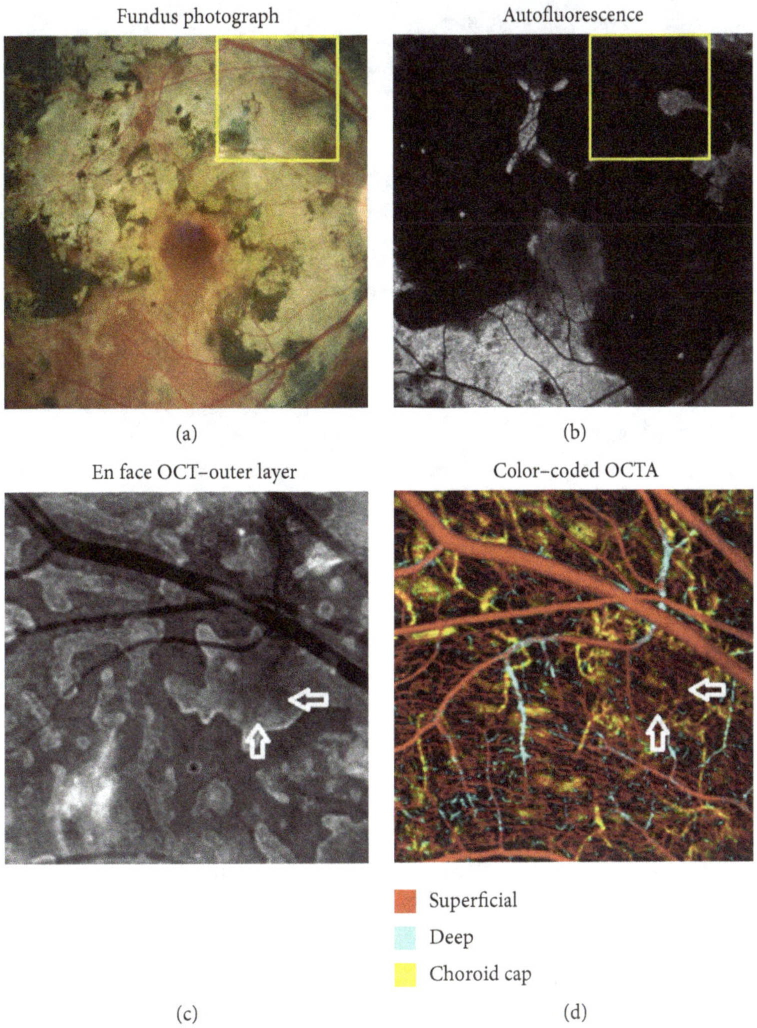

FIGURE 2: Composite images of the right eye: color fundus photo (a); fundus autofluorescence (b); magnified superficial en face OCT reflectance slab demonstrating ORT margins (c); and magnified color-coded OCTA of superficial, deep, and choriocapillaris vessels showing dropout beyond normal-appearing retina (d). White arrows demonstrate the corresponding area which is intact on fundus photo (a) and autofluorescence (b), lies within the border of the outer retinal tubules seen on en face imaging (c), but demonstrates patchy dropout of choriocapillaris identical to adjacent areas. Of note, there is increased visibility of choriocapillaris at the legion margins, seen as yellow-coded vessels and analogous to window defect.

serpiginous margins just adjacent to those areas of atrophic choriocapillaris on OCT which were normal-appearing on funduscopy and FA (Figure 2(c)). Cross-sectional OCT imaging confirmed the presence of ORT in areas of atrophic retina (Figure 3). To the best of our knowledge, only two reports of ORT in serpiginous choroidopathy exist [7, 8]. Our patient demonstrated outer retinal tubules adjacent to the serpiginous lesion borders between affected and nonaffected retina and choroid, but not within the atrophic areas themselves. Absence of ORT in areas of subclinical inflammation identified on OCTA indicates less chronic or severe inflammation in those areas, which would likely manifest without proper treatment. This may ultimately indicate inability of FA and OCT alone in identifying extent of risk in these patients and level of immunosuppression needed to preserve vision.

On SD-OCT imaging, outer retinal tubules appear as circular areas of hyporeflectivity with a ring of hyperreflectivity contained within the outer nuclear layer. Prior investigations of outer retinal tubules have centered around age-related macular degeneration (AMD) and spectral domain OCT (SD-OCT) but never reported in SC. Of the 69 eyes with outer retinal tubules identified in one study, 81% were attributable to AMD [9]. Other conditions observed with ORT included central serous chorioretinopathy, choroideremia, multifocal choroiditis with panuveitis, and Bietti crystalline dystrophy [9]. This finding is hypothesized to be secondary to reorganization of cone outer segments after loss of tight junction integrity. Histopathologic examinations of patients with outer retinal tubules have demonstrated ELM and inner segment mitochondria comprising the hyperreflective portion of the outer retinal tubules, with the luminal wall containing degenerated cone photoreceptors and RPE cells within the lumen [10, 11]. Given previously reported imaging and pathologic data of outer retinal tubules, this may indicate a shared anatomic pathway for SC and noninflammatory

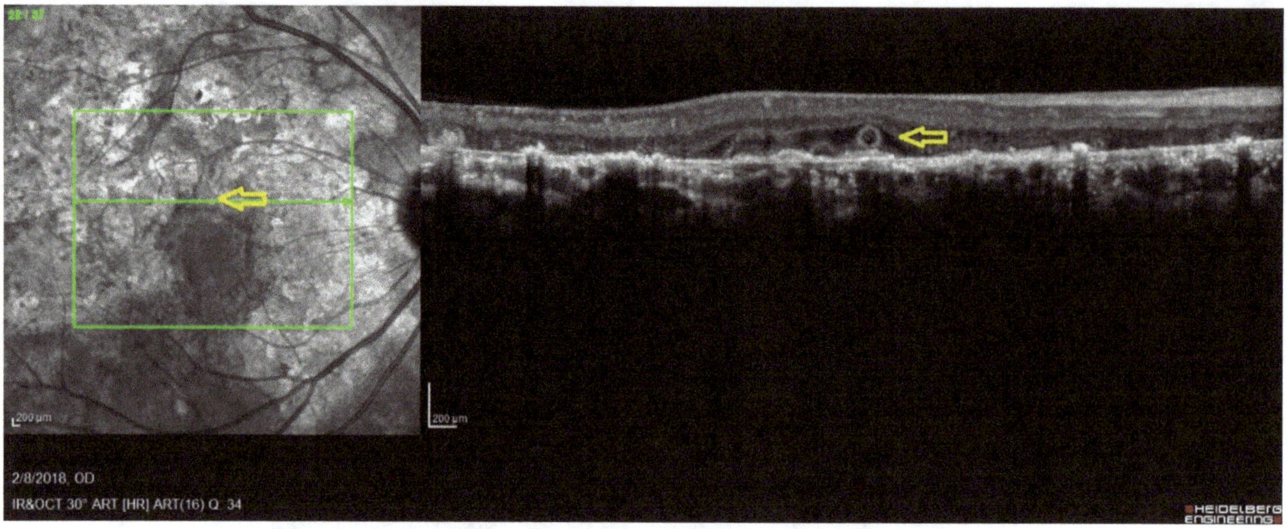

FIGURE 3: SD-OCT single-line raster of the right eye demonstrating superior parafoveal outer retinal tubule (yellow arrow).

retinal degenerations. Regardless of pathogenesis, this case demonstrates chronic inflammation at serpiginous borders as reflected by ORT and OCTA transition zones, and more importantly, those areas of relative deep retinal and choriocapillaris loss on OCTA occur beyond those lesion borders.

4. Conclusion

Severe choriocapillaris inflammation may be the cause of outer retinal atrophy in serpiginous choroidopathy, with the presence of ORT signifying reorganization of photoreceptors localizing inflammation to this area. Current multimodal imaging without use of OCTA is widely accepted for the diagnosis and monitoring of SC. In this report, we describe a patient with OCTA findings of choriocapillaris atrophy demonstrating subclinical disease beyond serpiginous lesion borders visible on standard imaging. Loss of choriocapillaris integrity in areas outside of the serpiginous borders suggests subclinical activity which, if followed with OCTA, may aid in earlier identification of progression or more targeted timing for tapering of immunomodulatory therapy if stable. This suggests that OCTA may be more sensitive than SD-OCT and FA in identifying activity in SC and should be more widely adopted in the long-term management of these patients.

Consent

Patient consent was not obtained for this manuscript as all images were kept anonymous in compliance with ICMJE standards. The patient's name, identity, and any unique characteristics were removed in compliance with patient privacy protection and HIPAA standards.

Disclosure

The content is solely the responsibility of the authors and does not necessarily represent the official views of the National Institutes of Health.

Acknowledgments

The authors would like to thank Dr. Giselle Lynch and the NYEEI Imaging Department for their contribution in obtaining clinical images. This study was supported by the National Eye Institute of the National Institutes of Health under award number R01EY027301. Additional funding for this study was provided by the New York Eye and Ear Infirmary Research Foundation and the Marrus Family Foundation.

References

[1] W. K. Lim, R. R. Buggage, and R. B. Nussenblatt, "Serpiginous Choroiditis," *Survey of Ophthalmology*, vol. 50, no. 3, pp. 231–244, 2005.

[2] H. N. Khanamiri and N. A. Rao, "Serpiginous Choroiditis and Infectious Multifocal Serpiginoid Choroiditis," *Survey of Ophthalmology*, vol. 58, no. 3, pp. 203–232, 2013.

[3] B. D. Krawitz, E. Phillips, R. D. Bavier et al., "Parafoveal Nonperfusion Analysis in Diabetic Retinopathy Using Optical Coherence Tomography Angiography," *Translational Vision Science & Technology*, vol. 7, no. 4, p. 4, 2018.

[4] G. Lynch, J. S. Andrade Romo, R. Linderman et al., "Within-subject assessment of foveal avascular zone enlargement in different stages of diabetic retinopathy using *en face* OCT reflectance and OCT angiography," *Biomedical Optics Express*, vol. 9, no. 12, pp. 5982–5996.

[5] R. Desai, P. Nesper, D. A. Goldstein, A. A. Fawzi, L. M. Jampol, and M. Gill, "OCT Angiography Imaging in Serpiginous Choroidopathy," *Ophthalmology Retina*, vol. 2, no. 4, pp. 351–359, 2018.

[6] K. Pakzad-Vaezi, K. Khaksari, Z. Chu, R. N. Van Gelder, R. K. Wang, and K. L. Pepple, "Swept-Source OCT Angiography of Serpiginous Choroiditis," *Ophthalmology Retina*, vol. 2, no. 7, pp. 712–719, 2018.

[7] A. Mateo-montoya, B. Wolff, J. A. Sahel, and M. Mauget-faÿsse, "Outer retinal tubulations in serpinginous choroiditis," *Graefe's Archive for Clinical and Experimental Ophthalmology*, vol. 251, no. 11, pp. 2657-2658, 2013.

[8] X. N. Wang, Q. S. You, H. Y. Zhao, and X. Y. Peng, "Optical Coherence Tomography Features of Tuberculous Serpiginous-like Choroiditis and Serpiginous Choroiditis," *Biomedical and Environmental Sciences*, vol. 31, no. 5, pp. 327–334, 2018.

[9] S. A. Zweifel, M. Engelbert, K. Laud, R. Margolis, R. F. Spaide, and K. B. Freund, "Outer Retinal Tubulation," *Archives of Ophthalmology*, vol. 127, no. 12, pp. 1596–1602, 2009.

[10] K. M. Litts, J. D. Messinger, K. Dellatorre, L. A. Yannuzzi, K. B. Freund, and C. A. Curcio, "Clinicopathological Correlation of Outer Retinal Tubulation in Age-Related Macular Degeneration," *JAMA Ophthalmology*, vol. 133, no. 5, pp. 609–612, 2015.

[11] K. B. Schaal, K. B. Freund, K. M. Litts, Y. Zhang, J. D. Messinger, and C. A. Curcio, "Outer retinal TUBULATION in advanced age-related macular DEGENERATION," *Retina.*, vol. 35, no. 7, pp. 1339–1350, 2015.

31

Combined *Rothia dentocariosa* and *Streptococcus viridans* Corneal Ulcer in an Immunocompromised Patient

Jamie Dietze and Thomas Mauger

WVU Medicine Department of Ophthalmology, USA

Correspondence should be addressed to Jamie Dietze; jamie.dietze@hsc.wvu.edu

Academic Editor: Alexander A. Bialasiewicz

Keratitis is a very common condition seen by ophthalmologists. However, many factors can complicate the treatment of this depending on the causative organism and other patient comorbid conditions. The objective of this clinical case report is to highlight the treatment of keratitis caused by *Rothia dentocariosa*. It also looks at the unique considerations in keratitis presentations for patients immunocompromised by chemotherapy agents. Our patient is a 58 yo female undergoing chemotherapy with folinic acid, fluorouracil, irinotecan, and panitumumab who presented with several days of a red, painful right eye with mucous discharge. Cultures were positive for *Rothia dentocariosa* and *Streptococcus viridans*. The patient ultimately underwent a conjunctival flap procedure as medical therapy with proper oral and topical antibiotics failed to resolve keratitis. This case is unique as previously, only a couple of cases of keratitis caused by *Rothia dentocariosa* have been reported and none of those patients were immunocompromised nor failed antibiotic therapy.

1. Introduction

Rothia dentocariosa is a gram-positive rod that was originally isolated from dental plaques and caries. It is commonly found in the oral cavity and pharynx as part of the normal microflora [1]. It has also been a source for transient bacteremia, endocarditis, and some meningitis, peritonitis, bone/joint infections, pneumonia, skin/soft tissue, endophthalmitis, and prosthetic device infections. Invasive disease of *Rothia* species occurs predominantly in immunocompromised hosts, and patients typically have periodontal disease or multiple carious teeth [2]. It is usually susceptible to penicillin, cephalosporin, erythromycin, and tetracycline, but there have been a few strains found that have developed B-lactamase [2]. Reported ocular infections of *Rothia* species typically are endophthalmitis following intravitreal injection or systemic bacteremia seeding [3]. We describe a case of keratitis due to *R. dentocariosa* in an immunocompromised host.

2. Case

A 58-year-old white female presented with a red, painful right eye. She had some photosensitivity and increasingly blurry vision. Her history was significant for daily wear soft contact lens use and stage IV colon cancer treated with partial bowel resection and was currently undergoing chemotherapy FOLFIRI (folinic acid, fluorouracil, and irinotecan) and panitumumab every other week. The exam was significant for hand motion visual acuity and moderate diffuse conjunctival injection with moderate mucous discharge (Figure 1). The cornea was diffusely opaque in the central 8 mm and an overlying epithelial defect. The far periphery had less dense anterior stromal corneal haze. The remainder of the exam was limited due to poor view into the anterior chamber. Ultrasound B scan showed no evidence of vitritis or endophthalmitis. Cultures for fungus, bacteria, and atypical microorganisms were taken, and the patient was started on fortified vancomycin (50 mg/ml) and fortified

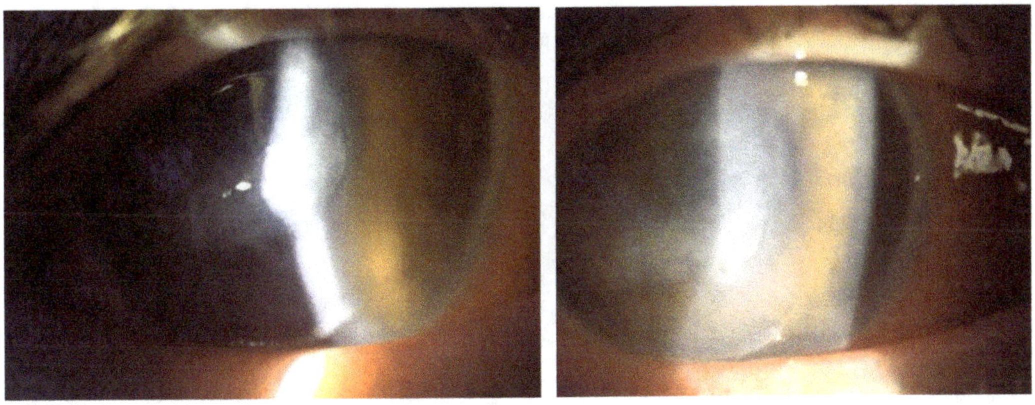

FIGURE 1: Slit lamp photos showing keratitis of patient's right eye three days after initial presentation. Central opacification with peripheral corneal clearing and diffuse conjunctival injection.

tobramycin (15 mg/ml) every hour, moxifloxacin every two hours, cyclopentolate three times per day, ciprofloxacin 500 mg by mouth twice daily, and vitamin C 500 mg by mouth twice daily. Bacteria cultures grew *Rothia dentocariosa* with sensitivities showing resistance to erythromycin and intermediate sensitivity to penicillin. *Strep viridans* also grew in the bacterial culture (Table 1). The treatment regimen was switched to moxifloxacin four times per day, fortified tobramycin four times per day, vancomycin every hour, cyclopentolate three times per day, vitamin C 500 mg by mouth twice daily, and doxycycline 100 mg by mouth twice daily. The patient continued to have an 8 mm epithelial corneal defect with irregular borders and central granular infiltrates but peripheral corneal clearing. The regimen was changed to fortified vancomycin every two hours, moxifloxacin every two hours, cefuroxime 50 mg/ml every hour while awake, and acyclovir 400 mg by mouth five times daily. The patient did not show further improvement, so cefixime 400 mg by mouth daily was added and acyclovir and doxycycline were discontinued. After six days on this regimen and still without significant improvement, the patient underwent a Gunderson conjunctival flap. A flap was taken from the superior bulbar conjunctiva and rotated over the cornea secured with 8-0 Vicryl sutures. The patient showed gradual improvement in symptoms, and the ocular inflammation was resolved. Six weeks postoperatively, the infection appeared to be resolved and the flap appeared to be well healed (Figure 2). The patient had been off antibiotic drops for four weeks, only using erythromycin ointment, and had total resolution of her ocular pain as well as no signs of recurrent infection. There is plan for keratoplasty in the future.

TABLE 1: Antibiotic sensitivity table from cornea bacterial culture performed.

Rothia dentocariosa Ceftriaxone	1 mcg/ml	Sensitive
Erythromycin	4 cg/ml	Resistant
Penicillin		Intermediate
Vancomycin	0.5 mcg/ml	Sensitive

3. Discussion

Georg and Brown first created the genus "Rothia" in 1967, which resembles both Nocardia and Actinomyces but differs in the physiology and cell wall constituents [4]. *Rothia dentocariosa* is a rod-shaped, nonsporogenic, nonmotile, catalase-positive, gram-positive bacterium that grows faster under aerobic rather than anaerobic conditions but can grow in either environment. Its colonies are either smooth and convex or rough with a "spoke-wheel" surface with scalloped edges [5]. *R. dentocariosa* is considered largely benign but can rarely cause infection, most commonly endocarditis in people with heart valve disorders. Typically, patients who get infections are predisposed by having poor dental hygiene or have had extensive dental procedures [1].

Rothia species tend to be widely susceptible to the penicillin class and other antibiotics covering gram-positive bacteria. However, there have been some recent reports of species with B-lactamase activity, therefore causing some penicillin resistance [6]. Despite this, the current accepted treatment for *Rothia* infections such as endocarditis is still treatment with penicillin [7].

Our patient presented with keratitis without any evidence of endophthalmitis. There have only been two previous cases reported of *R. dentocariosa* causing corneal ulceration. First was an 11-year-old boy with history of keratoplasty and was found to be licking his finger prior to eye rubbing [8]. The second was a 49-year-old South Asian female with history of recent dental procedure and a canine that frequently licked her face [9]. Both cases were treated with a cephalosporin and resolved. Our case, however, is the first one reported in an immunocompromised host that did not have a significant dental history.

Streptococcus viridans is an alpha group streptococcus that is a known pathogen for causing corneal ulceration and infectious crystalline keratopathy, especially in postkeratoplasty patients. It is thought to be of low-grade pathogenicity as it infects locally immunosuppressed hosts or those with surface damage due to contact lens wear. Infections are typically indolent, causing an anterior stromal

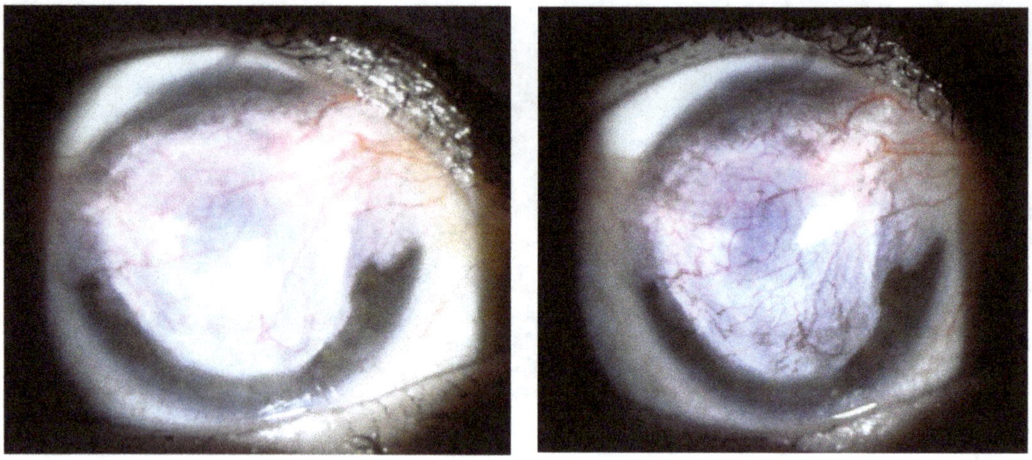

FIGURE 2: Slit lamp photos showing patient's right eye six weeks postoperatively from conjunctival flap placement. The flap appears to be in proper placement over previous corneal defect with good vascularization.

inflammatory reaction that is slow to progress with or without a mild anterior chamber reaction. When ulceration occurs, it is typically a well-circumscribed, gray white, "dry" appearing, and lying beneath a well-demarcated epithelial defect [10]. When seen as a crystalline keratopathy, it appears as discrete, white, crystalline/fernlike stromal opacities under an intact epithelium with little corneal inflammation. Typically, infections with *S. viridans* respond rapidly to proper antibiotic therapy [10]. *S. viridans* has continued to have good susceptibility to vancomycin in recent literature and is still considered a proper antimicrobial therapy for ocular infections [11, 12]. There have not been any reports of ocular coinfections with *Rothia* species, but *S. viridans* has been known to have coinfection with fungus, such as Candida and Acanthamoeba [13, 14]. We believe our patient had a true coinfection with *R. dentocariosa* and *S. viridans* rather than a superinfection based on her symptom timeline and the initial culture growing both species.

Our patient was immunocompromised due to ongoing FOLFIRI and panitumumab chemotherapy treatment. Panitumumab is one of the Epidermal Growth Factor Receptor (EGFR) inhibitor chemotherapies. EGFR inhibitors have been shown to cause poor healing of the corneal epithelial layer, corneal thinning, and melt. Some other chemotherapy agents can cause corneal deposits, verticillata, and tear film changes leading to both corneal and conjunctival epithelial damage [15]. While we know EGFR inhibitors can affect the corneal tissues, the actual mechanism is unclear as to which endogenous EGF-like ligand promotes corneal wound healing and therefore is disrupted by EGFR inhibitors. What is known is that having high level of basal EGF in tear fluid promotes EGFR-mediated corneal epithelial homeostasis and is the only ligand that is present in concentrations that would predict a significant level of receptor occupancy and therefore is the most likely mechanism that EGFR inhibitors influence the cornea [16].

Another aspect of interest about our patient was that the *R. dentocariosa* species was found to be erythromycin resistant and only intermediately sensitive to penicillin. She was treated with cefixime PO, ceftazidime drops QID, and vancomycin drops QID but only showed modest ocular improvement. She ultimately required a conjunctival flap to promote corneal healing, which was not needed in either of the previous two cases.

Conjunctival flaps were first started in the 1800s and used for corneal ulcerations and thinning disorders. Their purpose is to restore the integrity of the compromised corneal surface and provide metabolic and mechanical support for corneal healing [17, 18]. They can be used in cases where medical treatment has been exhausted to resolve infection such as our patient but are usually used for cases with marginal fungal ulcers but have also been shown to benefit in other infectious keratitis such as Acanthamoeba [19]. Flaps help improve comfort and ocular inflammation and promote healing [20]. Vascularized conjunctival tissues give both a rich blood supply and lymphatic vessels providing better nutrition to the corneal tissues, growth factors, an increased resistance to infection, and anticollagenolytic substances [17]. As long as the graft continues to stay healthy, these can be left in place. Once infection resolution is achieved, keratoplasty may be performed. Using a conjunctival flap as an intermediate step can lower the risk of keratoplasty graft rejection as compared to cases that do not use a conjunctival flap temporizing measure [20]. That is why a conjunctival flap intermediate step was chosen for our immunocompromised patient, so that she could continue chemotherapy treatment but reduce the risk of infection recurrence and graft failure of a keratoplasty procedure.

4. Conclusion

Rothia dentocariosa is a known part of the normal microflora of the oropharynx. It typically does not cause invasive disease, but when it does, it tends to cause endocarditis or pneumonia. Ocular infections with this organism are typically thought to be limited to post procedure endophthalmitis. Corneal ulceration is a rare presentation of *R. dentocariosa* infection and should be considered on the differential diagnosis in patients with recent extensive dental procedures and poor dental hygiene or those who are immunocompromised. While *R. dentocariosa* is still considered widely susceptible to penicillin, some resistance is starting to emerge. Treatment with a cephalosporin is the current recommendation for systemic infection when resistance is detected and therefore should be considered the treatment for ocular infection. In cases where ulceration or keratitis persists despite cephalosporin treatment, a conjunctival flap may be of benefit to resolve the infection prior to a keratoplasty procedure.

References

[1] A. V. Graevenitz, "*Rothia dentocariosa*: taxonomy and differential diagnosis," *Clinical Microbiology and Infection*, vol. 10, no. 5, pp. 399–402, 2004.

[2] P. Ramanan, J. N. Barreto, D. R. Osmon, and P. K. Tosh, "Rothia bacteremia: a 10-year experience at Mayo Clinic, Rochester, Minnesota," *Journal of Clinical Microbiology*, vol. 52, no. 9, pp. 3184–3189, 2014.

[3] R. A. Hayes, H. Y. Bennett, and S. O'Hagan, "*Rothia dentocariosa* endophthalmitis following intravitreal injection—a case report," *Journal of Ophthalmic Inflammation and Infection*, vol. 7, no. 24, 2017.

[4] S. Willner, Z. Imam, and I. Hader, "*Rothia dentocariosa* endocarditis in an unsuspecting host: a case report and literature review," *Case Reports in Cardiology*, vol. 2019, Article ID 7464251, 3 pages, 2019.

[5] D. Bratcher, "*Rothia dentocariosa*," 2012, https://www.sciencedirect.com/topics/immunology-and-microbiology/rothia-dentocariosa.

[6] K. Minato and Y. Abiko, "Beta-lactam antibiotics resistant *Rothia dentocariosa* from infected postoperative maxillary cyst: studies on R-plasmid and beta-lactamase," *General Pharmacology*, vol. 15, no. 4, pp. 287–292, 1984.

[7] R. Zbinden and S. Droz, "*Rothia dentocariosa*," 2010, http://www.antimicrobe.org/b230.asp.

[8] A. M. Morley and S. J. Tuft, "*Rothia dentocariosa* isolated from a corneal ulcer," *Cornea*, vol. 25, no. 9, pp. 1128-1129, 2006.

[9] B. Williams, M. Jafri, S. Arfeen, J. J. Reidy, S. M. Hariprasad, and A. V. Farooq, "Atypical keratitis caused by *Rothia dentocariosa*," *Ocular Immunology and Inflammation*, vol. 29, no. 1, pp. 26–28, 2021.

[10] R. Abbott, C. Halfpenny, M. Zegans, and P. Kremer, "Bacterial Corneal Ulcers," 2016, https://entokey.com/bacterial-corneal-ulcers/.

[11] K. Santin, P. Bispo, A. Hofling-Lima, and T. Laboratório de Microbiologia Ocular e Molecular, "Antimicrobial susceptibility profile of viridans group streptococci isolated from endophthalmitis," 2014, https://iovs.arvojournals.org/article.aspx?articleid=2268229.

[12] M. E. Marquart, A. H. Benton, R. C. Galloway, and L. M. Stempak, "Antibiotic susceptibility, cytotoxicity, and protease activity of viridans group streptococci causing endophthalmitis," *PLoS One*, vol. 13, no. 12, article e0209849, 2018.

[13] J. C. Pate, "Prevalence and spectrum of bacterial co-infection during fungal keratitis," *British Journal of Ophthalmology*, vol. 90, no. 3, pp. 289–292, 2006.

[14] E. Y. Tu, C. E. Joslin, L. M. Nijm, R. S. Feder, S. Jain, and M. E. Shoff, "Polymicrobial keratitis: Acanthamoeba and infectious crystalline keratopathy," *American Journal of Ophthalmology*, vol. 148, no. 1, pp. 13–19.e2, 2009.

[15] W. J. Kheir, M. C. Sniegowski, T. El-Sawy, A. Li, and B. Esmaeli, "Ophthalmic complications of targeted cancer therapy and recently recognized ophthalmic complications of traditional chemotherapy," *Survey of Ophthalmology*, vol. 59, no. 5, pp. 493–502, 2014.

[16] E. Shin, D. H. Lim, J. Han et al., "Markedly increased ocular side effect causing severe vision deterioration after chemotherapy using new or investigational epidermal or fibroblast growth factor receptor inhibitors," *BMC Ophthalmology*, vol. 20, no. 1, 2020.

[17] S. Mian and A. Sugar, "Chapter 33: conjunctival flaps for corneal disease," 2006, http://www.oculist.net/downaton502/prof/ebook/duanes/pages/v6/v6c033.html.

[18] T. D. Oostra and T. F. Mauger, "Conjunctival flaps: a case series and review of the literature," *Eye & Contact Lens*, vol. 46, no. 2, pp. 70–73, 2020.

[19] T. F. Mauger and E. Craig, "Combined acanthamoeba and Stenotrophomonas maltophilia keratitis treated with a conjunctival flap followed by penetrating keratoplasty," *Cornea*, vol. 25, no. 5, pp. 631–633, 2006.

[20] W. Y. Shi and S. X. Li, "The value of conjunctival flaps in the management of refractory corneal ulcer," *Chinese Journal of Ophthalmology*, vol. 43, no. 4, pp. 293–296, 2007.

32

Acute Posterior Multifocal Placoid Pigment Epitheliopathy Sharing Characteristic OCT Findings of Vogt-Koyanagi-Harada Disease

Yuta Kitamura,[1] Toshiyuki Oshitari ,[1,2] Masayasu Kitahashi,[1] Takayuki Baba ,[1] and Shuichi Yamamoto[1]

[1]*Department of Ophthalmology and Visual Science, Chiba University Graduate School of Medicine, Japan*
[2]*Department of Ophthalmology, International University of Health and Welfare, School of Medicine, Japan*

Correspondence should be addressed to Toshiyuki Oshitari; tarii@aol.com

Academic Editor: Maurizio Battaglia Parodi

A 17-year-old male presented with acute bilateral paracentral scotomata and blurred vision. Funduscopic examination showed bilateral macular serous retinal detachment and yellow-white placoid lesions at the level of retinal pigment epithelium. OCT study showed typical VKH disease findings with marked choroidal thickening and macular serous retinal detachment partly with subretinal septa in both eyes. FA demonstrated hypofluorescence at the placoid lesions in the early phase and hyperfluorescence in the late phase. Laboratory investigation showed negative result for HLA-DR4 serotype and the patient's cerebrospinal fluid test values were within normal range. We made the diagnosis of APMPPE from these results. At 2-month follow-up without the use of corticosteroids, OCT reexamination showed complete amelioration of subretinal fluid in both eyes. Patchy pigmentary lesions also resolved clinically with partial chorioretinal scars. The results in this case suggested OCT findings in APMPPE patients could be similar to characteristic features usually found in acute VKH disease. We recommend comprehensive assessments such as FA, cerebral spinal fluid analysis, and HLA typing which help in leading proper diagnosis.

1. Introduction

Acute posterior multifocal placoid pigment epitheliopathy (APMPPE) is a rare inflammatory eye disease typically affecting healthy young adults [1]. Patients typically present with bilateral rapid loss of central vision associated paracentral scotomata. Photopsias may occur prior to vision loss. Central nervous systems disorders such as headache and cerebrovascular vasculitis may be also observed [2]. Approximately 33% of APMPPE patients report flu-like symptoms prior to the onset of the disease [3]. The funduscopic examination typically shows bilateral multiple round, placoid, and gray-white lesions at the level of the retinal pigment epithelium (RPE) with distinctive findings of fluorescein angiography (FA) [1]. Visual outcome is normally good, with more than 80% of APMPPE patients without foveal involvement resolving visual acuity of 20/25 or better, but some patients experienced incomplete restoration of visual function [3]. Therefore, whether treatment should be done or not for the patients with APMPPE is still controversial issue. Although the pathogenesis of APMPPE is still under debate, it is currently thought to be secondary to an obstructive vasculitis, resulting in hypoperfusion of terminal choroidal lobules in the posterior pole with secondary impairment of RPE and retinal outer layer. To our knowledge, three studies have recently reported that APMPPE may share characteristic features with the acute phase of VKH disease, making it difficult to make the diagnosis of two diseases [4–6]. In this paper, we report a case of 17-year-old patient with APMPPE closely resembling OCT findings of acute VKH disease. Because there are still few cases reporting similar contents, we review the latest ocular imaging findings of two diseases and take some key points for proper diagnosis.

2. Case Report

A 17-year-old male high school student was referred to Chiba University Hospital because of rapid bilateral paracentral

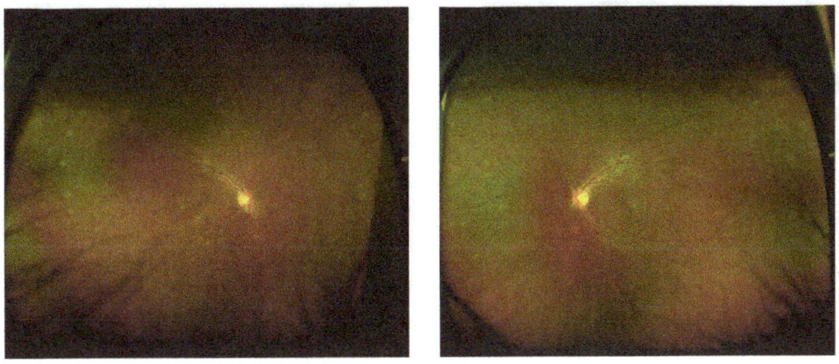

(a) (b)

FIGURE 1: Color fundus photographs with the 200Tx ultra-wide-field retinal imaging system (Optos) at the initial examination demonstrating multiple placoid subretinal lesions scattered from the posterior pole to the peripheral retina bilaterally. Foveal subretinal fluids are present in both eyes. (a) The right eye. (b) The left eye.

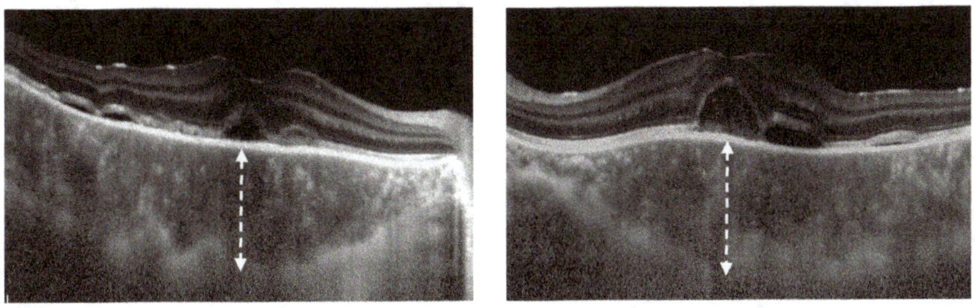

(a) (b)

FIGURE 2: Horizontal enhanced depth optical coherence tomographic (EDI-OCT) images at the initial examination showing marked choroidal thickening and subfoveal detachment with subretinal septa in both eyes. (a) The right eye. (b) The left eye. The choroidal thickness at the subfovea was 578 μm in the right eye and 642 μm in the left eye.

scotomata and blurred vision on awaking. He complained from a viral prodrome such as headache and nasal discharge 1 week before the onset of visual disturbance, although there were no symptoms of hearing loss or tinnitus. Medical history and family history were unremarkable. He took no medication. On examination, best-corrected visual acuity was 20/16 in both eyes. Intraocular pressure was normal. There were no light reflex disorders in both eyes. The ocular movements were normal. Slit-lamp examination showed 1+ anterior chamber cells in both eyes. Funduscopic examination showed bilateral macular serous retinal detachment, and the one-fourth to one-second disc diameter, placoid, multiple round, and yellow white lesions at the level of RPE from posterior pole to far peripheral retina (Figure 1). The placoid lesions were more obvious in the peripheral retina rather than posterior pole. The retinal vessels and optic disc were normal. Spectral domain OCT (SD-OCT) showed marked choroidal thickening and macular serous retinal detachment partly with subretinal septa in both eyes, which are known as characteristic OCT findings in VKH disease (Figure 2). FA of the both eyes revealed that the placoid lesions were hypofluorescence during early-phase FA images and subsequent progressive hyperfluorescence on late-phase FA images (Figure 3). Fundus autofluorescence (FAF) revealed the lesions were observed as increased fluorescence corresponding to the placoid lesions. Indocyanine green angiography (ICGA) revealed that the lesions were hypocyanescent in the early and late phases of the ICGA (Figure 4(a)). Visual fields analysis using by the Humphrey field analyzer 30-2 test showed bilateral paracentral scotomata. Laboratory investigation showed the absence of the HLA-DR4 serotype. Cerebrospinal fluid (CSF) examination was also normal. The laboratory screening was negative results for any known infectious or autoimmune cause. We made the diagnosis of APMPPE on the basis of these data. Because of good vision and absence of systemic neurological abnormalities, we did not administer oral prednisone. Instead, the patient was instructed to take Ibuprofen orally. At 1-month follow-up, OCT showed bilateral decrease of subretinal fluid. At 2 months' follow-up, OCT showed complete resolution of subretinal fluid and decrease of choroidal thickness in both eyes (Figure 5). Four months after the initial presentation, Patchy pigmentary lesions resolved clinically partly with chorioretinal scars and hypofluorescence lesions on ICGA images showed improvement in clinical findings (Figure 4(b)). There has been no recurrence until now.

3. Discussion

This case highlights the importance of detecting characteristic FA findings, absence of HLA-DR4, and absence of CSF lymphocytic pleocytosis to differentiate between APMPPE

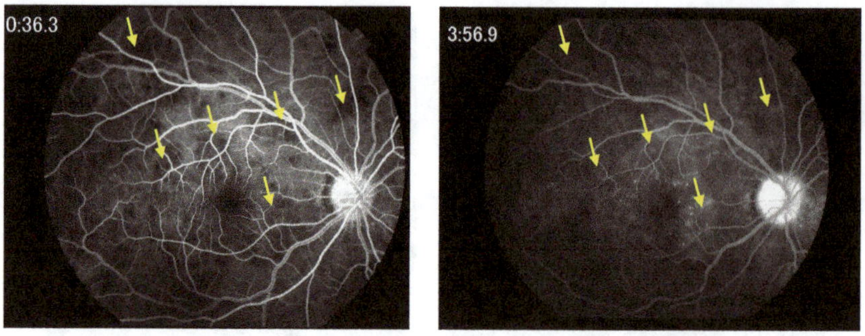

(a) (b)

Figure 3: Fluorescein angiography of the right eye at presentation. (a) Early-phase fluorescein angiogram shows areas of hypofluorescence corresponding to the placoid lesions. (b) Late-phase fluorescein angiogram shows the conversion of hypofluorescence to hyperfluorescence (arrows).

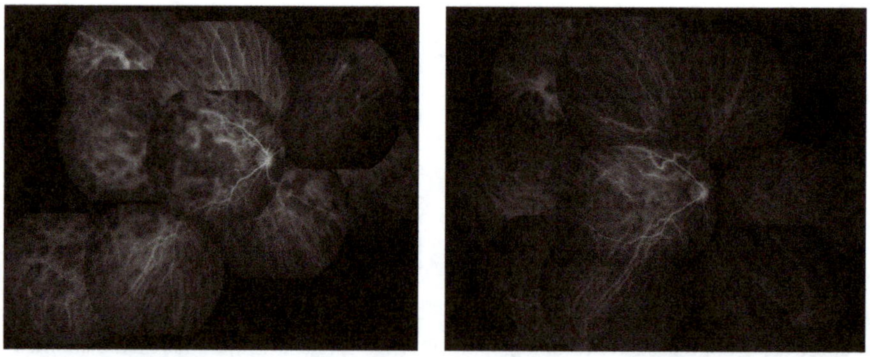

(a) (b)

Figure 4: Indocyanine green angiography (ICGA) of the right eye. (a) At presentation showing loss of choroidal circulation with lesions remaining hypofluorescent in the early and late phases and even into the very late phase. (b) At 4 months after the initial examination. ICGA shows an almost complete resolution of the choroidal hypofluorescence.

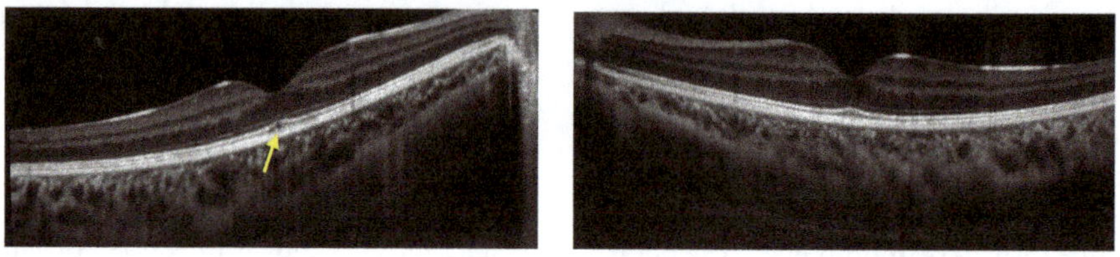

(a) (b)

Figure 5: Horizontal EDI-OCT images of the right (a) and left (b) eyes at 2 months after the initial presentation. Subretinal fluid disappeared completely and choroidal thickness recovered within normal range in both eyes. The external limiting membrane and ellipsoid zone (inner/outer segment junction) and retinal pigment epithelium are clearly recognized bilaterally, but there are unclear parts in the interdigitation zone (arrow). The choroidal thickness at the subfovea was 300 μm in the right eye and 275 μm in the left eye.

and VKH disease because, in some cases, APMPPE disease patients share some common clinical manifestations such as preceding viral prodrome, morphological changes on OCT such as subretinal fluid with multilobular spaces, marked choroidal thickening, and ICGA imaging study.

APMPPE is basically diagnosed with the characteristic fundus finding of multiple placoid yellow-white creamy deep retinal lesions, the typical pattern of early hypofluorescence and late hyperfluorescence corresponding to the placoid lesions on the FA images, and prolonged hypocyanescence on the ICGA imaging study [7]. Typical OCT findings observed in the APMPPE patients are slight irregularities in the inner segment ellipsoid layer and RPE, at early phase, subsequently evolving increased reflectance of the outer retinal layers and RPE with normal retinal thickness, and at later phase the thinning of the outer retina layer gradually occurs. Subretinal fluid may be observed in the APMPPE patients associated with large placoid lesions. [7]

Whereas the diagnosis of acute VKH disease is mainly based on typical fundus findings and OCT images, patient's history of preceding syndrome such as flu-like symptoms, headache, dysacusia, and tinnitus, lumbar puncture, and HLA typing are also useful diagnostic tests. CSF evaluation reveals lymphocytic pleocytosis in more than 80% of the VKH patients. HLA-DR4 is known to have strong association among Japanese patients with VKH syndrome. In acute phase of VKH disease, characteristic enhanced depth imaging OCT (EDI-OCT) features include multilobular serous retinal fluid, marked choroidal thickening, and choroidal folds (CFs) without pigment epithelial detachment [8]. The exact nature of serous detachment and septa was studied by Kishi et al. [9, 10], and they suggested the walls of cystoid spaces are made of inflammatory products, such as fibrin, and are located in the subretinal space. In acute phase of the disease, FA typically reveals a large number of spotted hyperfluorescent foci at the level of RPE in the early stage, followed by patchy pooling of dye in the subretinal space. ICGA study discloses an early choroidal stromal vessel hyperfluorescence and leakage, disc hyperfluorescence, multiple hypofluorescent dark, and fuzzy or lost pattern of large stromal vessel [11]. Among these imaging studies, OCT findings of characteristic exudate pooling with septa and marked choroidal thickening have been considered to highly valuable diagnostic findings associated with acute VKH disease.

In this case, the manifestations that teenage patient, with preceding flu-like symptoms, had acute onset of creamy multiple placoid deep retinal lesions, classic FA findings of "block early, stain late" angiographic pattern corresponding to the placoid lesions, persistent patchy hypocyanescence on the ICGA study, and negative findings of CSF lymphocytic pleocytosis and HLA-DR4 clearly suggest diagnosis of APMPPE. However, the most distinguishing feature in this case is that the patient demonstrated marked choroidal thickening and macular serous retinal detachment with subretinal septa on OCT imaging, not typical features in APMPPE but quite similar to characteristic features in acute VKH disease. According to a classification of the OCT findings observed in the APMPPE patients suggested by Goldenberg et al. [12], subretinal fluid have been reported at the very acute phase of the disease, but the nature of subretinal fluid and the frequency of septa formation are still controversial. In contrast with typical findings seen in VKH patients, choroidal thickening is not a typical OCT finding in patients with APMPPE. However, Lee et al. firstly reported this finding in the literature [6], and, more recently, two studies reported thickening imaging with EDI-OCT has been observed in APMPPE patients [13, 14].

Since the initial description by Gass in 1968, APMPPE was presumed to involve primarily RPE [1], whereas several researchers suggested that the underlying process in APMPPE is a focal inflammatory vasculitis affecting the choroidal vessels and that the RPE changes were a subsequent manifestation [15–17]. Recently, by using laser speckle flowgraphy (LSFG), Hirotaka et al. showed that the choroidal blood flow velocity decreased at the acute stage of APMPPE and subsequently increased with regression of the disease [13]. Moreover, with the advent of OCT-angiography (OCT-A), many researchers have noted choriocapillaris hypoperfusion, preceding the development of and corresponding anatomically to placoid lesions in the RPE [18, 19]. Bruke et al. proposed four characteristic sequential phases of APMPPE lesions by using multimodal imaging study including ten eyes of five APMPPE patients [7]. They concluded that choriocapillaris hypoperfusion is the primary event in the pathogenesis of APMPPE. These circulatory changes and choroidal thickening on EDI-OCT provided further evidence that inflammatory etiology was involved in the pathogenesis of choroidal circulatory disturbance in APMPPE [20]. From these viewpoints, anti-inflammatory agents such as systemic corticosteroid, intravitreal injection of triamcinolone acetonide have been used to treat APMPPE patients. In our case, subretinal fluid and choroidal thickening resolved spontaneously without taking oral corticosteroids, suggesting that there might be an unknown self-limit inflammatory process in the choroid.

Consistent with past reports, our patient showed the RPE line maintained almost flat on SD-OCT at the acute stage of disease although marked choroidal thickening was observed. In contrast, in 52-71% of VKH patients, choroidal folds (CFs), which are wave-like appearance in the RPE, Bruch's membrane and inner choroid, have been found on SD-OCT [21–23]. The recent study indicated that detection of both CFs and choroidal thickening is an effective method for diagnosing acute VKH disease [24]. However, another recent report has shown that the folds of RPE occurred less frequently in younger patients with VKH patients [25]. Therefore, in young patients, the lack of CFs on SD-OCT cannot clearly differentiate APMPPE from VKH. The reason why older patients with VKH disease developed CFs more frequently is still unknown.

As shown in this case, the choroidal hypofluorescence of ICGA image in eyes with APMPPE has been reported to result from a profound decrease in choroidal blood flow secondary to choroidal occlusive vasculitis [26, 27]. In VKH disease, one of the ICGA signs is known as multiple hypofluorescent spots, which are thought to correspond to foci of lymphocytic infiltration within the choroid. The hypofluorescent lesions detected by ICGA may persist even after the fundoscopic examination and FA are unremarkable [28, 29]. These reports indicate that ICGA findings of VKH disease may be similar to those of APMPPE because both show multiple hypofluorescent lesions.

In summary, we have reported some key points of distinguishing APMPPE from VKH.

In some cases, APMPPE and VKH disease may share some common clinical manifestations such as preceding viral prodrome and several imaging findings, which are morphological changes on OCT such as subretinal fluid, choroidal thickening, flat line of RPE (especially younger patients), and ICGA imaging study. Therefore, it is important for ophthalmologist to detect characteristic FA findings and HLA typing and investigate CSF evaluation to differentiate these two diseases.

Consent

Informed consent was obtained from the patient to use his medical records.

Acknowledgments

The authors thank Professor Emeritus Duco Hamasaki of the Bascom Palmer Eye Institute of the University of Miami, FL, for editing the manuscript. The case study is supported by a Grant-in-Aid from the Ministry of Education, Science, Sports and Culture of the Japanese Government.

References

[1] J. D. Gass, "Acute posterior multifocal placoid pigment epitheliopathy," *Archives of Ophthalmolgy*, vol. 80, no. 2, pp. 177–185, 1968.

[2] H. S. O'Halloran, J. R. Berger, W. B. Lee et al., "Acute multifocal placoid pigment epitheliopathy and central nervous system involvement: nine new cases and a review of the literature," *Ophthalmology*, vol. 108, no. 5, pp. 861–868, 2001.

[3] T. Fiore, B. Iaccheri, S. Androudi et al., "Acute posterior multifocal placoid pigment epitheliopathy: outcome and visual prognosis," *Retina*, vol. 29, no. 7, pp. 994–1001, 2009.

[4] B. Li, R. J. Bentham, and J. R. Gonder, "A case of unilateral and spontaneously resolving posterior uveitis with overlapping features of vogt–koyanagi–harada disease and acute posterior multifocal placoid pigment epitheliopathy," *Springer Plus*, vol. 5, no. 1, p. 1471, 2016.

[5] M. Tanigawa, Y. Tsukahara, and H. Yamanaka, "A case of acute posterior multifocal placoid pigment epitheliopathy demonstrating vogt-koyanagi-harada disease-like optical coherence tomography findings in the acute stage," *Case Reports in Ophthalmology*, vol. 4, no. 3, pp. 172–179, 2013.

[6] G. E. Lee, B. W. Lee, N. A. Rao, and A. A. Fawzi, "Spectral domain optical coherence tomography and autofluorescence in a case of acute posterior multifocal placoid pigment epitheliopathy mimicking vogt-koyanagi-harada disease: case report and review of literature," *Ocular Immunology and Inflammation*, vol. 19, no. 1, pp. 42–47, 2011.

[7] T. R. Burke, C. J. Chu, S. Salvatore et al., "Application of OCT-angiography to characterise the evolution of chorioretinal lesions in acute posterior multifocal placoid pigment epitheliopathy," *Eye*, vol. 31, no. 10, pp. 1399–1408, 2017.

[8] S. Silpa-archa, N. Silpa-archa, J. M. Preble, and C. S. Foster, "Vogt–koyanagi–harada syndrome: perspectives for immunogenetics, multimodal imaging, and therapeutic options," *Autoimmunity Reviews*, vol. 15, no. 8, pp. 809–819, 2016.

[9] Y. Maruyama and S. Kishi, "Tomographic features of serous retinal detachment in vogt-koyanagi-harada syndrome," *Ophthalmic Surgery, Lasers and Imaging Retina*, vol. 35, no. 3, pp. 239–242, 2004.

[10] Y. Yamaguchi, T. Otani, and S. Kishi, "Tomographic features of serous retinal detachment with multilobular dye pooling in acute Vogt-Koyanagi-Harada disease," *American Journal of Ophthalmology*, vol. 144, no. 2, pp. 260–265, 2007.

[11] M. Miyanaga, T. Kawaguchi, K. Miyata, S. Horie, M. Mochizuki, and C. P. Herbort, "Indocyanine green angiography findings in initial acute pretreatment Vogt-Koyanagi-Harada disease in Japanese patients," *Japanese Journal of Ophthalmology*, vol. 54, no. 5, pp. 377–382, 2010.

[12] D. Goldenberg, Z. Habot-Wilner, A. Loewenstein, and M. Goldstein, "Spectral domain optical coherence tomography classification of acute posterior multifocal placoid pigment epitheliopathy," *Retina*, vol. 32, no. 7, pp. 1403–1410, 2012.

[13] K. Hirooka, W. Saito, M. Saito et al., "Increased choroidal blood flow velocity with regression of acute posterior multifocal placoid pigment epitheliopathy," *Japanese Journal of Ophthalmology*, vol. 60, no. 3, pp. 172–178, 2016.

[14] S. Mrejen, D. Sarraf, S. Chexal, K. Wald, and K. B. Freund, "Choroidal involvement in acute posterior multifocal placoid pigment epitheliopathy," *Ophthalmic Surgery, Lasers and Imaging Retina*, vol. 47, no. 1, pp. 20–26, 2016.

[15] A. F. Deutman, J. A. Oosterhuis, T. N. Boen-Tan, and A. L. Aan de Kerk, "Acute posterior multifocal placoid pigment epitheliopathy. pigment epitheliopathy of choriocapillaritis?" *British Journal of Ophthalmology*, vol. 56, no. 12, pp. 863–874, 1972.

[16] A. F. Deutman and F. Lion, "Choriocapillaris nonperfusion in acute multifocal placoid pigment epitheliopathy," *American Journal of Ophthalmology*, vol. 84, no. 5, pp. 652–657, 1977.

[17] R. F. Spaide, L. A. Yannuzzi, and J. Slakter, "Choroidal vasculitis in acute posterior multifocal placoid pigment epitheliopathy," *British Journal of Ophthalmology*, vol. 75, no. 11, pp. 685–687, 1991.

[18] S. S. Park, S. Thinda, D. Y. Kim, R. J. Zawadzki, and J. S. Werner, "Phase-variance optical coherence tomographic angiography imaging of choroidal perfusion changes associated with acute posterior multifocal placoid pigment epitheliopathy," *JAMA Ophthalmology*, vol. 134, no. 8, pp. 943–945, 2016.

[19] M. J. Heiferman, S. Rahmani, L. M. Jampol et al., "Acute posterior multifocal placoid pigment epitheliopathy on optical coherence tomography angiography," *Retina*, vol. 37, no. 11, pp. 2084–2094, 2017.

[20] E. Maggio, A. Alfano, A. Polito, and G. Pertile, "Choroidal perfusion abnormalities associated with acute posterior multifocal placoid pigment epitheliopathy: a case report," *BMC Ophthalmology*, vol. 18, no. 1, p. 87, 2018.

[21] W. Wu, F. Wen, S. Huang, G. Luo, and D. Wu, "Choroidal folds in vogt-koyanagi-harada disease," *American Journal of Ophthalmology*, vol. 143, no. 5, pp. 900-901, 2007.

[22] V. Gupta, A. Gupta, P. Gupta, and A. Sharma, "Spectral-domain cirrus optical coherence tomography of choroidal striations seen in the acute stage of vogt-koyanagi-harada disease," *American Journal of Ophthalmology*, vol. 147, no. 1, pp. 148-153.e2, 2009.

[23] D. Lin, W. Chen, G. Zhang et al., "Comparison of the optical coherence tomographic characters between acute vogt-koyanagi-harada disease and acute central serous chorioretinopathy," *BMC Ophthalmology*, vol. 14, no. 1, p. 87, 2014.

[24] Y. Kato, Y. Yamamoto, H. Tabuchi, and A. Fukushima, "Retinal pigment epithelium folds as a diagnostic finding of Vogt-Koyanagi-Harada disease," *Japanese Journal of Ophthalmology*, vol. 57, no. 1, pp. 90–94, 2013.

[25] K. Tsuboi, K. Nakai, C. Iwahashi, F. Gomi, Y. Ikuno, and K. Nishida, "Analysis of choroidal folds in acute Vogt–Koyanagi–Harada disease using high-penetration optical coherence tomography," *Graefe's Archive for Clinical and Experimental Ophthalmology*, vol. 253, no. 6, pp. 959–964, 2015.

[26] C. T. Hsu, J. B. Harlan, M. F. Goldberg, and J. P. Dunn, "Acute posterior multifocal placoid pigment epitheliopathy associated with a systemic necrotizing vasculitis," *Retina*, vol. 23, no. 1, pp. 64–68, 2003.

[27] D. Park, H. Schatz, H. R. McDonald, and R. N. Johnson, "Indocyanine green angiography of acute mult-if-ocal posterior placoid pigment epitheliopathy," *Ophthalmology*, vol. 102, no. 12, pp. 1877–1883, 1995.

[28] Y. Oshima, S. Harino, Y. Hara, and Y. Tano, "Indocyanine green angiographic findings in Vogt-Koyanagi-Harada disease," *American Journal of Ophthalmology*, vol. 122, no. 1, pp. 58–66, 1996.

[29] N. Bouchenaki and C. P. Herbort, "The contribution of indocyanine green angiography to the appraisal and management of Vogt-Koyanagi-Harada disease," *Ophthalmology*, vol. 108, no. 1, pp. 54–64, 2001.

33

Sinoorbital Mucormycosis Associated with Corticosteroid Therapy in COVID-19 Infection

Zeinab Mehrabi,[1] Maryam Salimi,[2] Kianoush Niknam,[2] Farzaneh Mohammadi,[3] Hesan Jelodari Mamaghani,[4] Mohammad Reza Sasani,[5] Mohammad Javad Ashraf,[6] Amirhossein Salimi,[7] Mohammad Hassan Zahedroozegar,[8] and Zohreh Erfani[4]

[1]*Department of Internal Medicine, Namazi Hospital, Shiraz University of Medical Sciences, Shiraz, Iran*
[2]*Student Research Committee, Shiraz University of Medical Sciences, Shiraz, Iran*
[3]*Department of Surgery, Eastern Health, Victoria, Australia*
[4]*Students' Scientific Research Center (SSRC), Tehran University of Medical Sciences, Tehran, Iran*
[5]*Department of Radiology, Medical Imaging Research Center, Shiraz University of Medical Sciences, Shiraz, Iran*
[6]*Department of Pathology, Shiraz University of Medical Sciences, Shiraz, Iran*
[7]*Student Research Committee, Shahid Sadoughi University of Medical Sciences, Yazd, Iran*
[8]*Health Policy Research Center, Institute of Health, Shiraz University of Medical Sciences, Shiraz, Iran*

Correspondence should be addressed to Maryam Salimi; salimimaryam7496@gmail.com

Academic Editor: Huban Atilla

Background. Mucormycosis is a rare and invasive fungal infection, affecting almost exclusively immunocompromised individuals. Immunosuppressive effects of corticosteroids which are widely prescribed in COVID-19 patients might be a predisposing factor for opportunistic infections even though the other factors should also be considered. *Case Presentation.* A middle-aged man without any significant past medical history was admitted to the hospital due to a severe COVID-19 infection. He received a high dose of corticosteroids as a part of the treatment. Five days after discharge, he presents with a headache and fever. Eventually, orbital mucormycosis was diagnosed for him and he was treated with antifungal medications. *Conclusion.* Opportunistic infections should be considered during the current pandemic of COVID-19, during which corticosteroids are widely prescribed.

1. Background

Mucormycosis is a rare, potentially fatal infection caused by fungi from the order Mucorales. [1, 2]. It has various clinical presentations and predominantly affects immunocompromised patients, especially those with diabetes, renal failure, hematological malignancies, and transplant recipients [3, 4]. Because of the high mortality and morbidity rate, prompt diagnosis and intervention are essential [5]. In this case report, we present a male patient with no underlying disease who presented with orbital mucormycosis following hospitalization due to coronavirus disease 2019 (COVID-19) infection. We also aimed to find out the possible association between mucormycosis, COVID-19 infection, and/or medication used to treat them.

2. Case Presentation

A 51-year-old man without past medical or social history presented with fever and cough, followed by dyspnea. He was referred to the Khalije Fars Hospital, Busher, and admitted there with the impression of COVID-19 in July 2020. The patient's temperature was 39.4°C, and his pulse was 84/minute. Bilateral fine crackles were auscultated on both lungs. Chest computerized tomography (CT) revealed a patchy ground-glass appearance in both lungs, in favor of

COVID-19 (Figure 1). The real-time reverse transcription-polymerase chain reaction (RT-PCR) test was positive for COVID-19.

Laboratory evaluation revealed leukopenia with white blood cell counts (WBC) of 2700 per/μL and lymphocyte count of 864/μL. Additionally, mild thrombocytopenia (platelet: 128000 per/μL) and elevated qualitative C-reactive protein (+3) were detected.

Based on a definite diagnosis of COVID-19, he received dexamethasone 4 mg intravenous (IV) per day along with ceftriaxone 1 gram IV for the prevention of bacterial superinfection. After 5 days of treatment (20 mg dexamethasone totally), the patient (Pt) was discharged with stable vital signs, without leukopenia (WBC: 7200/μL) or any other complications. Prednisolone 25 mg, daily, was prescribed for him.

Seven days after the hospital discharge (20 mg dexamethasone and 175 mg prednisolone so far), the patient presented with severe headache, but without any significant findings in his physical exam. The brain magnetic resonance imaging (MRI) was in favor of sinusitis (Figure 2). Hence, oral amoxicillin-clavulanate 625 milligram (mg) every 8 hours (Q8h) was prescribed.

However, his condition did not improve, and he developed right (Rt) side preorbital edema (Figure 3) and redness that eventually spread to the left (Lt) side, so he was referred to an ophthalmologist for better evaluation.

In his physical examination, tenderness over the sinuses and bilateral preorbital edema were found. The paranasal sinus (PNS) CT scan showed osteomeatal obliteration associated with opacification of bilateral maxillary, ethmoid, frontal, and the Rt sphenoid sinus, suggestive of sinusitis (Figure 4). At this stage, the consumption of oral prednisolone was stopped (in total, 20 mg dexamethasone, and 300 mg prednisolone).

Levofloxacin was prescribed for him with the dosage of 750 mg orally, daily along with artificial tear 1 drop every 4 hours and ciprofloxacin eye drops 1 drop every 8 hours, but his condition worsened; therefore, the patient was referred to an otolaryngologist. The otolaryngologist found a palate lesion in the patient's mouth and took a biopsy from the palate lesion with suspicion of mucormycosis, but no evidence of mucormycosis was found in his pathology. After 5 days, the patient was transferred to Khalili hospital, Shiraz, which is the referral center of otolaryngology and ophthalmology, for anterior orbitotomy due to abscess development. Because of the dangerous condition of the Rt side-eye and the possible disruption of the orbital bones and spread of the infection to the Rt eye, the Lt eye underwent anterior orbitotomy and a cloudy liquid discharge with necrosis and oily component that extended to the orbital wall bone was seen in surgery. The patient was discharged with levofloxacin (750 mg, orally, daily) for sinusitis and prednisolone with a daily dose of 50 mg orally due to suspicion of autoimmune disease.

Three days after his discharge, the patient's condition did not improve, but also, he presented with reduced visual acuity of the Rt eye from 10/10 to 8/10; therefore, the patient has admitted again to Khalili hospital, and in a joint assessment by the ophthalmology and otolaryngology experts, a

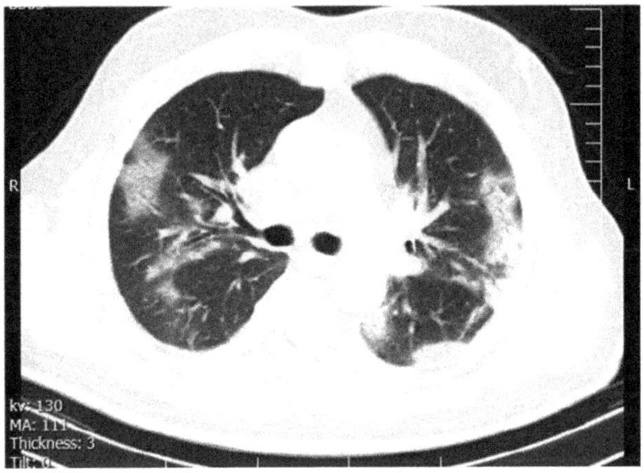

Figure 1: Axial chest CT image without contrast administration showed areas of ground-glass opacities and bilateral consolidations with the predominantly peripheral location.

functional endoscopic sinus surgery (Fess) along with another anterior orbitotomy was performed for the patient. During Fess, necrosis and pussy discharge were found in the paranasal sinuses, and samples from the orbital tissue, nasal cavity, and sinuses were obtained for pathological evaluation and sent to the laboratory of Khalili hospital, affiliated by Shiraz University of Medical Sciences.

Pathology evaluation of the paranasal sinus tissue showed heavy infiltration of acute and chronic inflammatory cells with an area of necrosis and hypha of the mucor fungus surrounded by polymorphonuclear leukocytes, which were in favor of mucormycosis (Figure 5).

The patient was evaluated for human immunodeficiency virus which was negative. Subsequently, antifungal therapy with Amphotericin B lipid complex (200 mg, IV, daily) was started for the patient. The patient was also transferred to Namazi hospital, a referral center affiliated with Shiraz University of Medical Sciences for continuing his antifungal therapy; this hospital has infectious disease specialists.

In Nemazi hospital, visual acuity was reduced to 1/10 and 4/10 in the Rt and Lt eye, respectively. The new PNS CT scan showed progression of the infection (Figure 6).

Therefore, his antifungal treatment regimen was adjusted to Caspofungin (80 mg, IV, daily) and Amphotericin B lipid complex (350 mg, IV, daily) which continued for about one month. Also, for reducing the chance of bacterial superimpose infection, piperacillin-tazobactam (4.5 gr, IV, Q12h) and teicoplanin (400 mg, IV, QD) were administered. During his treatment course, the patient developed hypokalemia, and increased blood urea nitrogen (BUN) and creatinine levels; therefore, Amphotericin dosage was adjusted to 200 mg, IV per day. Also, sixteen days after hospital admission, another Fess with Amphotericin irrigation was done for the patient. He was discharged after 59 days of hospitalization in Nemazi and Khalili hospitals after taking 15700 mg Amphotericin B lipid complex for 56 days, 2400 mg Caspofungin for 30 days, leading to favorable healing. At the time of discharge, the patient had better visual acuity in both eyes (6/10 in the Rt eye and 8/10 in the Lt eye), no orbital or preorbital edema, and tenderness.

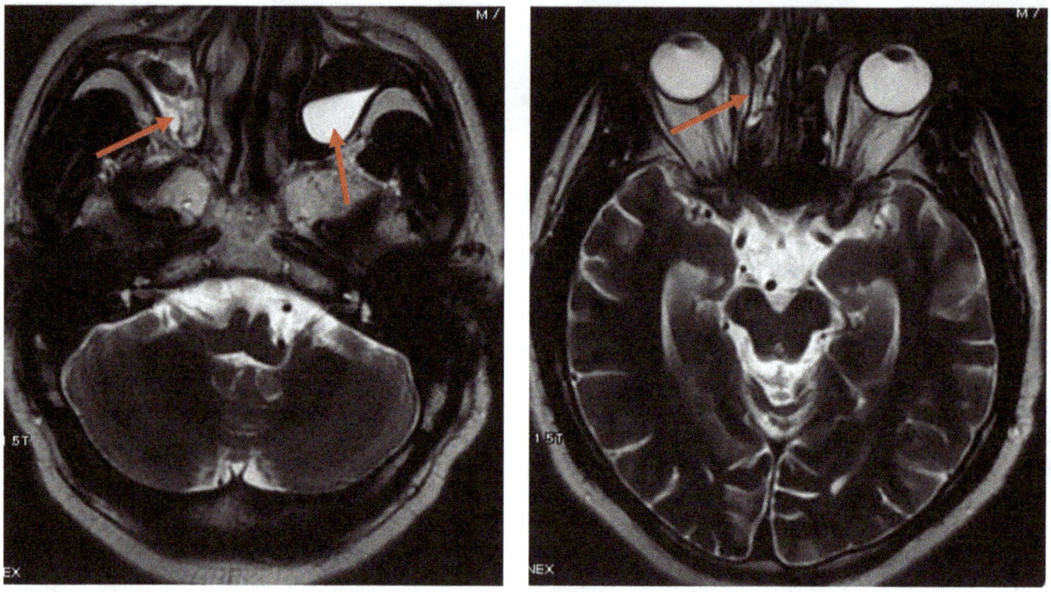

(a) (b)

Figure 2: Axial T2-weighted images without contrast administration show (a) mucosal thickening and secretion in the right maxillary sinus and a retention cyst in the left maxillary sinus and (b) mucosal thickening and secretion in the right ethmoid sinus with a lesser degree in the left ethmoid sinus.

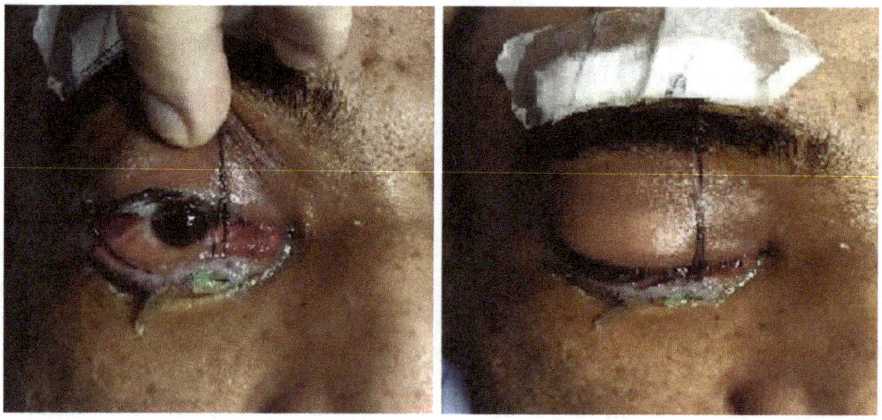

Figure 3: Rt side preorbital edema and redness.

3. Discussion

COVID-19 was recognized as a pandemic by the World Health Organization (WHO) on March 11, 2020. In the current context, with respect to the increase in the number of infected patients with COIVID-19 as well as the emergence of new species, corticosteroids have been prescribed widely for not only in critically ill patients but also some of the mild to moderate ones regardless of the potential rare adverse complications. In this case report, we described a sinoorbital mucormycosis in an immunocompetent middle age man that was previously treated with high doses of corticosteroid for the prevention of lung fibrosis following COVID-19 infection. In spite of the difficulties of diagnosing the disease, it was successfully managed with medical and surgical interventions.

Corticosteroids have a strong anti-inflammatory effect and are considered to have a role in treating immunologic complications of COVID-19 infection like cytokine storm, lung inflammation, fever, and abnormal laboratory indices of inflammation [5–7]. Observational studies showed that corticosteroid treatment was linked with higher mortality rates and nosocomial infections for influenza and delayed virus clearance for SARS-CoV and MERS-CoV; however, there is limited data regarding SARS-CoV-2 [8]. Also, corticosteroids have been associated with an increased risk of superinfection including bacterial, mycobacterial, and fungal infections [9–12]. Furthermore, several studies have particularly warned about the foregoing adverse effects of corticosteroids in patients with the comorbid disease, but there is little evidence of serious infectious complications in

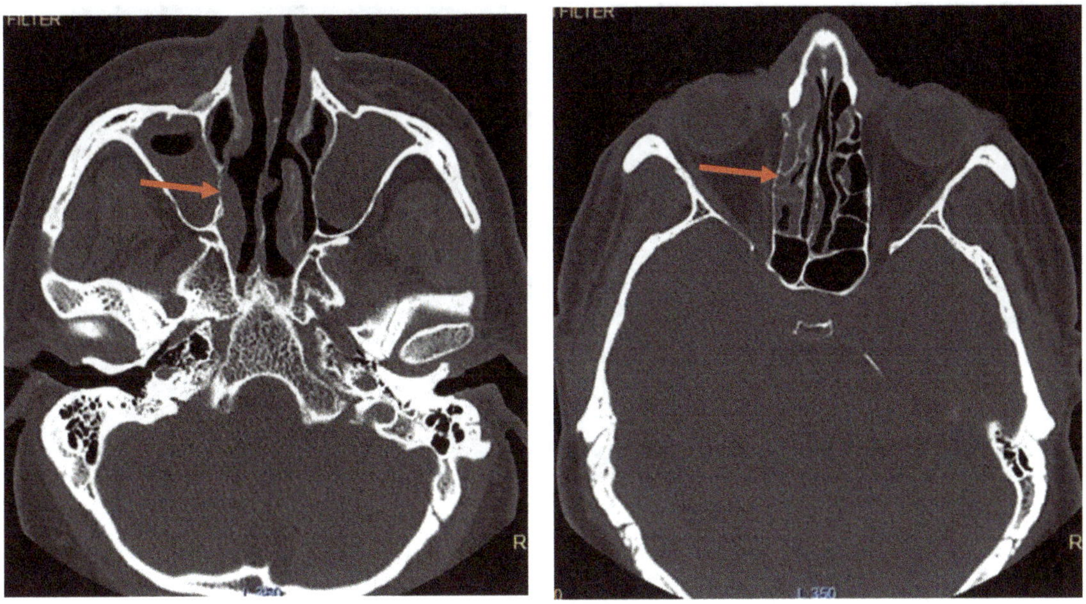

(a) (b)

Figure 4: Axial paranasal CT images without contrast administration showing (a) mucosal thickening and secretion in the right maxillary sinus and a retention cyst in the Lt maxillary sinus and (b) mucosal thickening and secretion in the right ethmoid sinus with a lesser degree in the Lt ethmoid sinus.

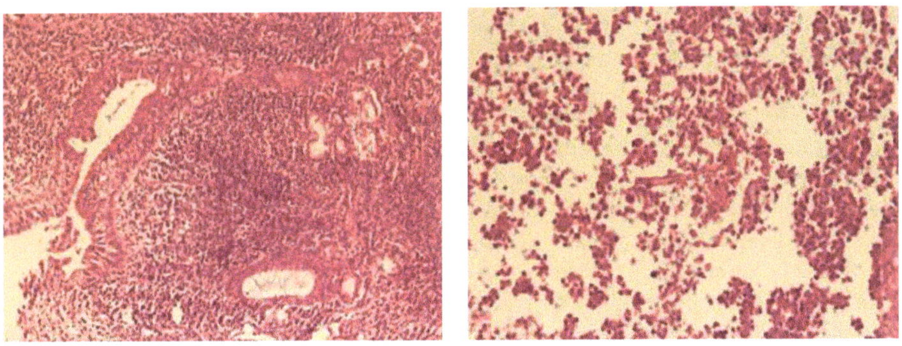

(a) (b)

Figure 5: (a) Paranasal sinus mucosa with heavy infiltration of acute and chronic inflammatory cells, H&E stain (×100). (b) Paranasal sinus mucosa with the area of necrosis and hypha which are in favor of the zygomycetes group of fungi, surrounded by polymorphonuclear leukocytes, H&E stain (×200).

immunocompetent patients without any comorbidities [13–15]. The aforementioned information did not mean to attribute this fungal infection to corticosteroid consumption accurately and purely or did not request corticosteroid elimination. It seeks to warn of the adverse and potentially fatal effects of steroids that may be overlooked because of their many benefits and also to give physicians a comprehensive overview of prescribing the drug.

Mucormycosis is a life-threatening fungal infection that primarily affects patients with immunosuppression [16]. In a study of 101 cases of mucormycosis reported by Lanternier et al., the median number of underlying medical conditions was 2 per patient [17]. Diabetes, hematological malignancies, transplantation, HIV infection, and systemic lupus erythematosus are examples of recognized conditions associated with mucormycosis [16, 18]. The fact that our patient lacked usual comorbidities was associated with a delayed diagnosis of the disease.

As indicated previously, treatment with corticosteroid causes immunosuppression in patients with COVID-19 infection; thus, mucormycosis should be considered as a potential infection affecting them. However, the role of SARS-CoV-2 infection on the cells of the innate immunity (macrophage and neutrophils) should be considered. Our review of the literature indicates that there have been reports of many cases of secondary cases of mucormycosis which is called COVID-19-Associated Mucormycosis (CAM). Those cases have orbital, rhinoorbital, gastrointestinal, and pulmonary involvement [12, 19–22]. In a

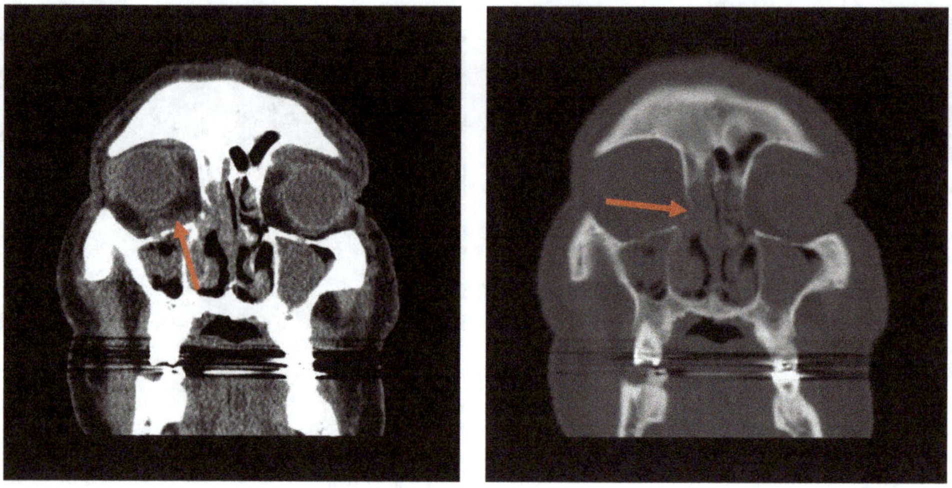

(a) (b)

Figure 6: Coronal paranasal CT images without contrast administration. Soft tissue window images: (a) area of increased density in the inferior aspect of right orbit suggestive of orbital inflammation. Mucosal thickening in the right maxillary sinus and a retention cyst in the Lt maxillary sinus was also demonstrated. Bone window image: (b) thinning in the medial aspect of the inferior orbital wall at the right side, suggestive of a small bony erosion (compared to the Lt one).

recent review, a significant percentage of patients with mucormycosis also had a bacterial or fungal coinfection [12]. In a study by Muthu et al., 2,568 cases of CAM are reported which most of them were also affected by diabetes mellitus [23]. Rudramurthy et al. also claimed that uncontrolled diabetes mellitus and inappropriate (high dose or not indicated) corticosteroid use are the major predisposing factors for this surge. Furthermore, a hyperglycaemic state leads to hyperferritinaemia and increased expression of the glucose-regulated protein (GRP-78) in endothelial cells that may help the entry of Mucorales into tissues [24]. The systematic review of literature reveals that there is a significant increase in mucormycosis due to COVID-19, in specific parts of the world, such as India. The reasons for this unprecedented increase remain unknown [25].

The patient was a healthy man that had received high doses of corticosteroids and broad-spectrum antibiotics due to COVID-19. The sign of orbital infection emerged 12 days after the first dose of corticosteroids. Given the lack of any underlying and previous disease or any proven coinfection (e.g., positive urine or blood culture) that usually leads to opportunistic fungal infections such as mucormycotic, we attributed the current infection to the condition called CAM as well as high dose and long duration of corticosteroid administration and its effects on systemic immunosuppression. However, the role of other factors such as iron and zinc metabolism, immunomodulatory effects of COVID-19, endothelial dysfunction which is met in COVID-19 infection, and overexpression of GRP78 should be considered. Our report further highlights the importance of paying attention to the serious complications of COVID-19 disease as well as its treatment of opportunistic infections.

To conclude, physicians should be mindful of the probability of secondary fungal infections in patients with COVID-19 who were managed by corticosteroids even in the absence of any comorbidities. Moreover, the importance of a multidisciplinary approach should be considered.

Abbreviations

CT:	Computerized tomography
RT-PCR:	Real-time reverse transcription-polymerase chain reaction
WBC:	White blood cell counts
IV:	Intravenous
Pt:	Patient
MRI:	Magnetic resonance imaging
mg:	Milligram
BUN:	Blood urea nitrogen
Rt:	Right
Lt:	Left
PNS:	Paranasal sinuses
Fess:	Functional endoscopic sinus surgery
COVID-19:	Coronavirus disease 2019
WHO:	World Health Organization.

Consent

Written informed consent was obtained from the patient for publication of this case report and any accompanying images. A copy of the written informed consent is available for review by the editor of this journal.

Authors' Contributions

ZM and MS conceived the idea for the manuscript. MRS contributed to reporting the radiological images. MJA made a definitive diagnosis by pathology and took tissue photographs. MHZ, FM, and KN drafted the manuscript. AS,

ZE, and HJM edited the manuscript. All authors read and approved the final manuscript. Zeinab Mehrabi is an Assistant Professor of Medicine, Infectious Diseases Shiraz University of Medical Sciences, Shiraz, Iran. Mohammad Reza Sasani is an Assistant Professor of Radiology, Shiraz University of Medical Sciences. Mohammad Javad Ashraf is an Associate Professor of Pathology, Shiraz University of Medical Sciences.

Acknowledgments

The authors would like to thank Shiraz University of Medical Sciences, Shiraz, Iran, and also the Center for Development of Clinical Research of Nemazee Hospital and Dr. Nasrin Shokrpour for editorial assistance.

References

[1] A. Skiada, C. Lass-Floerl, N. Klimko, A. Ibrahim, E. Roilides, and G. Petrikkos, "Challenges in the diagnosis and treatment of mucormycosis," *Medical Mycology*, vol. 56, Supplement 1, pp. 93–101, 2018.

[2] F. Salahshour, M.-M. Mehrabinejad, M. Nassiri Toosi et al., "Clinical and chest CT features as a predictive tool for COVID-19 clinical progress: introducing a novel semi-quantitative scoring system," *European Radiology*, vol. 31, no. 7, pp. 5178–5188, 2021.

[3] M. J. Zibaeenezhad, M. Sayadi, H. Bazrafshan et al., "The prevalence of cardiovascular risk factors in fatal cases of COVID-19 in Fars Province, Iran," *International Cardiovascular Research Journal*, vol. 15, no. 1, 2021.

[4] M. R. Hatamnejad, F. Fallah Tafti, A. Abdi Ardekani, S. Sadeghi Boogar, and H. Bazrafshan, "Coronary thrombosis in a patient with COVID-19 who was on anticoagulant therapy," *International Cardiovascular Research Journal*, vol. 15, no. 3, 2021.

[5] H. A. Fard, S. Mahmudi-Azer, S. Sefidbakht et al., "Evaluation of chest CT scan as a screening and diagnostic tool in trauma patients with coronavirus disease 2019 (COVID-19): a cross-sectional study," *Emergency Medicine International*, vol. 2021, Article ID 4188178, 2021.

[6] H. Abdolrahimzadeh Fard, R. Borazjani, G. Sabetian et al., "Establishment of a novel triage system for SARS-CoV-2 among trauma victims in trauma centers with limited facilities," *Trauma Surgery & Acute Care Open*, vol. 6, no. 1, article e000726, 2021.

[7] S. Fujishima, "COVID-19: stay cool toward corticosteroids," *The Keio Journal of Medicine*, vol. 69, no. 2, pp. 27–29, 2020.

[8] J.-W. Yang, L. Yang, R.-G. Luo, and J.-F. Xu, "Corticosteroid administration for viral pneumonia: COVID-19 and beyond," *Clinical Microbiology and Infection*, vol. 26, no. 9, pp. 1171–1177, 2020.

[9] P. Mattos-Silva, N. S. Felix, P. L. Silva et al., "Pros and cons of corticosteroid therapy for COVID-19 patients," *Respiratory Physiology & Neurobiology*, vol. 280, p. 103492, 2020.

[10] B. J. Langford, M. So, S. Raybardhan et al., "Bacterial co-infection and secondary infection in patients with COVID-19: a living rapid review and meta-analysis," *Clinical Microbiology and Infection*, vol. 26, no. 12, pp. 1622–1629, 2020.

[11] X. Chen, B. Liao, L. Cheng et al., "The microbial coinfection in COVID-19," *Applied Microbiology and Biotechnology*, vol. 104, no. 18, pp. 7777–7785, 2020.

[12] S. Mehta and A. Pandey, "Rhino-orbital mucormycosis associated with COVID-19," *Cureus*, vol. 12, no. 9, article e10726, 2020.

[13] Z. Yang, J. Liu, Y. Zhou, X. Zhao, Q. Zhao, and J. Liu, "The effect of corticosteroid treatment on patients with coronavirus infection: a systematic review and meta-analysis," *The Journal of Infection*, vol. 81, no. 1, pp. e13–e20, 2020.

[14] L. Zha, S. Li, L. Pan et al., "Corticosteroid treatment of patients with coronavirus disease 2019 (COVID-19)," *The Medical Journal of Australia*, vol. 212, no. 9, pp. 416–420, 2020.

[15] Y. Ma, H. Zeng, Z. Zhan et al., "Corticosteroid use in the treatment of COVID-19: a multicenter retrospective study in Hunan, China," *Frontiers in Pharmacology*, vol. 11, p. 1198, 2020.

[16] P. Badiee, Z. Jafarpour, A. Alborzi, P. Haddadi, M. Rasuli, and M. Kalani, "Orbital mucormycosis in an immunocompetent individual," *Iranian journal of microbiology*, vol. 4, no. 4, pp. 210–214, 2012.

[17] F. Lanternier, E. Dannaoui, G. Morizot et al., "A global analysis of mucormycosis in France: the RetroZygo Study (2005–2007)," *Clinical Infectious Diseases*, vol. 54, Supplement 1, pp. S35–S43, 2012.

[18] A. D. Castrejón-Pérez, E. C. Welsh, I. Miranda, J. Ocampo-Candiani, and O. Welsh, "Cutaneous mucormycosis," *Anais Brasileiros de Dermatologia*, vol. 92, no. 3, pp. 304–311, 2017.

[19] A. Werthman-Ehrenreich, "Mucormycosis with orbital compartment syndrome in a patient with COVID-19," *The American Journal of Emergency Medicine*, vol. S0735-6757, no. 20, pp. 30823–30826, 2020.

[20] Z. K. Mekonnen, D. C. Ashraf, T. Jankowski et al., "Acute invasive rhino-orbital mucormycosis in a patient with COVID-19-associated acute respiratory distress syndrome," *Ophthalmic Plastic & Reconstructive Surgery*, vol. 37, no. 2, pp. e40–e80, 2021.

[21] E. S. do Monte Junior, M. E. L. dos Santos, I. B. Ribeiro et al., "Rare and fatal gastrointestinal mucormycosis (zygomycosis) in a COVID-19 patient: a case report," *Clinical Endoscopy*, vol. 53, no. 6, pp. 746–749, 2020.

[22] D. Pasero, S. Sanna, C. Liperi et al., "A challenging complication following SARS-CoV-2 infection: a case of pulmonary mucormycosis," *Infection*, vol. 49, no. 5, pp. 1055–1060, 2021.

[23] V. Muthu, S. M. Rudramurthy, A. Chakrabarti, and R. Agarwal, "Epidemiology and pathophysiology of COVID-19-associated mucormycosis: India versus the rest of the world," *Mycopathologia*, pp. 1–16, 2021.

[24] S. M. Rudramurthy, M. Hoenigl, J. F. Meis et al., "ECMM/ISHAM recommendations for clinical management of COVID-19 associated mucormycosis in low-and middle-income countries," *Mycoses*, vol. 64, no. 9, pp. 1028–1037, 2021.

[25] A. Bhattacharyya, P. Sarma, D. J. Sharma et al., "Rhino-orbital-cerebral-mucormycosis in COVID-19: a systematic review," *Indian Journal of Pharmacology*, vol. 53, no. 4, pp. 317–327, 2021.

34

Peripheral Retinal Neovascularization in a Patient with Sarcoidosis and Cocaine-Associated Autoimmunity

Ramak Roohipourmoallai,[1] **Samaneh Davoudi,**[1] **Seyed Majid Hosseinian Benvidi,**[2] **and Siva S. R. Iyer**[1]

[1]*Department of Ophthalmology, University Of Florida, USA*
[2]*Department of Internal Medicine, University of Florida, USA*

Correspondence should be addressed to Siva S. R. Iyer; ssr@ufl.edu

Academic Editor: Winfried M. Amoaku

A 63-year-old African-American female with history of sarcoidosis (lymph node biopsy proven) and cocaine abuse for 8 years was referred to us because of new floater. Her ocular history was unremarkable except for vague complaints of visual disturbance during a hospital admission in 2016. On presentation, her visual acuity was 20/400 in the right eye and 20/30 in the left eye. Dilated fundus exam and multimodal imaging showed thick epiretinal membrane (ERM) superior to optic nerve head causing a lamellar macular hole and intra retinal edema in the right eye, a full thickness macular hole, and peripheral neovascularization in the left eye. Peripheral vasculitis was appreciated in both eyes and peripheral neovascularization in the left eye on fluorescein angiography. The patient underwent laser therapy, and the new vessels regressed in the left eye without any changes in systemic medications. Multiple factors may contribute to retinal vasculitis and neovascularization including sarcoidosis, cocaine abuse, and other undiagnosed systemic vasculitis, which makes this case a mystery.

1. Introduction

There are many reported etiologies for retinal vasculitis as described by Rosenbaum et al. [1], including systemic disease or as a part of an infectious process. In view of the significant potential morbidity of these conditions, ophthalmologists need to be aware of these entities when faced with patients presenting with retinal vasculitis.

Sometimes, the definite diagnosis is a mystery specifically when there are multiple reasons for the same objective findings. Here, we report a case of proven history of sarcoidosis, cocaine abuse, and some nonspecific immunologic serologic findings in a patient with maculopathy, retinal vasculitis, and retinal neovascularization.

1.1. Investigation. A 63-year-old African-American female with a past medical history of lymph node biopsy proven sarcoidosis in her early 40s was referred to us for new left eye floater assessment. Her medical history included sarcoidosis (diagnosed in 2008), COPD, pulmonary hypertension, smoking, and crack/cocaine abuse for eight years. She had a history of many neurologic episodes (TIA) with no obvious evidence of acute intracranial abnormality, brain perfusion abnormalities, or flow-limiting stenosis on workup. She had several admissions to the hospital over the years due to chronic hypoxic respiratory failure. The patient had been on oral prednisone 50 mg daily, but she stopped taking it years prior to presentation because of adverse side effects of nightmares and hirsutism. Her ocular history was unremarkable except vague complaints of a visual disturbance during one of her hospital admissions in 2016.

On presentation, her visual acuity was 20/400 in the right eye and 20/30 in the left eye. On dilated exam, a dense epiretinal membrane (ERM) was seen in the superior macula extending from the optic nerve head and peripheral retinal neovascularization in the temporal retina.

1.2. Diagnosis. Diagnostic testing including optical coherence tomography (OCT) showed a lamellar macular hole of the right eye and a full thickness macular hole in the left eye

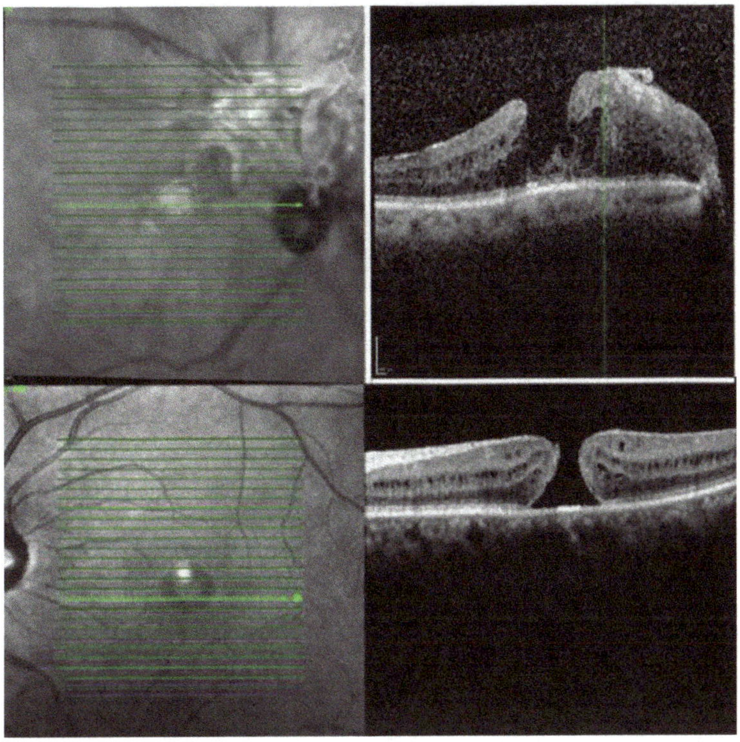

FIGURE 1: Macular OCT. Thick ERM on optic nerve head extending to the fovea causing lamellar macular hole and intra-retinal edema (OD). Full thickness macular hole (OS).

(Figure 1). Fluorescein angiography (FA) revealed peripheral vasculitis in both eyes in addition to a peripheral avascular area and temporal neovascularization in the left eye (Figure 2).

A review of systemic diagnostics included a chest CT six months prior that showed severe diffuse fibrosis bilaterally, emphysematous changes mostly prominently in the upper lobes along with cystic and honeycombing/reticulation changes. Her lab results were as follows: positive c-ANCA 1:320 (ref range < 1 : 20); positive PR3 41 (ref range 0-19 AU/ML); negative myeloperoxidase (MPO) Ab: 8 (ref range 0-19 AU/mL, negative angiotensin-converting enzyme (ACE): 26 (ref range 9-67 U/L), negative ANA and subsets DS DNA Ab (dsDNA) IgG < 1 : 10 (ref range < 1 : 10), negative ribonucleic protein (ENA) antibody 0 (ref range 0-40 AU/mL).

Peripheral retinal neovascularization could not be explained only with sarcoidosis alone, and another factor like cocaine use could be a contributing factor.

1.3. Treatment. Retinal photocoagulation was performed in the avascular area, and the neovascularization regressed completely (Figure 3). As the patient did not complain about vision impairment, a surgical option was not pursued for the full thickness macular hole per patient request.

1.4. Follow-Up. Though the patient's peripheral retinal neovascularization was controlled with laser only, the patient was started on azathioprine by her treating team for her systemic issues.

2. Discussion

Here, we report a case of an African-American patient with a history of sarcoidosis and substance abuse (cocaine) who had vague visual symptoms on presentation and was found to have findings of vasculitis and peripheral avascular retina with neovascularization and macular abnormalities in both eyes. She had a history of acute floaters which was related to intermittent vitreous hemorrhage in the left eye due to neovascularization.

The eye findings of vasculitis, ERM, peripheral avascular area, and neovascularization can be explained with different medical issues including sarcoidosis, cocaine abuse, sickle cell, or a history of FEVR. The patient also had no history of ROP and was not a diabetic, eliminating those additional theoretical causes of retinal ischemia. Patient's medical history was only positive for sarcoidosis and cocaine abuse.

Sarcoidosis is a systemic multiorgan inflammatory disorder typically involving the lungs and lymphatics. The disease course may be variable in different patients. It has symptoms that can involve the respiratory system, extrathoracic specifically lymph nodes, skin, or eye and constitutional symptoms such as fatigue, weight loss, fever or night sweats, and erythema nodosum. 30-60% of patients have ophthalmic involvement. All ocular structures may be involved, but uveitis is the most frequent form of ocular manifestation, and up to 20–30% of sarcoidosis patients may be affected. In a retrospective series by Jamilloux et al. of proven (histologically) sarcoidosis; symptomatic uveitis affects 20–50% of patients [2].

There are intraocular signs suggestive of ocular sarcoidosis explained by Herbort et al. as follows [3]:

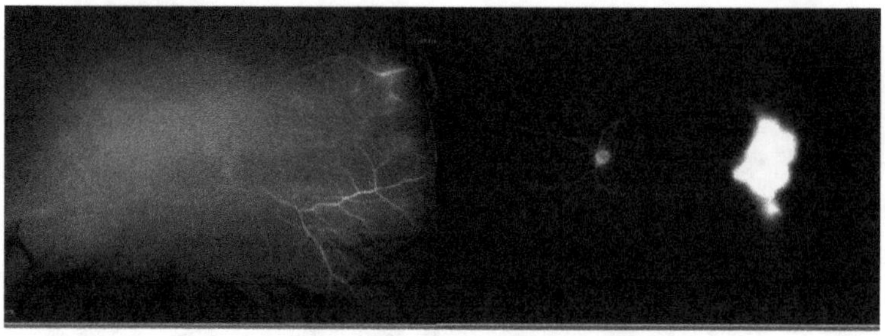

FIGURE 2: Fluorescein angiography showing peripheral vasculitis in the right eye and peripheral neovascularization in the left eye with significant leakage in temporal area.

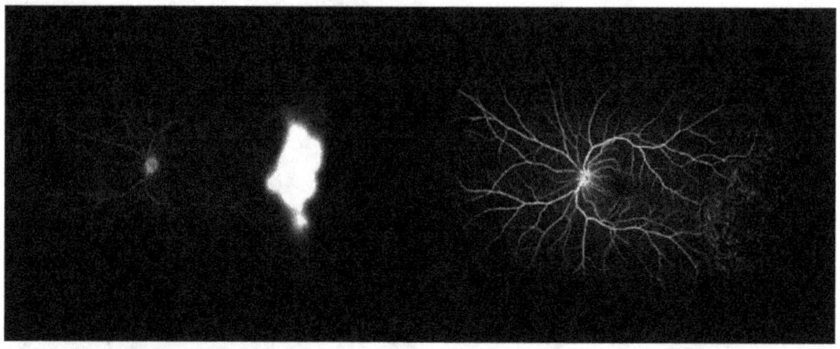

FIGURE 3: Neovascularization regressed after laser treatment in the left eye.

(1) Mutton-fat keratic precipitates (large or small) and/or iris nodules (Koeppe/Busacca)

(2) Trabecular meshwork nodules and/or tent-shaped peripheral anterior synechia

(3) Snowballs/strings of pearls' vitreous opacities

(4) Multiple chorioretinal peripheral lesions (active and/or atrophic)

(5) Nodular and/or segmental periphlebitis (±candle wax drippings) and/or retinal macroaneurysm in an inflamed eye

(6) Optic-disk nodule(s)/granuloma(s) and/or a solitary choroidal nodule

(7) Bilateral inflammation (evident on clinical examination or on investigational imaging) Rothova et al. described sarcoid uveitis is usually bilateral (80–90%). Anterior uveitis is the most common anatomical form of intraocular inflammation (41–75% of sarcoid uveitis) followed by posterior, intermediate uveitis and panuveitis [4]

Our patient was diagnosed with vitreous hemorrhage due to peripheral neovascularization in the left eye which was the reason for having the new floaters. There are some ocular findings that are not compatible with sarcoidosis as the cause in this patient. She did not report any signs of anterior uveitis such as eye pain, photophobia, or redness. Isolated posterior segment involvement has been reported in only 5% of patients with sarcoid disease as explained by Pasadhika and Rosenbaum [5]. The most common posterior findings are chorioretinitis and retinal periphlebitis with retinal hemorrhage. We could see only mild peripheral periphlebitis, in addition to ERM and a macular hole which can be explained with uveitis as one of the reason for development of these surface abnormalities although our patient did not report any symptoms of previous acute uveitis.

Our patient had peripheral retinal neovascularization and abrupt peripheral vessels drop out which occur very rarely in sarcoidosis patients but have been reported with other accompanying disease such as sickle cell or talc retinopathy as explained by Tran [6]. Our patient did not have any history of sickle cell trait or disease, but had history of cocaine abuse which could have caused the peripheral retinal neovascularization, but not the vitreoretinal surface abnormalities.

Neovascularization of the peripheral retina can be present in a number of systemic and ocular diseases and it can also be manifested in drug abusers. Retinal vascular emboli such as talc are common in drug abusers; however, the only reason for aforementioned findings in this patient with specific history could be sarcoidosis in a cocaine abuse patient. The macular and optic nerve findings can be explained with chronic inflammation due to sarcoidosis but not cocaine abuse.

The patient responded to laser only without the addition of any systemic medication, which makes sarcoidosis less probable as the sole reason for peripheral retinal neovascularization. ACE was tested several times which was within normal limits. This normal test cannot exclude a sarcoidosis diagnosis as sarcoidosis was proven with positive lymph node biopsy but can correlate with disease inactivity. In a large series of patients with uveitis; ACE had a sensitivity of 84% and a specificity of 95% for the diagnosis of sarcoidosis. In this study by Baarsma et al., lysozyme was a less-sensitive (60%) and specific (76%) test [7].

The patient had a positive test for c-ANCA and PR3. Given this, granulomatosis with polyangiitis (GPA) may be considered; however, the patient did not have known upper airway or kidney involvement and her lung parenchyma abnormalities did not include some of the more classic manifestations of GPA [8] such as cavitation explained by Yates and Watts.

Retinal vasculitis can be seen in ANCA-associated vasculitis (AAV) [8], although the patient denied joint pain, swelling, skin rashes, sinus disease, and a history of hemoptysis or kidney disease. Lab studies ruled out excessive proteinuria and/or hematuria.

We think this patient's positive c-ANCA and PR3 positive tests were due to a history of cocaine use, which has been reported by Morcos and Lood et al. before in a cocaine-associated autoimmunity syndrome (CLAAS) [9]. This diagnosis can explain the peripheral neovascularization in this patient, which is not explained only with sarcoidosis.

Her vitreous hemorrhage has been controlled with sectoral angiographic-guided retinal photocoagulation, and she has not required escalation of systemic immunosuppression from an ocular standpoint.

3. Conclusion

Our patient with history of sarcoidosis developed peripheral vasculitis, peripheral retinal neovascularization, and vitreoretinal surface abnormalities that could not be explained with sarcoidosis only but could be explained with both sarcoidosis and her cocaine abuse and/or cocaine immune-related reaction.

Acknowledgments

This work was supported in part by an unrestricted grant from research to prevent blindness.

References

[1] J. T. Rosenbaum, C. H. Sibley, and P. Lin, "Retinal vasculitis," *Current Opinion in Rheumatology*, vol. 28, no. 3, pp. 228–235, 2016.

[2] Y. Jamilloux, L. Kodjikian, C. Broussolle, and P. Sève, "Sarcoidosis and uveitis," *Autoimmunity Reviews*, vol. 13, no. 8, pp. 840–849, 2014.

[3] C. P. Herbort, N. A. Rao, M. Mochizuki, and the members of the Scientific Commi, "International criteria for the diagnosis of ocular sarcoidosis: results of the first International Workshop On Ocular Sarcoidosis (IWOS)," *Ocular Immunology and Inflammation*, vol. 17, no. 3, pp. 160–169, 2009.

[4] A. Rothova, C. Alberts, E. Glasius, A. Kijlstra, H. J. Buitenhuis, and A. C. Breebaart, "Risk factors for ocular sarcoidosis," *Documenta Ophthalmologica*, vol. 72, no. 3-4, pp. 287–296, 1989.

[5] S. Pasadhika and J. T. Rosenbaum, "Ocular sarcoidosis," *Clinics in Chest Medicine*, vol. 36, no. 4, pp. 669–683, 2015.

[6] K. H. Tran and P. F. Ilsen, "Peripheral retinal neovascularization in talc retinopathy," *Optometry - Journal of the American Optometric Association*, vol. 78, no. 8, pp. 409–414, 2007.

[7] G. S. Baarsma, E. La Hey, E. Glasius, J. de Vries, and A. Kijlstra, "The predictive value of serum angiotensin converting enzyme and lysozyme levels in the diagnosis of ocular sarcoidosis," *American Journal of Ophthalmology*, vol. 104, no. 3, pp. 211–217, 1987.

[8] M. Yates and R. Watts, "ANCA-associated vasculitis," *Clinical Medicine (London, England)*, vol. 17, no. 1, pp. 60–64, 2017.

[9] M. B. Morcos, C. Lood, and G. C. Hughes, "Demographic, clinical, and immunologic correlates among a cohort of 50 cocaine users demonstrating antineutrophil cytoplasmic antibodies," *The Journal of Rheumatology*, vol. 46, no. 9, pp. 1151–1156, 2019.

35

Long-Term Follow-Up Results of a Patient Undergoing Acute Retinal Necrosis: A Case Report and Literature Review

Büşra Köse,[1] Hidayet Erdöl,[2] and Dilek Uzlu[2]

[1]*The State Hospital of Bayburt, Bayburt, Turkey*
[2]*Karadeniz Technical University, Medical Faculty, Department of Ophthalmology, Trabzon, Turkey*

Correspondence should be addressed to Büşra Köse; busrakose-ktu@hotmail.com

Academic Editor: Stephen G. Schwartz

Purpose. To describe the follow-up and treatment approach of a patient with acute retinal necrosis. *Case Report.* A 44-year-old male patient, who had complaints of pain in the right eye and blurred vision, was referred to our clinic. Best-corrected visual acuity (BCVA) was 0.4. There was 2+ anterior chamber reaction and diffuse smooth-rounded keratic precipitates. Fundus examination revealed optic nerve and vascular involvement. Fundus fluorescein angiography revealed extensive ischemia in the periphery. Oral antiviral therapy was preferred. In addition, systemic steroid and laser photocoagulation were applied. Nonetheless, retinal detachment developed 2 months later. Detachment, silicon removal, and cataract surgery were performed sequentially. It was observed that the patient was followed for 4.5 years and did not have contralateral eye involvement. Best-corrected visual acuity remained stable at 0.3. *Conclusion.* Early diagnosis, appropriate treatment, accurate complication management, and frequent follow-up may provide useful vision in patients with acute retinal necrosis.

1. Introduction

Acute retinal necrosis is often unilateral, characterized by well-demarcated areas of necrosis in the retina deriving from Varicella zoster virus (VZV) or Herpes simplex virus (HSV) [1–4]. This entity is infectious uveitis in which vitreous and anterior chamber inflammation is added to the manifestation with retinitis exhibiting rapid and circumferential progression leading to occlusive retinal vasculopathy also involving the arteries [5, 6]. More rarely, cytomegalovirus and Epstein-Barr virus have also been shown to be capable of leading to the manifestation [4]. Visual outcomes are generally poor, with visual acuity decreasing to below 20/200 six months after onset in 48% of patients [7].

Treatment currently consists of intravenous acyclovir at a dosage of 10 mg/kg three times daily for 7-10 days, followed by long-term oral acyclovir therapy [3, 4, 8, 9]. Although antiviral therapy reduces the rate of involvement in the contralateral eye, the risk of severe loss of vision and retinal detachment in the affected eye is still high [3, 4, 7, 9–12]. Response to treatment varies from patient to patient, and the effect cannot be predicted.

Due to the high rates of acyclovir-related side effects, new antiviral drugs such as the prodrug valacyclovir, with higher oral bioavailability and a lower incidence of side effects, have been employed in clinical practice in recent years [11, 13, 14].

In this case report, we describe the clinical course of acute retinal necrosis in a patient under long-term follow-up.

2. Case

A 44-year-old man presented to our clinic due to reduced vision in May 2016. No characteristic associated with the manifestation was present in the patient's own or family history, and he had no history of chronic drug use or comorbid conditions such as severe influenza infection.

The patient was referred to us from another clinic with a preliminary diagnosis of uveitis with pain and blurred vision in the right eye for the previous week. Examination using a Snellen chart revealed visual acuity of 0.4 in the right eye. 2+ anterior chamber reaction was present in the anterior segment with diffuse smooth-rounded keratic precipitates. Fundus examination revealed edema and hyperemia in the head of the optic disk, 360-degree retinal hemorrhages in the peripheral retina, sheathing and occlusion of the vessels, and 2 + vitreous cells (Figures 1 and 2). Fundus fluorescein angiography (FFA) (Canon 60UVi, Tokyo, Japan) revealed ischemic areas in front of the equator in the peripheral retina and leakage associated with permeability impairment in vessels. No significant pathology was determined in the macular region on optical coherence tomography (OCT) (Optovue RTVue, RT 100, software version 6.3, Optovue, CA, USA). Acute retinal necrosis was diagnosed, and the patient was started on oral valacyclovir 1000 mg at 8 h intervals (3 ∗ 1000 mg), methylprednisolone 1 mg/kg/day, and topical steroid drops once every 2 h.

Visual acuity remained at the same level at the control examination one week later. Three hundred sixty-degree laser photocoagulation was applied to the posterior margin of the necrotized area in the peripheral fundus. The methylprednisolone dosage began being tapered to 8 mg once every three days, while valacyclovir and topical steroid therapy were maintained at the same dosages. Fluorescein angiography (Canon 60UVi, Tokyo, Japan) performed five days after laser photocoagulation revealed that laser application to the rear of the peripheral ischemic area had been effective, and leakage was detected in the optic disk (Figure 3).

Visual acuity using a Snellen chart at control examination after one month was 0.5, and the anterior segment reaction and fundus examination findings had regressed; valacyclovir was reduced to 2 ∗ 1000 mg due to diffuse eruption on the patient's body. Methylprednisolone continued to be tapered, and topical steroid therapy was reduced. At control examination on the sixth week, the patient's visual acuity using a Snellen chart was 10/10. The anterior segment findings had resolved entirely, fundus examination findings had regressed, and the retinal hemorrhage in the laser periphery had decreased. In addition, ghost vessels, perivascular sheathing, and mild vitreous condensation were present. Cystoid macular edema (CME) was detected at OCT evaluation. Treatment was modified to valacyclovir 2 ∗ 1000, nepafenac drops 4 ∗ 1, and oral indomethacin 2 ∗ 25 mg. At the end of the second month, the patient's vision had diminished to the hand movement level, and the retina was completely detached. In the peripheral retina, except for the superotemporal quadrant, there was grade B proliferative vitreoretinopathy (PVR) with prominent wrinkling of the inner retinal surface and increased vessel tortuosity on the diffuse retinal surface. In the inferonasal peripheral retina, several atrophic holes with irregular borders without operculum in front of and behind the laser field, horseshoe tears behind the laser field at 2 and 3 o'clock, and a well-circumscribed atrophic hole with operculum behind the laser field at 7 o'clock were present. The patient was started on single-dose 300 mg/day acetylsalicylic acid (ASA) therapy, maintained for three months. Pars plana vitrectomy and silicone tamponade were applied. The silicone was removed three months after detachment surgery, and cataract surgery was performed one month after that operation. Valacyclovir therapy was stopped at the end of nine months. The patient's visual acuity reached 0.3 at the end of 11 months, and no pathology was observed in the retina (Figure 4). No pathology was also detected in the other eye.

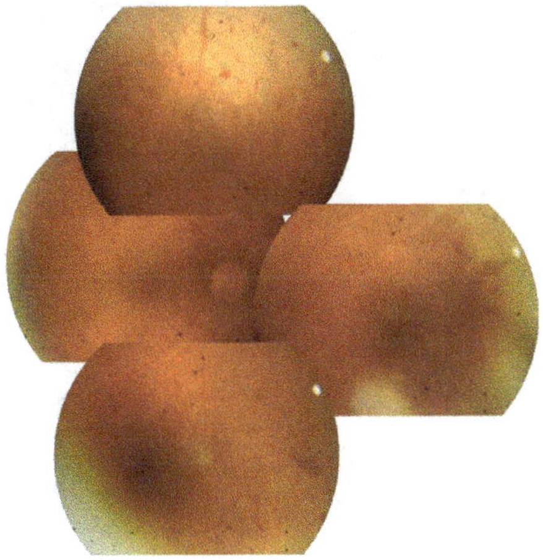

FIGURE 1: Montage of retinal photographs (Canon 60UVi, Tokyo, Japan) showing vitritis, areas of retinitis, retinal vasculitis, retinal hemorrhage, and hyperemia and edema in the head of the optic nerve at initial presentation examination.

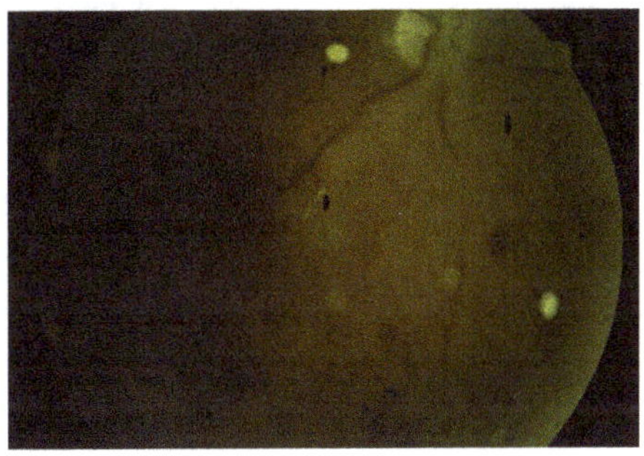

FIGURE 2: Red-free fundus photograph (Canon 60UVi, Tokyo, Japan) showing occlusive vasculopathy (black arrows).

On the 13th month of follow-up, the patient represented to our clinic due to mild redness and pain in the same eye. Visual acuity on a Snellen chart was 0.1, 1+ anterior chamber reaction and smooth-rounded keratic precipitates were present in the anterior segment, and posterior capsule opacities had developed. No activation was detected in retinal findings. The patient was started on 2 ∗ 500 mg valacyclovir, nepafenac drops 4 ∗ 1, and dexamethasone drops 4 ∗ 1. Right eye Nd-YAG laser capsulotomy was performed after one month. Valacyclovir was reduced to 1 ∗ 500 mg following laser therapy and was discontinued after one month. Visual acuity using a Snellen chart increased to 0.3 at the 16th month of follow-up, and no findings of inflammation were observed on the anterior segment or fundus. The patient represented to our clinic due to mild blurred vision one month after that examination, at which +1 anterior chamber reaction in the anterior segment and mild condensation in the vitreous were observed. Valacyclovir was restarted at 2 ∗ 500 mg. In order to avoid the tendency to recurrence of anterior segment inflammation when valacyclovir was stopped, we recommended that treatment be maintained at this dose for at least six months. Visual acuity on a Snellen chart following approximately the two-year follow-up was 0.4, and no

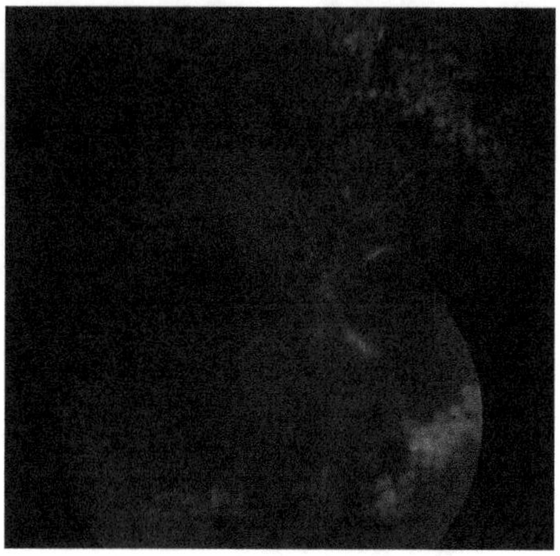

FIGURE 3: Fundus fluorescein angiography montage image (Canon 60UVi, Tokyo, Japan) showing ischemic areas in the laser periphery, leakage in the head of the optic disk, and vasculitis.

recurrence was observed. Valacyclovir therapy was maintained at 1 * 500 mg and was stopped after three months. No kidney function disorder or additional side effect, other than cutaneous eruption during the initial high-dose therapy, was observed during valacyclovir therapy. The patient was followed up for a total of 4.5 years, and no recurrence or other ocular involvement was observed after 1.5 years (Figures 5(a) and 5(b)). Although an epiretinal membrane, minimal cystoid changes, atrophy in the outer retinal layers, and impaired integrity of the ellipsoid zone were determined on macular OCT at the final examination (Figure 5(c)), the best-corrected visual acuity on a Snellen chart remained stable at 0.3.

3. Discussion

Acute retinal necrosis is a rare, vision-threatening, and difficult to treat retinal pathology. Oral valacyclovir has recently been preferred to intravenous acyclovir in treatment, the aim being to reduce both drug-related side effects and hospitalization rates. Advantages such as the high bioavailability of oral valacyclovir, the fact that it can achieve similar plasma concentrations to those of intravenous acyclovir, and that it involves lower costs and outpatient treatment have resulted in increasing recent use in the treatment of acute retinal necrosis [11, 15, 16]. Several small case-number studies in recent years have shown that oral valacyclovir produces good visual and anatomical results [14, 17–19]. One retrospective study comparing intravenous acyclovir and oral valacyclovir reported similar visual acuity and retinal detachment rates in both groups, consistent with Tibbetts et al. [9, 12]. However, it is difficult to compare the studies due to their retrospective natures and their being in a case report or case series form, fundamental differences in characteristics, and their being performed at different times (in the 1980s and 1990s for intravenous therapy and the 2000s for oral therapy). Nonetheless, studies have concluded that intravenous acyclovir and oral valacyclovir therapies achieve similar outcomes in terms of reducing ocular involvement rates and achieving regression of retinal pathologies [11]. We employed oral valacyclovir therapy in the present case and achieved a stable outcome with ambulatory vision.

Several studies have shown that similar plasma concentrations are achieved with 1000 mg oral valacyclovir and 5 mg/kg or 350 mg intravenous acyclovir [15, 20]. Huynh et al. compared vitreous drug concentrations and plasma concentrations following oral valacyclovir therapy in 10 noninflamed eyes undergoing elective vitrectomy. Those authors reported that oral 1000 mg application every 8 h achieved a half maximal inhibitor concentration (IC_{50}) for VZV, HSV-1, and HSV-2 [21]. Liu et al. compared different dosages of oral valacyclovir and reported that oral valacyclovir 1500 mg three times daily resulted in similar outcomes to 700 mg intravenous acyclovir three times daily [22]. Although the therapeutic intravenous acyclovir dosage has been standardized, there are still differences in the literature regarding the application of oral valacyclovir at therapeutic doses. Some studies have elected to apply 1000 mg three times daily [18, 19], while others have applied 2000 mg three times daily [12, 14]. There is also no consensus in previous studies regarding the duration of treatment. Age, additional diseases, and compliance with treatment have been described as factors affecting the duration, and individualized treatment regimens have been applied accordingly. While the duration of treatment may be only two weeks for some patients, it may last for months in others [6, 8, 10]. We also started oral valacyclovir therapy at 1000 mg three times daily in the present case but revised this to 1000 mg twice daily due to eruption in the first month. Treatment was stopped after nine months, but when the patient twice presented with findings of mild anterior uveitis, we decided to continue with long-term treatment and only discontinued antiviral therapy after 1.5 years. We encountered no recurrence, inflammatory findings, or additional retinal pathologies at subsequent follow-ups over three years.

Although systemic antiviral therapy has been reported to reduce contralateral eye involvement, severe loss of vision and retinal detachment rates have been reported in the affected eye [3, 4, 7, 9]. Retinal detachment is one of the most frequent complications of acute retinal necrosis, generally appearing in the first three months after diagnosis. The prevalence of detachment ranges in previous studies between 41% and 85% [3, 4, 8, 9, 23–26]. Laser photocoagulation to the posterior of the necrosed area is recommended in order to prevent retinal detachment. However, while some studies have described laser as beneficial and reducing the development of retinal detachment [4, 27, 28], others have reported no benefit [9, 12, 24, 29].

Studies have also recommended systemic and/or local steroid therapy and antiplatelet agents to reduce the damaging effect of host immunity in addition to systemic antiviral therapy and early pars plana vitrectomy to prevent retinal detachment [3, 9] Recently published case series have also shown that intravitreal foscarnet applied in addition to systemic antiviral therapy reduces the risk of severe vision loss and development of retinal detachment [30–32].

The most important outcome in patients undergoing acute retinal necrosis is the inability to preserve useful visual acuity. Several studies have reported visual acuity levels of 20/200 or below in 50% of cases [4, 7, 24]. Loss of visual

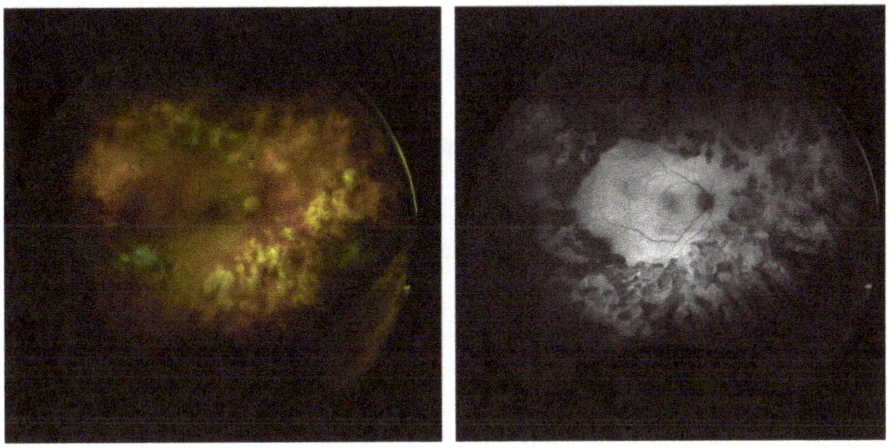

Figure 4: Wide-angle fundus photograph and fundus autofluorescence (FAF) images (Optos PLC, Dunfermline, UK). The laser photocoagulation therapy was effective, and no pathology was observed in the retina.

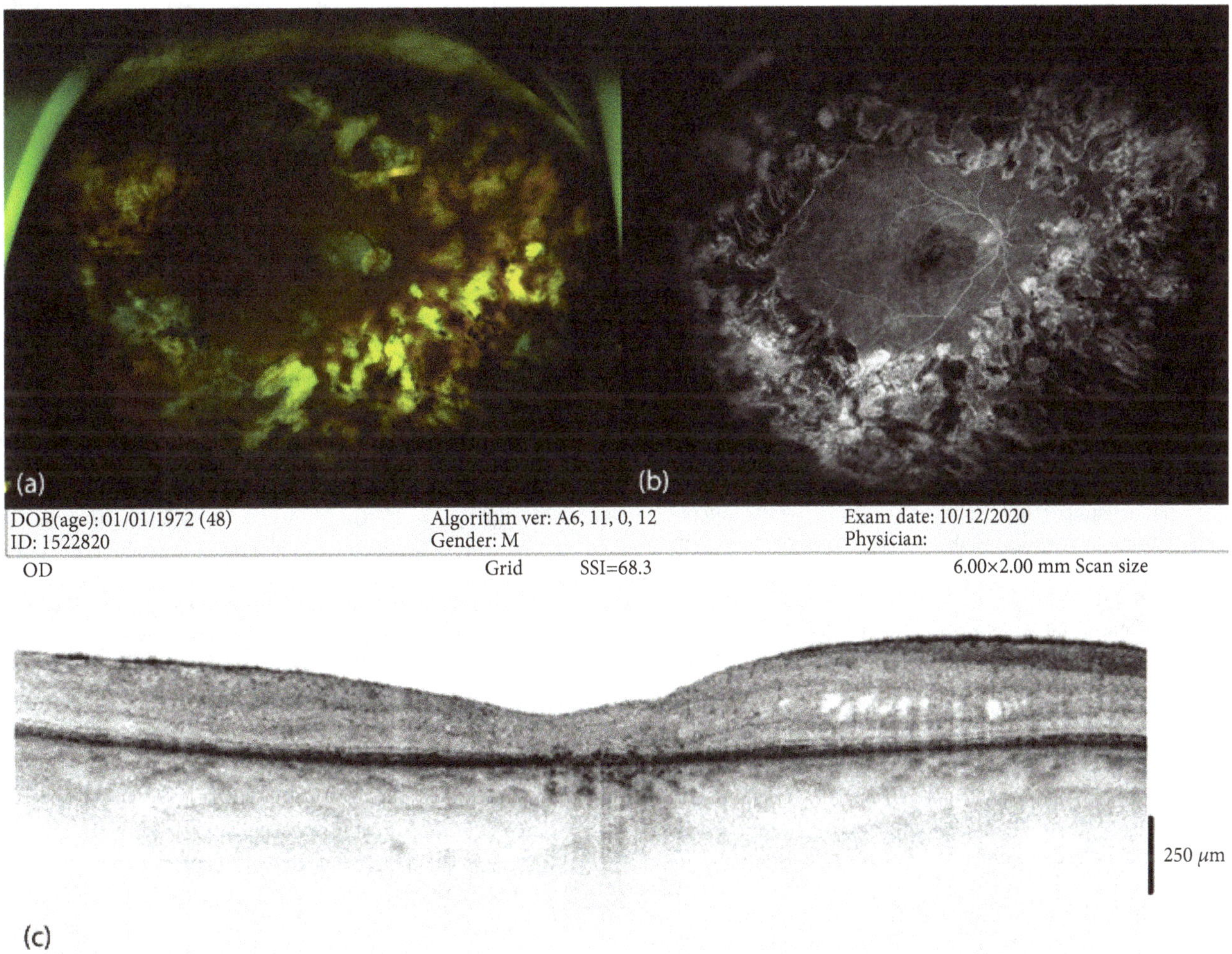

Figure 5: Right eye findings after 4.5 years: (a) wide-angle fundus photograph (Optos PLC, Dunfermline, UK), (b) fundus fluorescein angiography late phase image (Optos PLC, Dunfermline, UK), and (c) macular OCT image (Optovue RTVue, RT 100, software version 6.3, Optovue, CA, USA), atrophy in the outer retinal layers, irregularity in the ellipsoid zone, cystoid macular edema, and epiretinal membrane.

acuity has been linked to low initial visual acuity, development of retinal detachment, and late initiation of antiviral therapy [12].

In addition to retinal detachment in acute retinal necrosis, complications such as cataract, epiretinal membrane, cystoid macular edema, macular ischemia, recurrent anterior uveitis, chronic vitritis, optic neuropathy, optic atrophy, hypotonia, phthisis, rubeosis, and glaucoma may also develop [11, 33]. We observed consecutive retinal detachment, cataract, cystoid macular edema, and epiretinal membrane development in this case followed up for 4.5 years.

Due to its rarity, there is no standard therapeutic plan for acute retinal necrosis. However, the objective is to achieve early regression of the disease and to prevent involvement of the contralateral eye through early diagnosis and treatment. Achieving optimal visual acuity, the prime aim is possible with early diagnosis, appropriate treatment, and accurate complication management.

In conclusion, as reported in the literature and observed in the present case, since complications may occur at any time, frequent follow-up and an effective therapeutic approach may permit the preservation of useful vision in patients with acute retinal necrosis.

References

[1] J. B. Ganatra, D. Chandler, C. Santos, B. Kuppermann, and T. P. Margolis, "Viral causes of the acute retinal necrosis syndrome," *American Journal of Ophthalmology*, vol. 129, no. 2, pp. 166–172, 2000.

[2] M. N. Muthiah, M. Michaelides, C. S. Child, and S. M. Mittchell, "Acute retinal necrosis: a national population-based study to assess the incidence, methods of diagnosis, treatment strategies and outcomes in the UK," *The British Journal of Ophthalmology*, vol. 91, no. 11, pp. 1452–1455, 2007.

[3] J. Hillenkamp, B. Nölle, C. Bruns, P. Rautenberg, H. Fickenscher, and J. Roider, "Acute retinal necrosis: clinical features, early vitrectomy, and outcomes," *Ophthalmology*, vol. 116, no. 10, pp. 1971–1975.e2, 2009.

[4] C. H. Lau, T. Missotten, J. Salzmann, and S. L. Lightman, "Acute retinal necrosis: features, management, and outcomes," *Ophthalmology*, vol. 114, no. 4, pp. 756–762.e1, 2007.

[5] B. Wensing, J. D. F. De Groot-Mijnes, and A. Rothova, "Necrotizing and nonnecrotizing variants of herpetic uveitis with posterior segment involvement," *Archives of Ophthalmology*, vol. 129, no. 4, pp. 403–408, 2011.

[6] R. Margolis, O. F. M. Brasil, C. Y. Lowder et al., "Multifocal posterior necrotizing retinitis," *American Journal of Ophthalmology*, vol. 143, no. 6, pp. 1003–1008.e2, 2007.

[7] T. F. Cochrane, G. Silvestri, C. McDowell, B. Foot, and C. E. McAvoy, "Acute retinal necrosis in the United Kingdom: results of a prospective surveillance study," *Eye*, vol. 26, no. 3, pp. 370–378, 2012.

[8] M. S. Blumenkranz, W. W. Culbertson, J. G. Clarkson, and R. Dix, "Treatment of the acute retinal necrosis syndrome with intravenous acyclovir," *Ophthalmology*, vol. 93, no. 3, pp. 296–300, 1986.

[9] M. D. Tibbetts, C. P. Shah, L. H. Young, J. S. Duker, J. I. Maguire, and M. G. Morley, "Treatment of acute retinal necrosis," *Ophthalmology*, vol. 117, no. 4, pp. 818–824, 2010.

[10] D. A. Palay, P. Sternberg, J. Davis et al., "Decrease in the risk of bilateral acute retinal necrosis by acyclovir therapy," *American Journal of Ophthalmology*, vol. 112, no. 3, pp. 250–255, 1991.

[11] S. D. Schoenberger, S. J. Kim, J. E. Thorne et al., "Diagnosis and treatment of acute retinal necrosis: a report by the American Academy of Ophthalmology," *Ophthalmology*, vol. 124, no. 3, pp. 382–392, 2017.

[12] J. Baltinas, S. Lightman, and O. Tomkins-Netzer, "Comparing treatment of acute retinal necrosis with either oral valacyclovir or intravenous acyclovir," *American Journal of Ophthalmology*, vol. 188, pp. 173–180, 2018.

[13] R. W. Wong, J. M. Jumper, H. R. McDonald et al., "Emerging concepts in the management of acute retinal necrosis," *British Journal of Ophthalmology*, vol. 97, no. 5, pp. 545–552, 2013.

[14] S. R. Taylor, R. Hamilton, C. Y. Hooper et al., "Valacyclovir in the treatment of acute retinal necrosis," *BMC Ophthalmology*, vol. 12, no. 1, 2012.

[15] M. Höglund, P. Ljungman, and S. Weller, "Comparable aciclovir exposures produced by oral valaciclovir and intravenous aciclovir in immunocompromised cancer patients," *The Journal of Antimicrobial Chemotherapy*, vol. 47, no. 6, pp. 855–861, 2001.

[16] S. Weller, M. R. Blum, M. Doucette et al., "Pharmacokinetics of the acyclovir pro-drug valaciclovir after escalating single-and multiple-dose administration to normal volunteers," *Clinical Pharmacology and Therapeutics*, vol. 54, no. 6, pp. 595–605, 1993.

[17] I. M. Aslanides, S. De Souza, D. T. W. Wong et al., "Oral valacyclovir in the treatment of acute retinal necrosis syndrome," *Retina*, vol. 22, no. 3, pp. 352–354, 2002.

[18] A. Aizman, M. W. Johnson, and S. G. Elner, "Treatment of acute retinal necrosis syndrome with oral antiviral medications," *Ophthalmology*, vol. 114, no. 2, pp. 307–312, 2007.

[19] G. G. Emerson, J. R. Smith, D. J. Wilson, J. T. Rosenbaum, and C. J. Flaxel, "Primary treatment of acute retinal necrosis with oral antiviral therapy," *Ophthalmology*, vol. 113, no. 12, pp. 2259–2261, 2006.

[20] J. Soul-Lawton, E. Seaber, N. On, R. Wootton, P. Rolan, and J. Posner, "Absolute bioavailability and metabolic disposition of valaciclovir, the L- valyl ester of acyclovir, following oral administration to humans," *Antimicrobial Agents and Chemotherapy*, vol. 39, no. 12, pp. 2759–2764, 1995.

[21] T. H. Huynh, M. W. Johnson, G. M. Comer, and D. N. Fish, "Vitreous penetration of orally administered valacyclovir," *American Journal of Ophthalmology*, vol. 145, no. 4, pp. 682–686, 2008.

[22] T. Liu, A. Jain, M. Fung, C. Vinnard, and V. Ivaturi, "Valacyclovir as initial treatment for acute retinal necrosis: a pharmacokinetic modeling and simulation study," *Current Eye Research*, vol. 42, no. 7, pp. 1035–1038, 2017.

[23] R. Roy, B. P. Pal, G. Mathur, C. Rao, D. Das, and J. Biswas, "Acute retinal necrosis: clinical features, management and outcomes-a 10 year consecutive case series," *Ocular Immunology and Inflammation*, vol. 22, no. 3, pp. 170–174, 2014.

[24] J. L. Sims, J. Yeoh, and R. J. Stawell, "Acute retinal necrosis: a case series with clinical features and treatment outcomes," *Clinical & Experimental Ophthalmology*, vol. 37, no. 5, pp. 473–477, 2009.

[25] B. Meghpara, G. Sulkowski, M. R. Kesen, H. H. Tessler, and D. A. Goldstein, "Long-term follow-up of acute retinal necrosis," *Retina*, vol. 30, no. 5, pp. 795–800, 2010.

[26] J. G. Clarkson, M. S. Blumenkranz, W. W. Culbertson, H. W. Flynn, and M. Lewis, "Retinal detachment following the acute retinal necrosis syndrome," *Ophthalmology*, vol. 91, no. 12, pp. 1665–1668, 1984.

[27] T. Hudde, C. Althaus, and R. Sundmacher, "Argon laser photocoagulation to prevent rhegmatogenous retinal detachment in patients with acute retinal necrosis (ARN) syndrome," *Der Ophthalmologe*, vol. 95, no. 7, pp. 473–477, 1998.

[28] D. P. Han, H. Lewis, G. A. Williams, W. F. Mieler, G. W. Abrams, and T. M. Aaberg, "Laser photocoagulation in the acute retinal necrosis syndrome," *Archives of Ophthalmology*, vol. 105, no. 8, pp. 1051–1054, 1987.

[29] H. R. McDonald, H. Lewis, A. E. Kreiger, Y. Sidikaro, and J. Heckenlively, "Surgical management of retinal detachment associated with the acute retinal necrosis syndrome," *The British Journal of Ophthalmology*, vol. 75, no. 8, pp. 455–458, 1991.

[30] S. Yeh, E. B. Suhler, J. R. Smith et al., "Combination systemic and intravitreal antiviral therapy in the management of acute retinal necrosis syndrome," *Ophthalmic Surgery, Lasers and Imaging Retina*, vol. 45, no. 5, pp. 399–407, 2014.

[31] C. J. Flaxel, S. Yeh, and A. K. Lauer, "Combination systemic and intravitreal antiviral therapy in the management of acute retinal necrosis syndrome (an American Ophthalmological Society thesis)," *Transactions of the American Ophthalmological Society*, vol. 111, pp. 133–144, 2013.

[32] R. Wong, C. E. Pavesio, D. A. H. Laidlaw, T. H. Williamson, E. M. Graham, and M. R. Stanford, "Acute retinal necrosis: the effects of intravitreal foscarnet and virus type on outcome," *Ophthalmology*, vol. 117, no. 3, pp. 556–560, 2010.

[33] S. Winterhalter, N. Stuebiger, A. K. Maier et al., "Acute retinal necrosis: diagnostic and treatment strategies in Germany," *Ocular Immunology and Inflammation*, vol. 24, no. 5, pp. 537–543, 2016.

36

Central Retinal Artery Occlusion after Rhinoplasty Surgery: A Case Report and Literature Review

Mohammad-Reza Ansari-Astaneh, Fereshteh Raoufi, Saeed Shokoohirad, Naser Shoeibi, and Mojtaba Abrishami

Eye Research Center, Mashhad University of Medical Sciences, Mashhad, Iran

Correspondence should be addressed to Mohammad-Reza Ansari-Astaneh; m_ansariastaneh@yahoo.com

Academic Editor: Maurizio Battaglia Parodi

Aim. This study was aimed at reporting a case of central retinal artery occlusion (CRAO) after rhinoplasty. *Case Report.* Unilateral blindness occurred in a 22-year-old woman after rhinoplasty with a history of transient visual loss due to migraine aura and vasospasm. The physical examination of the patient revealed a visual acuity of no light perception in the right eye, a 4^+ relative afferent pupillary defect, disc swelling, cherry-red spot in the macula, and ischemic retina in the right eye. Based on the diagnosis of CRAO, the patient underwent anterior chamber paracentesis (AC tap) along with treatment with mannitol and intravenous hydrocortisone. Visual acuity improved to 1/10 after a two-month follow-up. *Conclusion.* Taking history is very important in rhinoplasty surgery, and vasoconstrictors should be limited in the patients with a suspected history of vasospasm.

1. Introduction

Rhinoplasty is a historical surgery mainly conducted for aesthetic issues and functional problems. This surgery is a risky procedure, as the aesthetic outcome is not fully predictable and many acute, chronic, and functional complications have been reported in the literature [1–3]. Orbital and ophthalmic complications are rare. The orbit may be involved through trauma and infection. Swelling may impair lacrimal drainage and subsequently cause purulent dacryocystitis. Moreover, enophthalmos may be developed [1, 2]. Even in an extremely rare condition, blindness may happen. This blindness is mainly due to orbital compartment syndrome, direct trauma to the optic nerve, or central retinal artery occlusion (CRAO). The role of embolization in the case of intranasal injection of local anesthetics should be considered [1, 3]. Herein, we report a case of CRAO in a 22-year-old female one day after rhinoplasty.

2. Case Presentation

A 22-year-old woman presented with sudden visual loss the day after rhinoplasty surgery for aesthetic reasons to the emergency room of Khatam Hospital affiliated to Mashhad University of Medical Sciences, Mashhad, Iran. The surgery was conducted under general anesthesia by an ENT surgeon without reported complications during surgery. The surgeon used a topical and local injection of vasoconstrictors (epinephrine) for reducing bleeding and maintaining a good surgical field which is a common practice in nasal surgery. Regarding past medical history, the patient reported intermittently reduced vision since two years ago with a negative cardiologic and neurologic workup. The reason for the transient decrease in vision was stated to be migraine aura due to vasospasm. The visual acuity of the left eye was 20/20, and no light perception was in the right eye. Relative afferent pupillary defect (RAPD) was 4^+ for the right eye. The anterior segment examination with a slit lamp was normal for both eyes. The posterior segment examination showed nerve fiber layer swelling, cherry-red spot in the macula, vessel attenuation, and ischemic retina in the right eye. It should be mentioned that the left eye was normal. Clinically, the patient was a CRAO case, and the treatment was initiated as soon as possible. Considering this, anterior chamber paracentesis (AC tap) was conducted for the patient. Immediately, 300 cc of 20% serum mannitol infusion was started. Following that, the patient received intravenous 250 mg prednisolone QID and 10,000 units Eprex BID for 3 days. Complementary imaging including optical coherence tomography (OCT), fluorescein angiography (FAG), and fundus photography further confirmed the diagnosis (Figures 1(a)–1(e)).

In order to find the underlying cause of CRAO, different specialists were consulted. All rheumatologic workups were negative, and the nailfold capillaroscopy reported nonspecific morphology abnormalities. Routine laboratory exams, the cardiac system evaluation, and color Doppler ultrasound of carotid vessels were normal. The only positive finding in the studies was the patient's history of transient visual loss with negative workup, which was the reason for the patient's delay in timely visits to the emergency room as the patient experienced vision loss and improvement. The patient received the previously mentioned treatments and was followed for two months. In fact, after AC tap and mannitol therapy, she had a hand motion visual acuity, and a 1/10 visual acuity was achieved at the end of the follow-up.

3. Discussion

CRAO is not a common condition in itself; moreover, it may be transient/permanent and happen due to a variety of causes. Among the vast list of etiologies, perirhinoplasty CRAO is an extremely rare condition. The underlying pathology that causes rhinoplasty-related CRAO is not fully investigated. Direct trauma to the orbital apex or compartment-related syndrome is a more common cause in sinus surgeries but not rhinoplasty. Furthermore, in close approaches, such as filler injection, the emboli from filler may cause the obstruction in the central retinal artery as reported by Lin et al. [4].

Local anesthetic and epinephrine injection have been reported as the causes of vasospasm along with hypoperfusion and ischemia for the central retinal artery in the rhinoplasty surgery in the literature. Cheney and Blair [5] reported a case of CRAO in a 37-year-old man who underwent rhinoplasty and experienced decreased visual acuity and pain in the right eye eight hours after the surgery. However, unlike our case, the case of this study had no change in visual acuity even after supportive treatments. They reported that the condition was developed mainly due to the use of epinephrine and vasospasm. Another case of CRAO after rhinoplasty was reported by Alis et al. [1] in a 32-year-old female with complaints of decreased visual acuity in the left eye. A combination of possible etiologies was assumed for this case including direct mechanical trauma, vasospastic/embolic vascular events, and vasospasm by epinephrine.

The literature review revealed that CRAO can also be found after sinus surgeries. Byrd et al. [6] reported a case of CRAO after endoscopic sinus surgery in a 41-year-old female. The patient developed eye pain along with blurry vision in the left eye 12 h after the surgery. Ophthalmology was immediately consulted, and the fundoscopic exam showed pallor of the left retina and optic disk with an inferior visual loss and an afferent pupillary defect. However, after receiving nitroglycerin treatment, the patient had normal-appearing retina and optic disk. They also reported vasoconstriction in the background of epinephrine usage and the presence of autoimmune disease as the main cause of this problem, which was reversed by nitroglycerine. Similarly, Chowdhary et al. [7] discussed a case of CRAO after sinus surgery in a 25-year-old healthy Caucasian male, with painless loss of vision in the left eye. Their case also received hyperbaric oxygen and showed improvement in visual acuity. Fat embolism was proposed to be the cause of CRAO in this patient.

CRAO is still not the only cause of blindness after surgery. It is reported that in an extremely rare condition, a direct injury to the optic nerve or compartment-induced syndrome may be the cause of blindness. However, this usually happens in sinus surgeries, such as ethmoidectomy [8, 9], and has not been reported in rhinoplasty. Monteiro [10] reported another case of blindness related to septoplasty. The cause of blindness was direct trauma to the medial orbital wall, as was evident from the computed tomography scan.

Whatever the cause of CRAO is, the timely diagnosis and treatment affect the prognosis of the patient. The diagnosis mostly relies on the history and physical examination. Cherry-red spots along with the development of retinal opacity are the earliest signs found in fundoscopy. Furthermore, FAG shows a delay or absence of filling in occluded vessels during the arterial phase. OCT can also demonstrate edema in parts of the macula. All these findings were evident in our case in this study.

There are a few things to mention about our patient. First of all, the rhinoplasty surgery has been completed without any complications, and therefore, direct trauma to the optic nerve or compartment syndrome could not be considered the reason. The second point is that all rheumatologic, cardiologic, and neurological workups were negative, and therefore, the systemic problems are not relevant. Third, the issue of embolism cannot be discussed in this patient because no trace of embolization has been observed in the retinal examination, since the use of vasoconstrictors is common in rhinoplasty surgery, and as mentioned in several previous reports, the authors believe that the cause of this rare and severe complication in our patient was related to these vasoconstrictors.

The amount and type of adrenaline used in rhinoplasty surgery vary according to the need of the surgeon, time of surgery, and amount of bleeding from the nasal mucosa. One of the important points in this case that made it unique was the history of transient vision loss in the past, which is important in two ways. First of all, this history has prevented the patient from going to the medical center immediately.

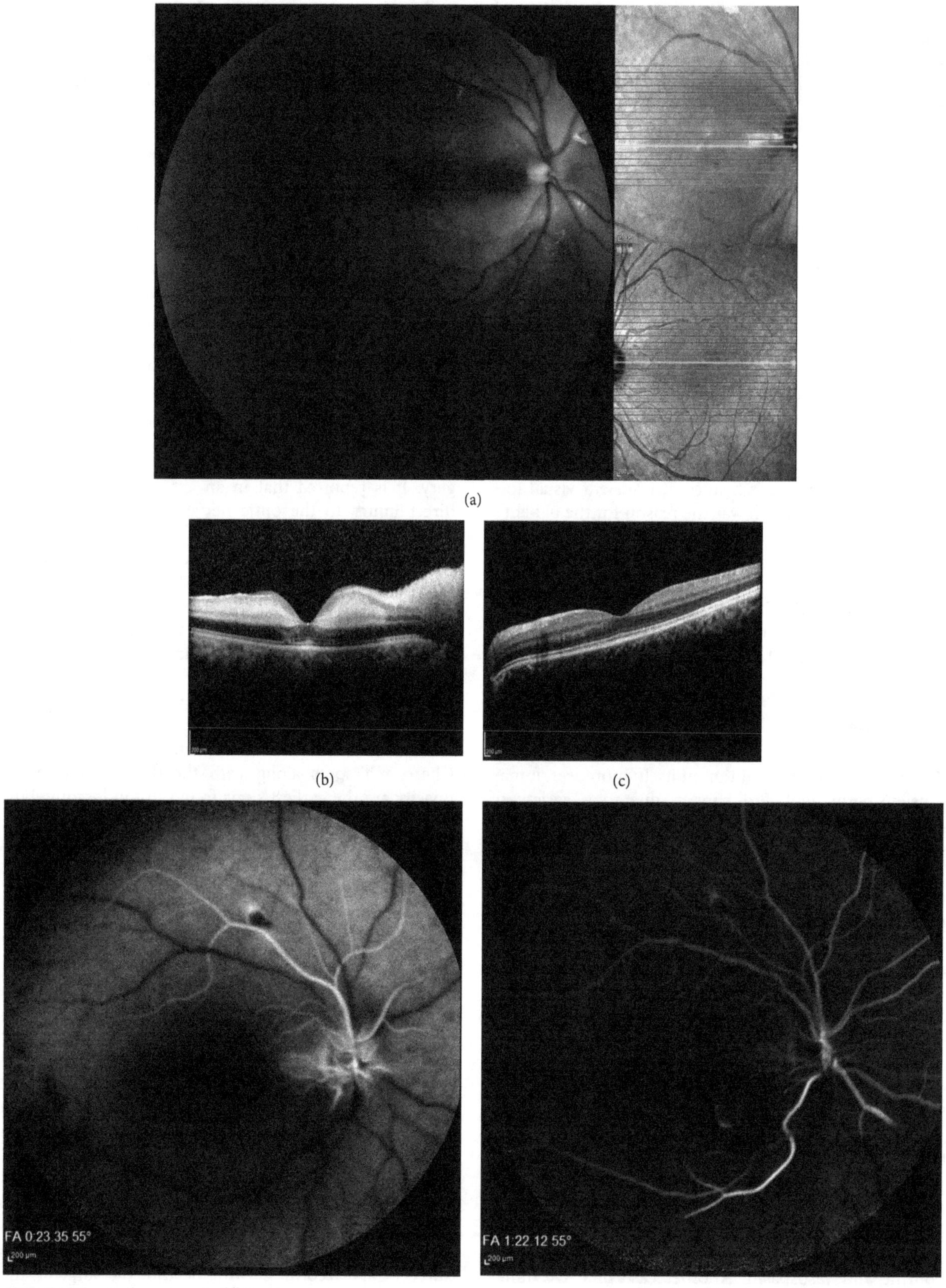

FIGURE 1: Fundus photography (a), optical coherence tomography (c, d), and fluorescein angiography (f, f) of the patient. Arterial vessel attenuation, cherry-red spot, and edematous nerve fiber layer are seen in the fundus photo (a). Thickening and edema of inner retinal layers in the right eye (b) and normal OCT in the left eye (c).Note: no perfused vessels in FAG still after 0′ 23″ (d) and 1′ 23″ of dye injection (e).

The reason was that the patient considered this symptom similar to her previous experiences and expected her vision to improve after a few hours. Second, the cause of reduced vision in migraine, which is often observed in young people, is vasospasm and temporary loss of blood supply to retinal or choroid tissue. The question of whether people with symptoms of migraine are more sensitive to vasoconstriction can logically be raised. Therefore, the authors consider vasospasm to be the cause of this event in this patient and have considered the presence of a history of migraine a predisposing factor although other unknown factors can be considered predisposing factors.

Unfortunately, there is no consensus in the treatment of CRAO; however, many believe that decompression should be made with lowering intraocular pressure using techniques, such as AC tap and infusion of mannitol [11, 12]. Moreover, the use of corticosteroid and vasodilators seems to be efficient in these patients. However, the use of thrombolytic is still controversial and seems not to be related to better prognosis in the CRAO case; nonetheless, it should be used within 6-50 h after CRAO development [13, 14]. Hyperbaric oxygen therapy is another treatment that has been used in the literature; however, further investigation of this treatment is needed.

In the end, it should be mentioned that although CRAO in the background of a rhinoplasty is a very rare disorder, it is a very catastrophic complication for a surgery conducted in case of aesthetic reasons. Moreover, most of the cases that underwent this type of surgery are young people, and this gives higher importance to the condition. Our case in this study developed an acuity of 1/10 at the final follow-up. Surgeons should be more experienced in this type of surgery and have a full vision of the anatomy of the region. Moreover, the use of local anesthetics and vasoconstrictors should be restricted [1]. Our case reported amaurosis fugax attacks before surgery which can predispose the patient for vasospasm attacks and should be considered an important finding, which was not indicated in any of the reviewed cases in the literature.

4. Conclusion

In conclusion, CRAO is a rare complication of rhinoplasty. Surgeons should consider and avoid vasospasm and retrograde emboli during rhinoplasty surgery. Taking history is very important, and vasoconstrictors should be limited in the patients with a suspected history of vasospasm. Furthermore, ophthalmologists should keep this etiology in mind, and prompt treatment should be started as soon as possible.

Consent

The authors give their consent for the publication including photographs and case history within the text.

References

[1] M. G. Alis, B. Acikalin, A. Alis, and Y. O. Ucal, "Transient retinal artery occlusion after uncomplicated rhinoplasty," *Journal of Craniofacial Surgery*, vol. 30, no. 3, pp. e221–e224, 2019.

[2] R. K. Daniel and P. Pálházi, *The Preservation Rhinoplasty: A New Rhinoplasty Revolution*, Oxford University Press US, 2018.

[3] B. Sahil Aggarwal, R. H. Gensure, and M. Paul Bernstein, *Branched Retinal Artery Occlusion after Rhinoplasty*, Moran Eye Center in partnership with the Eccles Library, 2018, Identifier: Moran_CORE_26767.

[4] Y.-C. Lin, W.-C. Chen, W.-C. Liao, and T.-C. Hsia, "Central retinal artery occlusion and brain infarctions after nasal filler injection," *QJM: An International Journal of Medicine*, vol. 108, no. 9, pp. 731-732, 2015.

[5] M. L. Cheney and P. A. Blair, "Blindness as a complication of rhinoplasty," *Archives of Otolaryngology-Head & Neck Surgery*, vol. 113, no. 7, pp. 768-769, 1987.

[6] S. Byrd, A. S. Hussaini, and J. Antisdel, "Acute vision loss following endoscopic sinus surgery," *Case Reports in Otolaryngology*, vol. 2017, 3 pages, 2017.

[7] S. Chowdhary, V. Sawhney, A. Pandya, K. Sambhav, and S. K. Gupta, "Central retinal artery occlusion after nasosinal surgery–an insight," *International Medical Case Reports Journal.*, vol. 13, pp. 211–215, 2020.

[8] G. N. Rao, K. Rout, and A. Pal, "Central retinal artery occlusion and third cranial nerve palsy following nasal septoplasty," *Case reports in Ophthalmology*, vol. 3, no. 3, pp. 321–326, 2012.

[9] S. Plate and S. Asboe, "Blindness as a complication of rhinosurgery," *The Journal of Laryngology & Otology*, vol. 95, no. 3, pp. 317–322, 1981.

[10] M. L. R. Monteiro, "Unilateral blindness as a complication of nasal septoplasty: case report," *Arquivos brasileiros de oftalmologia*, vol. 69, no. 2, pp. 249-250, 2006.

[11] S. G. Schwartz, M. Hickey, and C. A. Puliafito, "Bilateral CRAO and CRVO from thrombotic thrombocytopenic purpura: OCT findings and treatment with triamcinolone acetonide and bevacizumab," *Ophthalmic Surgery, Lasers and Imaging Retina*, vol. 37, no. 5, pp. 420–422, 2006.

[12] S. Cugati, D. D. Varma, C. S. Chen, and A. W. Lee, "Treatment options for central retinal artery occlusion," *Current Treatment Options in Neurology*, vol. 15, no. 1, pp. 63–77, 2013.

[13] C. Framme, D. Spiegel, J. Roider et al., "Central retinal artery occlusion. Importance of selective intra-arterial fibrinolysis," *Der Ophthalmologe: Zeitschrift der Deutschen Ophthalmologischen Gesellschaft*, vol. 98, no. 8, pp. 725–730, 2001.

[14] J. Noble, N. Weizblit, M. Baerlocher, and K. Eng, "Intra-arterial thrombolysis for central retinal artery occlusion: a systematic review," *British Journal of Ophthalmology*, vol. 92, no. 5, pp. 588–593, 2008.

Permissions

All chapters in this book were first published by Hindawi Publishing Corporation; hereby published with permission under the Creative Commons Attribution License or equivalent. Every chapter published in this book has been scrutinized by our experts. Their significance has been extensively debated. The topics covered herein carry significant findings which will fuel the growth of the discipline. They may even be implemented as practical applications or may be referred to as a beginning point for another development.

The contributors of this book come from diverse backgrounds, making this book a truly international effort. This book will bring forth new frontiers with its revolutionizing research information and detailed analysis of the nascent developments around the world.

We would like to thank all the contributing authors for lending their expertise to make the book truly unique. They have played a crucial role in the development of this book. Without their invaluable contributions this book wouldn't have been possible. They have made vital efforts to compile up to date information on the varied aspects of this subject to make this book a valuable addition to the collection of many professionals and students.

This book was conceptualized with the vision of imparting up-to-date information and advanced data in this field. To ensure the same, a matchless editorial board was set up. Every individual on the board went through rigorous rounds of assessment to prove their worth. After which they invested a large part of their time researching and compiling the most relevant data for our readers.

The editorial board has been involved in producing this book since its inception. They have spent rigorous hours researching and exploring the diverse topics which have resulted in the successful publishing of this book. They have passed on their knowledge of decades through this book. To expedite this challenging task, the publisher supported the team at every step. A small team of assistant editors was also appointed to further simplify the editing procedure and attain best results for the readers.

Apart from the editorial board, the designing team has also invested a significant amount of their time in understanding the subject and creating the most relevant covers. They scrutinized every image to scout for the most suitable representation of the subject and create an appropriate cover for the book.

The publishing team has been an ardent support to the editorial, designing and production team. Their endless efforts to recruit the best for this project, has resulted in the accomplishment of this book. They are a veteran in the field of academics and their pool of knowledge is as vast as their experience in printing. Their expertise and guidance has proved useful at every step. Their uncompromising quality standards have made this book an exceptional effort. Their encouragement from time to time has been an inspiration for everyone.

The publisher and the editorial board hope that this book will prove to be a valuable piece of knowledge for researchers, students, practitioners and scholars across the globe.

List of Contributors

Ali Mahdavi Fard and Jeffrey Desilets
Ross Eye Institute, Department of Ophthalmology, Jacobs School of Medicine and Biomedical Sciences, State University at Buffalo, Buffalo, New York, USA

Sangita Patel
Ross Eye Institute, Department of Ophthalmology, Jacobs School of Medicine and Biomedical Sciences, State University at Buffalo, Buffalo, New York, USA
Research and Ophthalmology Services, Veterans Administration of Western New York Healthcare System, Buffalo, NY, USA

Luis Izquierdo
Head of Department of Cornea and Anterior Segment, Instituto de Ojos Oftalmosalud, Lima, Peru

Josefina A.Mej-as Smith, Jose R. Lievano and Ramón Sarquis
Research Department, Instituto de Ojos Oftalmosalud, Lima, Peru

Maria A. Henriquez
Head of Research Department, Instituto de Ojos Oftalmosalud, Av. Javier Prado Este 1142, San Isidro, Lima, Peru

Monica P. Gonzalez, Radames Rios, Mariella Pappaterr, Carmen Santos and Armando L. Oliver
University of Puerto Rico, Medical Sciences Campus, Department of Ophthalmology, Paseo Dr. Jose Celso Barbosa, San Juan 00921, USA

Andres Emanuelli
University of Puerto Rico, Medical Sciences Campus, Department of Ophthalmology, Paseo Dr. Jose Celso Barbosa, San Juan 00921, USA
Emanuelli Research and Development Center, 452 Dr R Rivera Aulet Avenue, Suite 45 Arecibo, PR 00612-4368, USA

Shree K. Kurup
University of Puerto Rico, Medical Sciences Campus, Department of Ophthalmology, Paseo Dr. Jose Celso Barbosa, San Juan 00921, USA
Department of Ophthalmology & Visual Sciences, Case Western Reserve University, University Hospitals Cleveland Medical Center, 11100 Euclid Avenue, Cleveland, OH 44106, USA

Miguel Hernandez
Ponce Health Sciences University School of Medicine, 388 Zona Industrial Reparada 2, Ponce, PR 00716, USA

Allison Toledo
Emanuelli Research and Development Center, 452 Dr R Rivera Aulet Avenue, Suite 45 Arecibo, PR 00612-4368, USA

Sofie Van der Auwera
Department of Ophthalmology, Antwerp University Hospital, Edegem, Belgium

Oscar Kallay
Centre Médical de l'Alliance, Braine l'Alleud, Belgium

Alastair David Bezzina and Isaac Bertuello
Ophthalmology Department, Mater Dei General Teaching Hospital, Malta

Ping Huang, Tal Ben Ami and Weiye Li
Department of Ophthalmology, Drexel University College of Medicine, 219 N. Broad Street, Philadelphia, PA 19107, USA

Angelica Pedraza-Concha
Faculty of Medicine, Universidad Autónoma de Bucaramanga, Bucaramanga 680003, Colombia

Karin Brandauer and Christian Scheib
Augenklinik am Diakonissenkrankenhaus, Karlsruhe 76199, Germany

Alejandro Tello
Cornea and Anterior Segment Division, Centro Oftalmológico Virgilio Galvis, Bucaramanga 680003, Colombia

Carlos Mario Rangel
Retina and Posterior Segment Division, Centro Oftalmológico Virgilio Galvis, Bucaramanga 680003, Colombia

Jessica Ruzicki
Department of Ophthalmology, Kingston Health Sciences Centre, Queen's University, Kingston, ON, Canada

Eric K. Chin
Private Practice, Retina Consultants of Southern California, Redlands, California, USA

David Almeida
Private Practice, Metrolina Eye Associates, Charlotte, North Carolina, USA

G. Aloe, C.M. De Sanctis, F. Missiroli, M. Cesareo and F. Ricci
Unit Retinal Pathology PTV Foundation, Tor Vergata University, Rome, Italy

C. Strafella and E. Giardina
Department of Biomedicine and Prevention, Tor Vergata University, Rome, Italy
Molecular Genetics Laboratory UILDM, Santa Lucia Foundation, Rome, Italy

R. Cascella
Molecular Genetics Laboratory UILDM, Santa Lucia Foundation, Rome, Italy
Department of Biomedical Sciences, Catholic University Our Lady of Good Counsel, Tirana, Albania

Anastasia Tsiogka, Apostolos Gkartzonikas, Konstantinos Markopoulos and Iordanis Georgiou
Department of Ophthalmology, 401 General Military Hospital, 3 P. Kanellopoulou Street, Athens 11525, Greece

George L. Spaeth
Department of Ophthalmology, Wills Eye Hospital, 840 Walnut St, Philadelphia, PA 19107, USA

A. Altun
Department of Ophthalmology, Bahcesehir University, Faculty of Medicine, Istanbul, Turkey

Mingkwan Lumyongsatien
Department of Ophthalmology, Mettapracharak Hospital, Sampran District, 52 moo2 Rhikhing, Sampran, Nakhon Pathom, Thailand

Pimkwan Jaru-ampornpan
Department of Ophthalmology, Faculty of Medicine, Siriraj Hospital, Mahidol University, 2 Arun Amarin Road, Siriraj, Bangkoknoi, Bangkok, Thailand

Mongkol Uiprasertkul
Department of Pathology, Faculty of Medicine, Siriraj Hospital, Mahidol University, 2 Arun Amarin road, Siriraj, Bangkoknoi, Bangkok, Thailand

Dinesh Selva
Department of Ophthalmology and Visual Sciences, South Australian Institute of Ophthalmology, University of Adelaide, Adelaide, South Australia, Australia

Chase A. Liaboe, Michael S. Lee and Justin J. Y. Yamanuha
University of Minnesota, Department of Ophthalmology and Visual Neurosciences, Phillips Wangensteen Building, 9th Floor, 516 Delaware St SE, Minneapolis, MN 55455, USA

Simanta Khadka, Raghunandan Byanju, Sangita Pradhan and Suchan Poon
Bharatpur Eye Hospital, Bharatpur, Chitwan, Nepal

Rinkal Suwal
BP Eye Foundation, Hospital for Children, Eye, ENT, and Rehabilitation Services (CHEERS), Madhyapur Thimi, Bhaktapur, Nepal

Mariama Touray, Victoria Ando and Jean-Philippe Zuber
Etablissements Hospitaliers du Nord Vaudois, Internal Medicine, Saint-Loup Hospital, Pompaples, Switzerland

Erwin Samutelel
Jules-Gonin Ophthalmic Hospital, Lausanne, Switzerland

Madiha Huq
University Hospitals Parma Medical Center, Cleveland, Ohio, USA

Neha Sanan
University Hospitals, Cleveland Medical Center, Cleveland, Ohio, USA

Phuong Daniels
Lake Erie College of Osteopathic Medicine, Erie, Pennsylvania, USA

Robert Hostoffer
Allergy/Immunology Associates Inc., Mayfield Heights, Ohio, USA

Pranav Shrestha and Sadhana Sharma
Mechi Eye Hospital, Jhapa 57200, Nepal

Ranju Kharel
Department of Uveitis, B. P. Koirala Lions Center for Ophthalmic Studies (BPKLCOS), Institute of Medicine, Maharajgunj, Kathmandu 44600, Nepal

Katsuya Yagisawa, Tomomi Kaiho, Hirotaka Yokouchi and Shuichi Yamamoto
Department of Ophthalmology and Visual Science, Chiba University Graduate School of Medicine, Chiba, Japan

Geraldine P. B. M. Accou, Fanny Nerinckx and Julie De Zaeytijd
Department of Ophthalmology, Ghent University Hospital, Ghent, Belgium

Bart P. Leroy
Department of Ophthalmology & Center for Medical Genetics, Ghent University Hospital, Ghent, Belgium
Children's Hospital of Philadelphia, Philadelphia, PA, USA

Elcin Suren, Ersan Cetinkaya, Mustafa Kalayci, Mehmet Fatih Kucuk and Muhammet Kazim Erol
University of Health Sciences, Antalya Training and Research Hospital, Department of Ophthalmology, Antalya, Turkey

Sariye Elif Özyazıcı Özkan
University of Health Sciences, Antalya Training and Research Hospital, Department of Pediatrics, Antalya, Turkey

Adam Goldman, Michael Bivona and Sinan Albear
Department of Ophthalmology, SUNY Downstate, Brooklyn, NY 11203, USA

Stephen A. LoBue
Department of Ophthalmology, SUNY Downstate, Brooklyn, NY 11203, USA
LoBue Laser & Eye Medical Centers, Murrieta, CA 92562, USA

Thomas D. LoBue
LoBue Laser & Eye Medical Centers, Murrieta, CA 92562, USA

Richard A. Giovane
LV Stabler Hospital, Greenville, AL 36037, USA

Stacy M. Carlson
Montefiore Medical Center, Bronx, NY 10467, USA

Yoko Takatsuna
Department of Ophthalmology, Chiba Rosai Hospital, Ichihara, Chiba, Japan
Department of Ophthalmology and Visual Science, Chiba University Graduate School of Medicine, Chiba, Japan

Tomoaki Tatsumi and Shuichi Yamamoto
Department of Ophthalmology and Visual Science, Chiba University Graduate School of Medicine, Chiba, Japan

Ryoichi Ishibashi
Department of Medicine, Division of Diabetes, Endocrinology and Metabolism, Kimitsu Chuo Hospital, Kisarazu, Chiba, Japan
Department of Endocrinology, Hematology and Gerontology, Graduate School of Medicine, Chiba University, Chiba, Japan

Koutaro Yokote
Department of Endocrinology, Hematology and Gerontology, Graduate School of Medicine, Chiba University, Chiba, Japan
Division of Diabetes, Metabolism and Endocrinology, Chiba University Hospital, Chiba, Japan

Masaya Koshizaka
Division of Diabetes, Metabolism and Endocrinology, Chiba University Hospital, Chiba, Japan

Ana Marta, Paula Costa, Virgínia Lopes, Miguel Mesquita Neves, Miguel Gomes and Luís Oliveira
Department of Ophthalmology, Centro Hospitalar e Universitário do Porto, Oporto, Portugal

Rachel A. Sabol
Tulane University School of Medicine, New Orleans, LA, USA

Virginia Bubenzer, Audrey Dang, Carol Boyd and Kendra Harris
Department of Radiation Oncology, Tulane University School of Medicine, New Orleans, LA, USA

Krzysztof Moroz and Shams Halat
Department of Pathology, Tulane University School of Medicine, New Orleans, LA, USA

Keith Ferdinand
Department of Cardiology, Tulane University School of Medicine, New Orleans, LA, USA

Angela Traylor
Department of Psychiatry and Neurology, Tulane University School of Medicine, New Orleans, LA, USA

Ana Maria Cunha, Marta Silva and Ana Catarina Pedrosa
Department of Ophthalmology, Centro Hospitalar Universitário de São João, Porto, Portugal

Fernando Falcão-Reis
Department of Ophthalmology, Centro Hospitalar Universitário de São João, Porto, Portugal
Department of Surgery and Physiology, Faculty of Medicine, University of Porto, Porto, Portugal

S. Cutting
East Kent University Hospitals NHS Trust, UK

C. Davies-Husband
Brighton and Sussex University Hospitals NHS Trust, UK

Luís Figueira
Department of Ophthalmology, Centro Hospitalar Universitário de São João, Porto, Portugal
Department of Pharmacology and Therapeutics, Faculty of Medicine of the University of Porto, Porto, Portugal
Center for Drug Discovery and Innovative Medicines (MedInUP), University of Porto, Porto, Portugal

C. Poitelea
Western Sussex Hospitals NHS Trust, UK

Ning-Yi Hsia and Chun-Ting Lai
Department of Ophthalmology, China Medical University Hospital, China Medical University, Taichung, Taiwan

Chun-Ju Lin, Cheng-Hsien Chang, Jane-Ming Lin and Yi-Yu Tsai
Department of Ophthalmology, China Medical University Hospital, China Medical University, Taichung, Taiwan
School of Medicine, College of Medicine, China Medical University, Taichung, Taiwan
Department of Optometry, Asia University, Taichung, Taiwan

Henry Bair
Department of Ophthalmology, China Medical University Hospital, China Medical University, Taichung, Taiwan
Stanford University School of Medicine, Stanford, CA, USA

Prashanth G. Iyer, Stephen G. Schwartz, Jonathan F. Russell and Harry W. Flynn Jr.
Department of Ophthalmology, Bascom Palmer Eye Institute, University of Miami Miller School of Medicine, Miami, Florida, USA

Maria Fernanda Flores Herrera, Hind El Ouardighi, François Willermain and Dorine Makhoul
Department of Ophthalmology, CHU Saint-Pierre, Université Libre de Bruxelles (ULB), Brussels, Belgium

Nicolas Dauby and Agnes Libois
Department of Infectious Diseases, CHU Brugmann, Université Libre de Bruxelles (ULB), Brussels, Belgium

Evelyne Maillart and Alberto Papaleo
Department of Infectious Diseases, CHU Saint-Pierre, Université Libre de Bruxelles (ULB), Brussels, Belgium

Laurence Postelmans
Department of Ophthalmology, CHU Brugmann, Université Libre de Bruxelles (ULB), Brussels, Belgium

Carl S. Wilkins, Jorge S. Andrade Romo, Toco Y. P. Chui, Richard B. Rosen and Stephanie Llop
Department of Ophthalmology, New York Eye and Ear Infirmary of Mount Sinai, 310 East 14th Street, New York, NY 10003, USA

Jamie Dietze and Thomas Mauger
WVU Medicine Department of Ophthalmology, USA

Yuta Kitamura, Masayasu Kitahashi
Department of Ophthalmology and Visual Science, Chiba University Graduate School of Medicine, Japan

Takayuki Baba
Department of Ophthalmology and Visual Science, Chiba University Graduate School of Medicine, Chiba, Japan
Department of Ophthalmology and Visual Science, Chiba University Graduate School of Medicine, Japan

Toshiyuki Oshitari
Department of Ophthalmology and Visual Science, Chiba University Graduate School of Medicine, Japan
Department of Ophthalmology, International University of Health andWelfare, School of Medicine, Japan

Zeinab Mehrabi
Department of Internal Medicine, Namazi Hospital, Shiraz University of Medical Sciences, Shiraz, Iran

Maryam Salimi and Kianoush Niknam
Student Research Committee, Shiraz University of Medical Sciences, Shiraz, Iran

Farzaneh Mohammadi
Department of Surgery, Eastern Health, Victoria, Australia

Hesan Jelodari Mamaghani and Zohreh Erfani
Students' Scientific Research Center (SSRC), Tehran University of Medical Sciences, Tehran, Iran

Mohammad Reza Sasani
Department of Radiology, Medical Imaging Research Center, Shiraz University of Medical Sciences, Shiraz, Iran

Mohammad Javad Ashraf
Department of Pathology, Shiraz University of Medical Sciences, Shiraz, Iran

Amirhossein Salimi
Student Research Committee, Shahid Sadoughi University of Medical Sciences, Yazd, Iran

Mohammad Hassan Zahedroozegar
Health Policy Research Center, Institute of Health, Shiraz University of Medical Sciences, Shiraz, Iran

Ramak Roohipourmoallai, Samaneh Davoudi and Siva S. R. Iyer
Department of Ophthalmology, University Of Florida, USA

Seyed Majid Hosseinian Benvidi
Department of Internal Medicine, University of Florida, USA

Büşra Köse
The State Hospital of Bayburt, Bayburt, Turkey

Hidayet Erdöl and Dilek Uzlu
Karadeniz Technical University, Medical Faculty, Department of Ophthalmology, Trabzon, Turkey

Mohammad-Reza Ansari-Astaneh, Fereshteh Raoufi, Saeed Shokoohirad, Naser Shoeib and Mojtaba Abrishami
Eye Research Center, Mashhad University of Medical Sciences, Mashhad, Iran

Index

www.ingramcontent.com/pod-product-compliance
Lightning Source LLC
LaVergne TN
LVHW082232200926
848484LV00008B/2344